Totally Implantable Venous Access Devices

Isidoro Di Carlo • Roberto Biffi
Editors

Totally Implantable Venous Access Devices

Management in Mid- and Long-term Clinical Setting

Foreword by
John E. Niederhuber

Springer

Editors
Isidoro Di Carlo
Department of Surgical Sciences
Organ Transplantation
and Advanced Technologies
University of Catania
Cannizzaro Hospital
Catania, Italy

Roberto Biffi
Division of Abdomino Pelvic Surgery
European Institute of Oncology
Milan, Italy

ISBN 978-88-470-5811-8 ISBN 978-88-470-2373-4 (eBook)

DOI 10.1007/978-88-470-2373-4

Springer Milan Dordrecht Heidelberg London New York

Softcover re-print of the Hardcover 1st edition 2012

9 8 7 6 5 4 3 2 1 2012 2013 2014

Cover design: Ikona S.r.l., Milan, Italy
Typesetting: Graphostudio, Milan, Italy

Springer-Verlag Italia S.r.l. – Via Decembrio 28 – I-20137 Milan
Springer is a part of Springer Science+Business Media (www.springer.com)

To our wives and sons,
thanking them for their endearment

Foreword

A few personal reflections

When asked by the editors to contribute a few words to introduce the reader to this important new reference text on "Totally Implanted Venous Access Devices", my mind of course drifted back in time to those initial port placements in 1981 but also to two personal experiences validating for me the great benefit to our patients. In reliving for a moment those days of designing the first "Ports" as well as my surgeon angst as to whether this idea would really work – concerns of port site infection and skin breakdown from repeated needle access of the port – I could not help but think of how much this has impacted vascular access and patient quality of life. And in that regard, my thoughts quickly went to two individuals in my life that because of the closeness of our relationship I was even more aware of the very significant benefit these small implanted devices had on their lives.

The first individual was a distinguished surgeon colleague and mentor who suffered from bouts of bacterial endocarditis requiring prolonged administration of antibiotics and who came to me each time asking that I place a port. The second was my wife who required extensive chemotherapy, repeated venous sampling and occasional administration of fluids and other support during a two year battle with cancer. One only needs to care for even a few cancer patients receiving chemotherapy to quickly understand how extremely important to their care is a well-positioned and well-functioning totally implanted central venous access. The value, safety and durability of these implanted port devices have certainly been well documented over the years since their introduction in 1982 (Niederhuber J et al., Surgery 1982, 92:706-712).

As with most advances in medicine, several prior accomplishments set the stage for developing totally implanted devices. There was of course, extensive experience using external catheters to access the central venous circulation on a chronic basis and the introduction of silicon rubber (Broviac JW et al., Surg. Gynecol. Obstet. 1973, 136, 602) as the material for making these catheters was obviously a critical step in their evolution. The introduction of the Seldinger technique with the peel away sheath for accessing the central venous system was also important to the rapid expansion of the use of vascular access devices.

It was within this background and with my personal experience of perfecting the technical aspects of surgically implanting subcutaneous, percutaneously accessible, continuous infusion pumps for the administration of hepatic arterial chemotherapy (5-fluorodeoxyuridine) that triggered the design of the "totally implantable venous access devices" frequently called "ports". The design of the original totally implanted infusion pumps had, at our request, a "side-port" that bypassed the pumping mechanism and the main drug reservoir providing direct catheter access for radio nucleotide scans to confirm drug distribution and for the bolus administration of chemotherapy agents whose mechanism of action was better suited to bolus administration (Metal Bellows Corp., Sharron, Mass.). The central pump drug reservoir and the side port were accessed percutaneously through their small self-sealing silicone rubber septum using a special non-coring deflected point needle.

An interesting aside (see Chapter 4) is the use of the non-coring deflected point needle invented by a dentist in Seattle, Washington by the name of Ralph Lee Huber. Dr. Huber was a rather prolific inventor and in 1946 patented a modification of the original Tuohy hypodermic needle. His redesign of the needle tip resulted in a needle that would enter the tissue with less pain and more importantly would not remove a core of tissue. The Huber needle quickly became the mainstay of regional and obstetric spinal anesthesia.

As a result, the University of Michigan team had considerable experience with repeated percutaneous access of the totally implanted continuous infusion pumps through the small silicon rubber septum. I can remember sitting around one day in the hospital and talking about what if we just had the "side port" without the pump? Could we use such a device for central venous access and perhaps even for arterial access when we did not wish to use the implanted pump? We sketched out the small reservoir and the attached catheter and asked the company if they would make a few for testing. It is interesting to note that the first few, six as I recall, were actually machined from titanium metal. It was only after their initial successful use that the material of choice was of course plastic. And thus the story began and the text you have before you superbly documents their use, management and patient benefits. My thanks to the editors for their confidence in seeking my thoughts and reflections to introduce their special contribution to the literature of implanted vascular access devices.

September 2011

John E. Niederhuber, MD
Professor of Oncology & Surgery
Johns Hopkins University School of Medicine
EVP and CEO Inova Translational Medicine Institute
Inova Health System, Falls Church, VA, USA

Preface

Almost 30 years have passed since the first TIVAD insertion, and now approximately one million TIVADs are implanted each year throughout the world. Since their first clinical use, these devices have had an enormous and incommensurable impact on quality of life, especially in cancer patients, by offering them the opportunity of continuous venous access and allowing more reliable and effective treatment. To a certain extent TIVADs have also changed the approach to patients suffering from cancer, as new and more active therapies have been developed. After many years these devices are not only used for cancer patients, as they have now found a place in the treatment of many diseases where continuous intravenous therapies are required.

As with all medical fields, TIVADs evolved over time. Some aspects of TIVADs have been well studied and the problematic features solved, while others remain controversial. It is with this aim that we decided to write this book, to fully describe the consolidated aspects of TIVADs and to clarify as much as possible the controversial or debated areas.

To accomplish this goal, we invited many colleagues with tremendous experience and skill to cooperate with us. We sincerely thank all these colleagues for their highly valued support.

Last but not least, we would personally like to express our appreciation along with the co-authors for the foreword by Prof. John Niederhuber. He was the first surgeon to implant a TIVAD in the world, and by writing the foreword to this book he has bestowed upon us a great honor.

September 2011

Isidoro Di Carlo
Roberto Biffi

Contents

Part V Late Complications

Contributors

Luca Aldrighetti Department of Surgery, Hepatobiliary Surgery Unit, San Raffaele Hospital, Vita-Salute San Raffaele University, Milan, Italy

Roberto Biffi Division of Abdomino Pelvic Surgery, European Institute of Oncology, Milan, Italy

Paul L. Blackburn Clinical Education, Bard Access Systems, Salt Lake City, Utah, USA

Kathleen Bubb Department of Anatomical Sciences, St. George's University, School of Medicine, Grenada, West Indies

Markus W. Büchler Department of General Visceral and Transplantation Surgery, University of Heidelberg, Heidelberg, Germany

Marco Catena Department of Surgery, Hepatobiliary Surgery Unit, San Raffaele Hospital, Vita-Salute San Raffaele University, Milan, Italy

Rita Celli Medico Legal Institute. University of Turin, Turin, Italy

Pierre A. Clavien Department of Surgery, University Hospital Zürich, Zürich, Switzerland

Johan Coolen Department of Radiology, UZ, Leuven, Belgium

Eric Desruennes Department of Anesthesiology, Gustave Roussy Cancer Institute, Villejuif, France

Bree D. Dewing University of North Dakota School of Medicine and Health Sciences, North Dakota, USA

Isidoro Di Carlo Department of Surgical Sciences, Organ Transplantation and Advanced Technologies, University of Catania, Cannizzaro Hospital, Catania, Italy

Markus K. Diener Department of General Visceral and Transplantation Surgery, University of Heidelberg, Heidelberg, Germany

Lisa Dougherty Nurse Consultant IV Therapy, The Royal Marsden NHS Foundation Trust, Surrey, UK

Walid Faraj American University of Beirut, Medical Center, Department of Surgery, Beirut, Lebanon

José Luis Fougo Breast Centre and Department of General Surgery, Hospital de São João, Porto, Portugal

Joel D. Harris Department of Surgery, Aurora Wilkinson Clinic, Summit, Wisconsin, USA

Roland Hennes Department of General Visceral and Transplantation Surgery, University of Heidelberg, Heidelberg, Germany

Hasan Karanlik Department of Surgery, Institute of Oncology, Istanbul University, Istanbul, Turkey

Phillip Knebel Department of General Visceral and Transplantation Surgery, University of Heidelberg, Heidelberg, Germany

Sidika Kurul Department of Surgery, Institute of Oncology, Istanbul University, Istanbul, Turkey

Gennaro D. LaBella Hatton Research Center, Good Samaritan Hospital, Department of Medical Education, Cincinnati, OH, USA

Hong-Shiee Lai Department of Surgery, National Taiwan University Hospital, Taipei, Taiwan

Marios Loukas Department of Anatomical Sciences, St. George's University, School of Medicine, Grenada, West Indies

Jason Malenfant Department of Anatomical Sciences, St. George's University, School of Medicine, Grenada, West Indies

Antonio Nocito Department of Surgery, University Hospital Zürich, Zürich, Switzerland

Franco Orsi Unit of Interventional Radiology, European Institute of Oncology, Milan, Italy

Alexandra Ozimek Department of Surgery, University Hospital Zürich, Zürich, Switzerland

Michele Paganelli Department of Surgery, Hepatobiliary Surgery Unit, San Raffaele Hospital, Vita-Salute San Raffaele University, Milan, Italy

Zhang Qinming Pediatric Surgery, Beijing Children's Hospital affiliated to Capital University of Medicine, Beijing, China

Francesca Ratti Department of Surgery, Hepatobiliary Surgery Unit, San Raffaele Hospital, Vita-Salute San Raffaele University, Milan, Italy

Marguerite Stas Department of Surgical Oncology, UZ Leuven, Leuven, Belgium

Christoph M. Seiler Department of General Visceral and Transplantation Surgery, University of Heidelberg, Heidelberg, Germany

Makoto Sonobe Department of Thoracic Surgery, Kyoto University Hospital, Kyoto, Japan

Robert P. Sticca University of North Dakota School of Medicine and Health Sciences, North Dakota, USA

Julius Tang Department of General Surgery, Good Samaritan Hospital, Cincinnati, OH, USA

Adriana Toro Department of Surgical Sciences, Organ Transplantation, and Advanced Technologies, University of Catania, Cannizzaro Hospital, Catania, Italy

R. Shane Tubbs Section of Pediatric Neurosurgery, Children's Hospital, Birmingham, AL, USA

Ton J. H. van Boxtel Training and Consultancy, Infusion Innovations (infu-In), Bilthoven, The Netherlands

Alena Wade Department of Anatomical Sciences, St. George's University, School of Medicine, Grenada, West Indies

Rik Willems Cardiovascular Diseases, UZ Leuven, Leuven, Belgium

Ahmad Zaghal American University of Beirut, Medical Center, Department of Surgery, Beirut, Lebanon

Part I

Introduction

History of Vascular Access

1

Roberto Biffi

Abstract

Milestones in the history of the development of vascular access and the subsequent advances in practical clinical applications are here described. The original achievements are presented and discussed. Fundamental steps to achieve a safe and effective IV access and management are pointed out.

Keywords

Totally implantable central venous access device • Tunneled central venous catheters • Total parenteral nutrition • Chemotherapy • Supportive care in cancer

Chronic hemodialysis and parenteral nutrition (PN), both in the hospital and the outpatient setting, are the most common and lifesaving methods of therapy made possible by modern technical advances in achieving and maintaining safe vascular access.

More recently, long-term totally implantable central venous access devices (TIVAD) have been shown to be safe and effective for repeated administration of chemotherapy, blood, nutrients and blood drawing for testing in oncology patients, and their use has been advocated to improve venous access reliability, reduce the discomfort and anxiety associated with repetitive venous access and improve overall quality of life.

Venesection and transfusion have long histories, the latter following the recognition of the circulation of blood by William Harvey in 1616 (Table 1.1), although the Egyptians in the Edwin Smith and Ebers papyri (circa 1550 BC) described 22 blood vessels which carried air, liquids and waste material, and were connected to the heart.

R. Biffi (✉)
Division of Abdomino Pelvic Surgery, European Institute of Oncology,
Milan, Italy
e-mail: roberto.biffi@ieo.it

I. Di Carlo, R. Biffi (eds.), *Totally Implantable Venous Access Devices*,

Table 1.1 Highlights in the development of venous access

Year	Development	Pioneer(s)
1616	First description of the circulation in *Excercitatio Anatomica de Moto Cordis et Sanguinis in Animalibus*.	Harvey
1654	First animal-to-animal transfusion using a silver tube inserted into the artery of the donor and a cannula of bone inserted into the vein of the recipient.	Folly
1665	Transfusion of blood from one live dog to another using quills to transfer blood from a carotid artery of the donor to a jugular vein of the recipient.	Lower
1669	Description of IV injections of drugs and medications into dogs in *Tractatus de Corde*.	Lower
1818	First successful blood transfusion into a woman dying of severe postpartum hemorrhage with blood obtained from a man using 8-oz syringes.	Blundell
1831	IV infusion of water and saline for successful treatment of cholera in humans.	O'Shaughnessy, Latta
1877	First creation of a fistula between the canine portal vein and inferior vena cava using a continuous silk suture. This was probably the first direct vascular anastomosis.	Eck
1912	Carrel presented with a Nobel Prize for a work published in 1902 dealing with technical aspects of vascular anastomoses.	Carrel
1944	Infusion of hypertonic dextrose, insulin and plasma protein by peripheral vein in high-risk surgical patients.	Dennis
1945	First polyethylene plastic catheter for IV infusion introduced into a vein by passing it through the lumen of a needle. Later developed and made available commercially as Intracath (BD Worldwide, Franklin Lakes, NJ).	Zimmermann
1950	Development of the Rochester plastic needle by an anesthesiology resident at the Mayo Clinic. Rubber tubing replaced by plastic tubing for routine IV administration.	Massa
1952	First description of subclavian percutaneous venipuncture to achieve rapid transfusion in severely injured war victims.	Aubaniac
1952	First description of the technique of inserting and advancing catheters for interventional radiology over a flexible J-wire inserted into an artery or vein through a needle.	Seldinger
1960	Central venous catheters inserted peripherally in upper and lower extremity veins for monitoring central venous pressure primarily in cardiac surgery patients and critically ill patients.	Wilson
1963	First description of a subcutaneous reservoir for repeated intrathecal injections (later modified for venous access).	Ommaya
1966	Creation of an arterio-venous fistula in the forearm to ensure a venous blood flow of 250-300 mL per minute is reported.	Brescia, Cimino, Appel, Hunvich
1966	Central venous polyvinyl catheters inserted into superior vena cava of beagle puppies *via* jugular veins. Puppies grew and developed normally for up to 256 days fed entirely by hypertonic parenteral nutrition solutions infused continuously into the central vein.	Dudrick, Vars, Rhoads

(*cont.*) →

Table 1.1 (continued)

1967	First comprehensive technique for long-term parenteral nutrition (PN) *via* central venous catheters inserted by percutaneous puncture of an external jugular or internal jugular vein and advanced into the superior vena cava of malnourished adult surgical patients.	Dudrick
1968	First patient supported entirely by infusion of long-term PN at home *via* an infraclavicular subclavian vein catheter for 6 months.	Dudrick, Steiger
1973	Silicone rubber catheter with attached Dacron cuff (for fixation by ingrowth of tissue) developed for insertion into superior vena cava for infusion and tunneled subcutaneously to exit on the chest; 9 of 18 patients received infusions by this catheter in hospitals; 9 patients were trained in appropriate techniques to allow them to undergo PN therapy in their homes.	Broviac, Cole, Scribner
1974	Replacement of subclavian vein catheters without venipuncture using Seldinger J wire technique.	Blewitt, Kyger, Patterson
1979	Broviac catheter modified by increasing wall thickness and lumen diameter. Double lumen silicone rubber Dacron cuffed catheter developed for ambulatory home PN and chemotherapy. Triple-lumen version was also designed to allow blood sampling in addition to infusions.	Hickman, Buckner, Clift, Sanders, Stewart, Thomas
1982	Introduction of implantable infusion chambers (ports or TIVAD) or chronic venous access devices (CVAD), placed surgically in subcutaneous pockets. Specially ground needles (Huber) designed to prevent coring of the entry site, intermittently placed through a self-sealing silicone rubber diaphragm after appropriate antimicrobial skin preparation.	Niederhuber, Ensminger, Gyves, Liepman, Doan, Cozzi
1984	Percutaneous translumbar and transhepatic inferior vena caval catheters inserted for prolonged vascular access for both inpatient and ambulatory home PN.	Dudrick, O'Donnell, Englert
1985-2011	Development of uncommon central venous access sites (Table 1.2)	

Before the 17th century, scientists and physicians did not understand the physiology of blood vessels and body fluids, until Harvey introduced them to the concepts of experimentation and biologic research. As physician and investigator, he first described the circulatory system in 1616 after experimenting with deer carcasses. Later, in conducting research on vivisected animals, he discovered that the heart circulates the blood throughout the body, acting as both a muscle and a pump and producing a continuous circulation of the blood. Until that time, it was believed that, although arteries and veins contained blood, the blood flowed like *human breath*. Indeed, until Harvey subsequently identified the capillary network, the liver was regarded as the center of the circulatory system. Well into the 19th century, many physicians believed that a *useless abundance of blood* was a principal cause of all disease, and accordingly, blood was commonly removed with lancets, cupping, and leeches.

Bloodletting was a common practice in the past, and venesection was performed by specialists for the treatment of fevers and apoplexy. Hippocrates describes the best method of venesection in his book Regimen in Acute Diseases: "... *if the vein is to be cut, do so at the elbow and draw plenty of blood*". A small Attic red-figure cup in the Louvre in Paris shows a physician about to perform a venesection.

The Romans had precision tools, which can be clearly identified in a surgeon's house in Pompeii devastated by the eruption of Vesuvius in AD 67. These instruments included scalpels, forceps, probes, needles, syringes and catheters. Many illustrations and woodcuts depicting bloodletting in medieval literature also show patients having blood let from the antecubital fossa.

After the pioneering activity of Harvey, in February 1665 Dr Richard Lower demonstrated successful blood transfusion from a cervical artery of one dog to a jugular vein of another. Previous vein-to-vein experiments had been unsuccessful because of the clotting of the slow movement of the venous blood. Cannulation was achieved by the use of sharpened quills and ligature using the same operative technique as in modem vascular access.

In 1877 Nicolai Vladimirovich Eck reported his experience with the creation of a fistula between the canine portal vein and inferior vena cava using a continuous silk suture. This was probably the first direct vascular anastomosis. Vascular anastomoses were then performed in Europe by Jassinowsky in 1889 and Jaboulay in 1896. Alexis Carrel in association with Charles G. Guthrie were to be the most acknowledged for early vascular surgery. Carrel was presented with a Nobel Prize in 1912 for a work published in 1902 dealing with technical aspects of vascular anastomoses.

Single needle dialysis, described by Kopp in 1972, has been replaced by double lumen needle dialysis because of superior blood flow and clearance characteristics. In most cases hemodialysis by catheter is reserved for acute and short-term use, particularly during the period of maturation of an internal fistula. The subclavian vein, the most convenient site, is frequently injured. Subsequent stenosis may be corrected with balloon angioplasty, but can result in incapacitating arm edema and compromise future access. Cuffed double lumen catheters can be used for permanent access.

In 1966, Brescia et al. [1] reported the creation of an arteriovenous fistula in the forearm to ensure a venous blood flow of 250-300 mL per minute. They had found cannula morbidity, revisions and clotting were a frequent cause of hospitalization of dialysis patients.

The pivotal development in providing opportunity for successful long-term infusion of hypertonic PN solutions was the accomplishment of consistently safe and effective central venous access by percutaneous infraclavicular subclavian vein catheterization. Although methods for gaining vascular access have been evolving and have been recorded for three and a half centuries (and likely were attempted even much earlier), practical central venous access is a relatively recent achievement of the past 60 years (Table 1.1). The primary development in the most frequently used route of central venous access today was the first successful percutaneous catheterization of the subclavian vein for blood transfusion in critically wounded French military personnel in 1952 by Aubaniac [2]. Within the next two years, this novel technique was subsequently used and developed further as a means of emergency central venous access for rapid volume resuscitation. Subclavian vein catheterization was not used initially for these purposes in the United States. However, it was used as a means of vascular access for central venous pressure monitoring in seriously ill patients, especially those undergoing open heart surgery, as reported by Wilson and Owens about a decade after Aubaniac's original report. The supraclavicular approach to percutaneous subclavian vein catheterization as a means of access for rapid fluid resuscitation was first described a few years later by Yoffa in 1965. During this time period, various percutaneous external and internal jugular vein catheter insertion techniques had also been used for venous access for fluid resuscitation in adults and for transfusion in infants before being used by Dudrick et al. [3] and Wilmore and Dudrick [4] as the initial route of central venous access for infusion of PN solutions both in adults and infants.

The first plastic (polyethylene) catheter for IV infusion was inserted into a vein either as a cutdown or by passing it through the lumen of a needle percutaneously [5]. A needle guard was added later to the needle catheter combination to prevent inadvertent transaction and embolization of the catheter. The decision to abandon peripheral venous infusion in favor of central venous infusion as the preferred route for providing all required nutrients entirely by vein was a key factor leading to the successful development and clinical application of PN. The quantity of high-quality nutrients required to achieve and maintain positive nitrogen balance and its associated clinical benefits in a critically ill patient had to be concentrated in a volume of water that could be tolerated without untoward complications. The resulting hypertonic nutrient solutions exceeded the normal osmolarity of the circulating blood approximately 6-fold (1800 mOsm/L) or more. The infusion of hypertonic solutions of this magnitude into peripheral veins caused an intolerable degree of pain, together with an inevitable and unjustifiable inflammation of the intima of the vein and damage to the formed elements of the blood, resulting in inordinate phlebitis and thrombophlebitis and associated adverse secondary consequences and complications. However, it was discovered and demonstrated in the animal laboratory, and subsequently confirmed in human subjects and patients, that hypertonic solutions, when infused at a constant rate over the 24 hours of each day through a catheter with its tip in a large central vein, such as the superior vena cava, were rapidly diluted virtually to iso-osmolarity by the high blood flow (50% of cardiac output) in this major vein.

In 1979, the Hickman catheter, a long-term venous access device, was used for chemotherapy for the first time [6]. The introduction of totally implantable devices (TIVAD) started in the early 1980s [7] (Table 1.2). By the 1990s, 85% of hospitalized patients received IV therapy at some point in their hospitalization, and the practice of IV therapy expanded to physicians' offices and other outpatient services while developing into a major home care modality. Today, these devices provide easy vascular access for the delivery of

Table 1.2 Uncommon vascular access sites

Common facial vein
Percutaneous right atrium
Right atrial appendage
Azygous vein
Hemiazygous vein
Umbilical vein
Splenic vein
Mesenteric vein
Gonadal vein
Common iliac vein (retroperitoneal)
Percutaneous translumbar vena cava
Percutaneous transhepatic vena cava

chemotherapy, fluids, medications, blood products and PN solutions. Over the last few decades, many management changes in oncology have occurred, particularly with respect to new chemotherapy combinations and more complex application schemes. Cancer patients usually require repeated venous punctures for treatment monitoring, application of chemotherapy or blood transfusions. Central venous catheters and implantable port systems have therefore substantially facilitated the problem of vascular access. To date, safe and easy-to-handle port systems have become an integral part of daily clinical routine in oncology. The use of vascular access devices (VADs) is an integral aspect of health care for neonates, children and adults, and has moved beyond the acute care setting to chronic, long-term care. VADs have a paramount role throughout the management of the oncology patient, as they are needed in the initial phases for surgery or chemotherapy, in the advanced stages for chronic treatment, and in the end stages for palliative measures. According to US data, approximately 150 million intravenous catheters are purchased, and at least 5 million central venous catheters (CVCs) are inserted every year. It is difficult to estimate how many of these VADs are actually used for oncology patients. However, it is reasonable to assume that the proportion is high, as most surgery, chemotherapy, and radiotherapy protocols for the management of neoplastic disease require intravenous infusions, including even those for palliative care, for which a long-term VAD is usually the best route of administration. Technological advancements in the future will inevitably produce devices for long term vascular access, which will be even safer, more reliable, and more cost-effective.

References

1. Brescia MJ, Cimino JE, Appel K, Hunvich BJ (1966) Chronic haemodialysis using venepuncture and a surgically created arteriovenous fistula. N Engl J Med 275:1089–1092

2. Aubaniac R (1952) Subclavian intravenous injection: advantages and technic. Presse Med 60:1456
3. Dudrick SJ, Wilmore DW, Vars HM, Rhoads JE (1968) Long-term total parenteral nutrition with growth, development, and positive nitrogen balance. Surgery 64:134–142
4. Wilmore DW, Dudrick SJ (1968) Growth and development of an infant receiving all nutrients exclusively by vein. JAMA 203:860–864
5. Massa DJ, Lundy JS, Faulconer A Jr, Ridley RW (1950) A plastic needle. Proc Staff Meet Mayo Clin 25:413–415
6. Hickman RO, Buckner CD, Clift RA et al (1979) A modified right atrial catheter for access to the venous system in marrow transplant recipients. Surg Gynecol Obstet 148:871–875
7. Niederhuber JE, Ensminger W, Gyves JW et al (1982) Totally implanted venous and arterial access system to replace external catheters in cancer treatment. Surgery 92:706–712

Vascular Anatomy of Central and Peripheral Veins

2

Jason Malenfant, Kathleen Bubb, Alena Wade, R. Shane Tubbs
and Marios Loukas

Abstract

Any practitioner dealing with a vascular access device requires a comprehensive knowledge and understanding of the anatomy of the venous system. For central venous access, catheters are most frequently inserted into the internal jugular vein or subclavian vein, but a wide variety of other options exists when these vessels cannot be used. The external jugular vein of the neck, cephalic and basilic veins of the upper limb, and the posterior intercostal veins of the thorax can also be used to access the superior vena cava which leads to the right atrium of the heart. The femoral vein is another route used to access the inferior vena cava which also leads to the right atrium. Other vessels that provide access to the inferior vena cava include the inferior epigastric vein, gonadal vein, and long saphenous vein. This chapter outlines the anatomy of the central and peripheral venous system with an emphasis on the commonly used routes for venous access.

Keywords

Vein cannulation • Subclavian vein • Axillary vein • Internal jugular vein • Femoral vein • Inferior vena cava

Any practitioner dealing with a vascular access device requires comprehensive knowledge and understanding of the anatomy of the venous system [1, 2]. This is critical to ensure successful access as well as to minimize the risk of complications for the patient [3, 4].

M. Loukas (✉)
Department of Anatomical Sciences, St. George's University, School of Medicine,
Grenada, West Indies
e-mail: mloukas@sgu.edu

I. Di Carlo, R. Biffi (eds.), *Totally Implantable Venous Access Devices*,

The general function of veins is to return low-oxygen blood from the capillary beds to the heart [5]. The venous system has a much lower blood pressure than its counterpart arterial system, which accounts for its thinner walls, specifically a thinner tunica media [5, 6]. This is also why blood does not spurt out if a vein is punctured [5].

Veins are more abundant within the body than arteries, and usually have a larger luminal diameter despite the thinner walls [5, 6]. Although the arteries and veins make up a circuit throughout the body, veins are known as the capacitance vessels because they carry about 80% of total blood volume at any given time [5]. Veins often contain bicuspid valves, most commonly in peripheral vessels that lie inferior to the heart; these act to facilitate blood flow towards the heart [6]. For central venous access, catheters are most frequently inserted into the internal jugular vein or subclavian vein, but a wide variety of other options exist when these choices are unavailable [7, 8].

The internal jugular vein runs anterior and lateral to the internal carotid and vertebral arteries. The vagus nerve is also found in close association, lying posteriorly in the groove between the internal jugular vein and internal carotid artery. The internal jugular vein receives blood from the brain at the base of the skull and receives branches from the face, mouth and upper neck [2, 9]. It is a dilated continuation of the sigmoid sinus, a dural venous sinus [6]. This vein lies just posterior to the sternocleidomastoid muscle. Once at the base of the neck, it runs over the subclavian artery, phrenic and vagus nerves, and thoracic duct or right lymphatic duct (on the left and right sides, respectively), joining the subclavian vein. This union of the internal jugular and subclavian vein marks the beginning of the brachiocephalic vein [9]. The right brachiocephalic vein is approximately 2.5 cm long and runs nearly vertically downward, while the left brachiocephalic vein crosses over to the right side of the chest to join with the right vein. The merging of these veins creates a single trunk, the superior vena cava, which runs approximately 3-10 cm long depending on the height of the patient and is 20-30 mm in diameter [1-3]. The superior vena cava also receives the azygos vein and other small veins of the mediastinum. This trunk serves as the main route of entry of venous blood from the upper body into the right atrium of the heart [2]. The right internal jugular vein is usually given preference for catheterization because of the almost straight course of that vein and the right brachiocephalic vein into the superior vena cava and right atrium [4, 9, 10].

The external jugular vein lies superficial to the internal and is smaller in size (Fig. 2.1). It receives drainage from the temporal and occipital veins of the scalp and some parts of the shoulder vessels. It runs from the angle of the mandible over the sternocleidomastoid muscle to the base of the neck, just lateral to the muscle. It is quite superficial during its course down the sternocleidomastoid, lying just beneath the platysma. At the base of the neck it usually joins with the superior portion of the internal jugular vein or with the subclavian vein [2, 9].

The subclavian vein is the continuation of the axillary vein and begins at

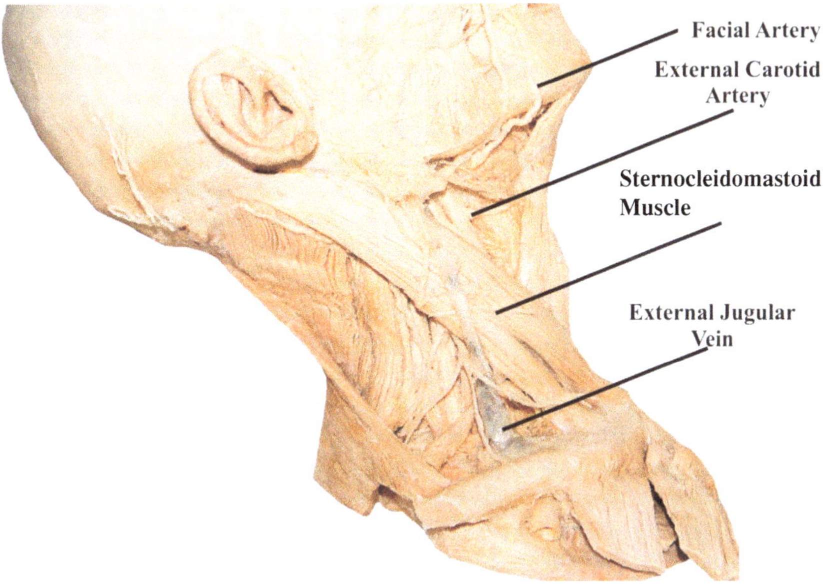

Fig. 2.1 In this cadaveric specimen the external jugular vein is exposed crossing over the sternocleidomastoid muscle

the lateral border of the first rib anterior to the insertion point of the anterior scalene muscle [6, 9]. This muscle, which is 10-15 mm thick in adults and 5-8 mm thick in children, separates the subclavian vein from the subclavian artery and brachial plexus, thereby protecting these two structures during catheterization of the vein [1]. The medial portion of the anterior scalene muscle is where the brachiocephalic vein is formed by the union of the subclavian vein and internal jugular vein [9]. The subclavian vein varies between 3-4 cm in length and 10-20 mm in diameter [1, 3, 11]. As the vein runs over the first rib to arch behind the clavicle, it reaches its largest diameter of 12-25 mm. Anteriorly, the vein rests on the first rib laterally and the apex of the lung medially. This has important significance because in instances of increased inflation of the lung, such as in diseases like chronic emphysema, the subclavian vein becomes elevated above its normal position. This could increase the risk for pneumothorax during cannulation of this vein [9]. It should also be noted that on the left side, the thoracic duct crosses over the anterior scalene muscle above the subclavian vein to join with the internal jugular vein. This also creates the risk of damage to the thoracic duct upon subclavian vein catheterization [9].

The upper extremities contain both superficial and deep veins. Deep veins in the hand and lower arm accompany the radial and ulnar arteries. Other smaller branches from the lower arm join to form the brachial veins approximately at the level of the elbow, and then again join to form the axillary vein at the shoulder [2]. The axillary vein begins at the lower border of the teres

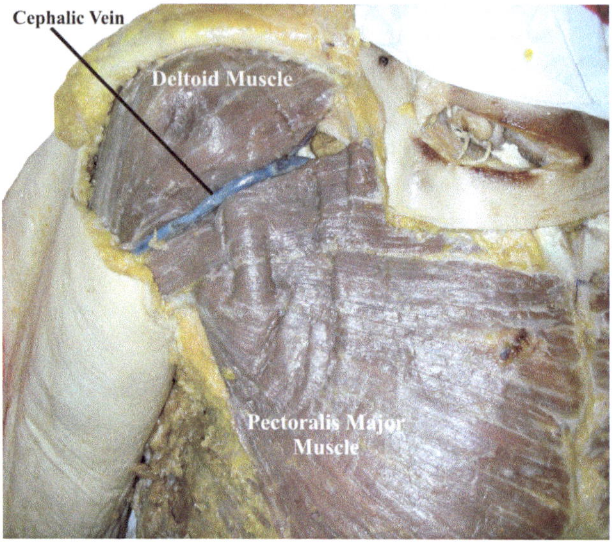

Fig. 2.2 In this cadaveric specimen the skin over the deltopectoral triangle has been reflected and the cephalic vein is exposed

major and runs until it enters the chest at the border of the first rib when it becomes the subclavian vein. The superficial veins of the upper extremities are usually visible and palpable as they lie in the superficial fascia just below the skin. The cephalic, basilic, and median antebrachial veins are among these [2].

The cephalic vein is approximately 6 mm in diameter (Fig. 2.2) [2]. It begins at the base of the thumb and crosses over the anatomical snuff box, passing laterally around the distal forearm and ascending the limb on the anterior border of the brachioradialis muscle. In most cases, at the level of the elbow, it anastomoses with the basilic vein via the obliquely crossing median cubital vein [6, 12-14]. Once it leaves the antecubital fossa, it ascends along the lateral border of the biceps brachii until the proximal third of the arm where it passes through the deltopectoral triangle between the deltoid and pectoralis muscles [12, 13]. The cephalic vein enters the terminal portion of the axillary vein at a right angle, which sometimes creates a barrier preventing further catheter advancement [2].

The basilic vein is approximately 8 mm in diameter, the largest of the upper limb vessels. It also offers the benefit of a non-tortuous entry through to the subclavian vein [2]. Similarly to the cephalic vein, it originates in the dorsal venous network on the back of the hand. It originates on the medial side and ascends the posteromedial surface of the forearm, before coming anterior just below the elbow [6]. It is usually palpable both inferior and superior to the antecubital fossa, where it continues proximally to penetrate the deep fascia approximately midway up the arm [2, 6]. This vein then continues medially to form the larger axillary vein [9].

Lastly, the long saphenous vein runs upwards and backwards across the medial surface of the tibia, superiorly and anteriorly to the medial malleolus

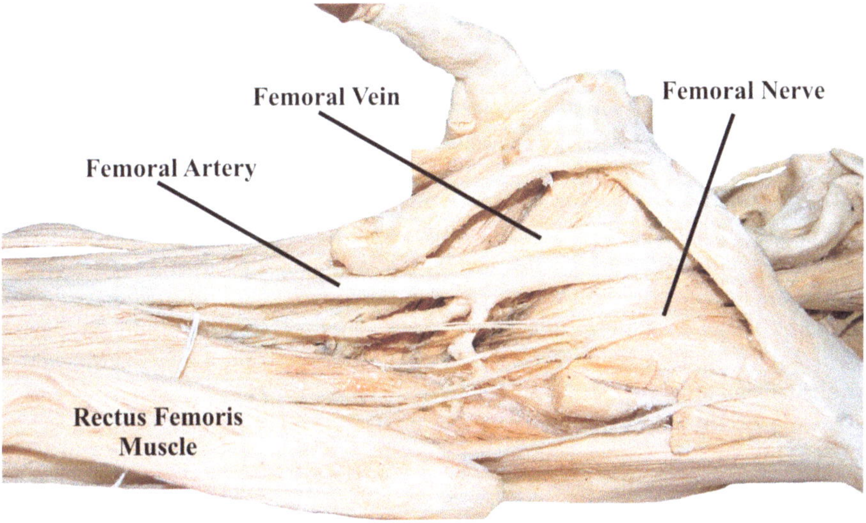

Fig. 2.3 In this cadaveric specimen the femoral artery and vein are exposed

[5, 6]. The long saphenous vein is accompanied by the saphenous nerve. The position of the nerve in relationship to the vein is usually anterolateral, but it could also be found posteriorly [5, 6]. The long saphenous vein eventually drains into the femoral vein.

In special circumstances when none of the above described veins can provide central venous access, other vessels are used. For example, these main veins of some children requiring total parenteral nutrition for long periods of time become no longer available for cannulation. In such instances, the central venous system can still be accessed via the azygos vein by placing the catheter through one of the right posterior intercostal veins. These veins lie above the intercostal artery and nerve in the subcostal groove. There are 12 intercostal veins in total. While the first vein drains directly into the right brachiocephalic vein, the second and third veins unite to form the right superior intercostal vein. This drains into the azygos vein which ascends from the abdomen [6, 15, 16]. These second and third veins are the preferred sites of access to use in these patients [15]. At approximately the level of T4, the azygos vein arches over the right lung to enter the posterior wall of the superior vena cava, allowing access to the right atrium [6, 15, 16].

In instances where the veins of the upper extremity or thorax cannot be used for central venous access, such as in cases of thrombosis, the inferior vena cava is used as the access route. The femoral vein is the major deep vein draining the lower limb and is the most common vein used to access the inferior vena cava (Fig. 2.3) [6, 9]. The vein lies just medial to the femoral artery, which is the palpable landmark used in these procedures [9]. The femoral vein becomes the external iliac vein when passing under the inguinal ligament to enter the abdomen. The external iliac joins with the internal iliac to form the common iliac vein. The inferior vena cava is formed from the union of both common iliac veins at the level of vertebra L5 and is present just to the right of the midline. It is responsible for draining blood from all structures below the diaphragm. The inferior vena cava ascends the posterior abdominal region immediately to the right of the abdominal aorta. It leaves the abdomen at the level of vertebra T8 by piercing the central tendon of the diaphragm [6]. There are several structures in close association with the inferior vena cava. Over its course, its anterior portion is crossed by the right common iliac artery, the root of the mesentery, the right testicular or ovarian artery, the inferior and superior parts of the duodenum, the head of the pancreas, the bile duct, the portal vein, and the liver, which overlaps and in some cases completely surrounds the inferior vena cava [6].

The inferior epigastric vein can also be used if no other better option exists [17]. This vein lies posterior to the rectus abdominis muscle throughout its course, as it follows the artery of the same name. It drains to the external iliac vein, leading to the inferior vena cava and subsequently the right atrium [6].

The gonadal vein (testicular or ovarian vein in males or females, respectively) is also used as an alternative for access to the right atrium in cases of thrombosis of the iliofemoral system or lower inferior vena cava [17, 18]. The right gonadal vein is the optimal choice because it drains directly into the inferior vena cava, whereas the left gonadal vein drains to the renal vein which then joins the inferior vena cava [17].

While the internal jugular and subclavian veins are the preferred routes for venous access [7, 8], the venous system runs in a network that allows for many other available routes to the superior or inferior venae cavae. Healthcare worker should always be aware of variation in the anatomy of the venous system among patients. A variety of genetic and environmental causes, such as collateral vein development or previous injury, can create differences in the size, length, and location of these veins [2]. With several forms of variation possible, it is crucial to be mindful of this possibility when performing cannulation procedures in order to achieve the best possible outcome for the patient.

References

1. Mitchell SE, Clark RA (1979) Complications of central venous catheterization. AJR 133:467-476
2. Sansivero GE (1998) Venous anatomy and physiology. Considerations for vascular access device placement and function. J Intraven Nurs 21:S107-114
3. Boon JM, Van Schoor AN, Abrahams PH et al (2007) Central venous catheterization - an anatomical review of a clinical skill - Part 1: subclavian vein via the infraclavicular approach. Clin Anat 20:602-611
4. Boon JM, Van Schoor AN, Abrahams PH et al (2008) Central venous catheterization - an anatomical review of a clinical skill - Part 2: internal jugular vein via the supraclavicular approach. Clin Anat 21:15-22

5. Moore KL, Dalley AF, Agur AMR (2010) Clinically oriented anatomy, 6th edn. Lippincott Williams & Wilkins, Baltimore
6. Drake RL, Vogl AW, Mitchell AWM (2010) Gray's anatomy for students, 2nd edn. Churchill Livingstone, Philadelphia
7. Felleiter P, Gustorff B, Lierz P, Hörauf K (1999) Use of electrocardiographic placement control of central venous catheters in Austria. Acta Med Austriaca 26:109-113
8. Ruesch S, Walder B, Tramèr MR (2002) Complications of central venous catheters: internal jugular versus subclavian access - a systematic review. Crit Care Med 30:454-460
9. Grant JP (2006) Anatomy and physiology of venous system vascular access: implications. J Parenter Enteral Nutr 30:S7-S12
10. Mathers LH Jr, Smith DW, Frankel L (1992) Anatomic considerations in placement of central venous catheters. Clin Anat 5:89-106
11. Moosman DA (1973) The anatomy of infraclavicular subclavian vein catheterization and its complications. Surg Gynecol Obstet 136:71
12. Loukas M, Myers CS, Wartmann ChT et al (2008) The clinical anatomy of the cephalic vein in the deltopectoral triangle. Folia Morphol (Warsz) 67:72-77
13. Au FC (1989) The anatomy of the cephalic vein. Am Surg 55:638-639
14. Bergman R, Thompson SA, Afifi AK (1988) Compendium of human anatomic variation. Urban and Schwarzenberg, Inc., Baltimore
15. Tannuri U, Tannuri AC, Maksoud JG (2005) The second and third right posterior intercostal veins: an alternate route for central venous access with an implantable port in children. J Pediatr Surg 40:E27-E30
16. Sansivero GE (2010) Features and selection of vascular access devices. Semin Oncol Nurs 26:88-101
17. Saleh HM, Abdelaziz AS, Hefnawy E, Mansour O (2008) Alternate routes for children with difficult central venous access. Acta Chir Belg 108:563-568
18. Coit DG, Turnbull AD (1992) Long term central vascular access through the gonadal vein. Surg Gynecol Obstet 175:362-364

Type of Devices for Mid- and Long-term Venous Access

3

Eric Desruennes

Abstract

This chapter describes the principal devices used for mid- and long-term venous access: midlines, central venous catheters, and implanted ports.

Midline catheters can be classified between peripheral short catheters and central venous catheters, but should not be used for periods exceeding 15 days nor for drips of irritating products or hyperosmolar infusions.

Central venous catheters (CVCs) are ideal for frequent or continuous venous access over mid- and long-term periods. CVCs can be cuffed or non-cuffed, tunnelled or non-tunnelled, implanted in a central vein or a peripheral vein (PICCs).

Implanted ports carry a very low risk of catheter-related bloodstream infection. Some of them can now be used for high-pressure contrast media injection.

Keywords

Mid- and long-term venous access • Midlines • Central venous catheters • Implanted ports • Tunnellization • Bloodstream infection • Cuffed central venous catheters • PICCs • Groshong • Contrast media injection • Catheter tip position

3.1 Introduction

Safe and reliable venous access is an important issue for various and complex therapies in the hospital or in the home, such as parenteral antibiotic therapy,

E. Desruennes (✉)
Department of Anesthesiology, Gustave Roussy Cancer Institute, Villejuif, France
e-mail: desruen@igr.fr

I. Di Carlo, R. Biffi (eds.), *Totally Implantable Venous Access Devices*,

cancer treatments, parenteral nutrition and blood products administration. We can consider that short-term venous access corresponds to a period less than 10-15 days, mid-term between 2 weeks and 3 months, and long term more than 3 months. Different devices are adapted to mid- and long-term venous access: midlines, central venous catheters and implanted ports [1, 2].

Implantation procedures are performed by many different specialties: surgeons, anesthesiologists, vascular radiologists, oncologists, and for some devices by nurses.

3.2 Midline Catheters

Midline catheters are peripheral catheters usually inserted into antecubital veins. They can be classified between peripheral short catheters and central venous catheters. These devices are little used in Europe. The best indications for midline catheter insertion are short term and not irritating infusion, short antibiotic therapy. Patients requiring 6 or more days of IV therapy should be assessed for a peripherally inserted central catheter (PICC) or a midline [3]. The mean duration of catheterization of midline catheters is usually 8 to 14 days and sometimes up to 1 month. Midline catheters are made of silicone or polyurethane. Some allergic adverse reactions with polyurethane have been reported by Mermel [4]. In the same study the incidences of catheter colonization and midline-associated bloodstream infection were low, respectively 5.0 and 0.8 per 1000 catheter days. However the major problem with a midline catheter is its tip, which is too short and rests below the axillary fold in the cephalic or the basilic vein; this location is very different from the position of a central catheter tip in the superior vena cava or the upper right atrium. When the catheter is long and central it is less likely to be in contact with the vein wall and there is a strong relationship between catheter malfunction, catheter-related thrombosis and catheter tip position [5-7]. For these reasons midline catheters should not be used for periods exceeding 15 days nor for drips of irritating products or hyperosmolar infusions.

3.3 Central Venous Catheters

Central venous catheters (CVCs) are ideal for frequent or continuous venous access over mid- and long-term periods. The catheter should be chemically inert, radio-opaque and non thrombogenic. The best materials for CVCs are silicone elastomer and polyurethane [1]. All types of CVCs are available in different lengths and sizes for adults, children and infants.

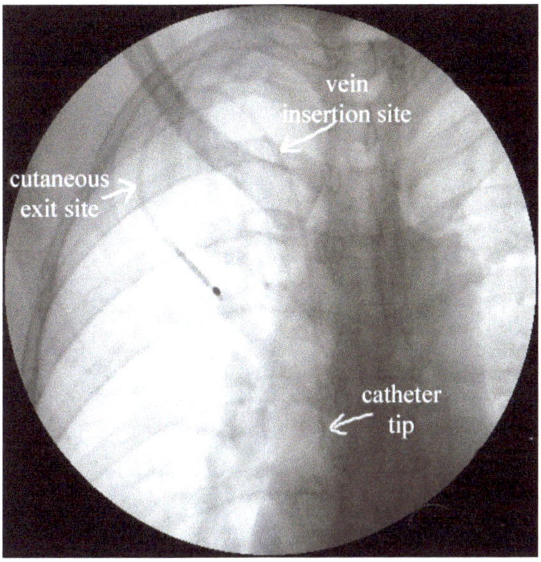

Fig. 3.1 Non-cuffed tunneled internal jugular catheter; because of the subcutaneous tunnel the cutaneous exit site is below the clavicle and approximately 6-8 cm of the vein insertion site. The tip of the catheter is located at the junction of the lower superior vena cava with the atrium

3.3.1 Non-cuffed Central Venous Catheters

Available in single or multiple lumen configuration, non-cuffed CVCs are suitable for short to long-term venous access. One and two-lumen CVCs may be tunneled to take away the cutaneous exit site from the vein insertion site (Fig. 3.1). The efficacy of tunnelization on catheter-related infections has been demonstrated for internal jugular and femoral vein accesses in critically ill patients, not for subclavian access [8-10]. Non-cuffed CVCs require stabilization with sutures or securement devices which are more efficient at reducing infection. CVCs coated with antibiotics or antiseptics have been used in critical care, but there is no evidence to support their use for mid- and long-term access. In Maki's review the risk of bloodstream infection associated with tunneled CVCs was around 1.7 per 1000 catheter days [11].

3.3.2 Cuffed Central Venous Catheters

The first cuffed CVCs were developed by Broviac and Hickman in the 1970s [12, 13]. Hickman-Broviac catheters have a Dacron cuff which provides an anchorage of the catheter in the subcutaneous tissue, eliminates the need for sutures and may act as a barrier for microorganisms (Fig. 3.2). Long-term total parenteral nutrition at home is a good indication of a cuffed CVC. The risk of bloodstream infection (BSI) associated with a cuffed CVC is around 1.6 per 1000 catheter days [11].

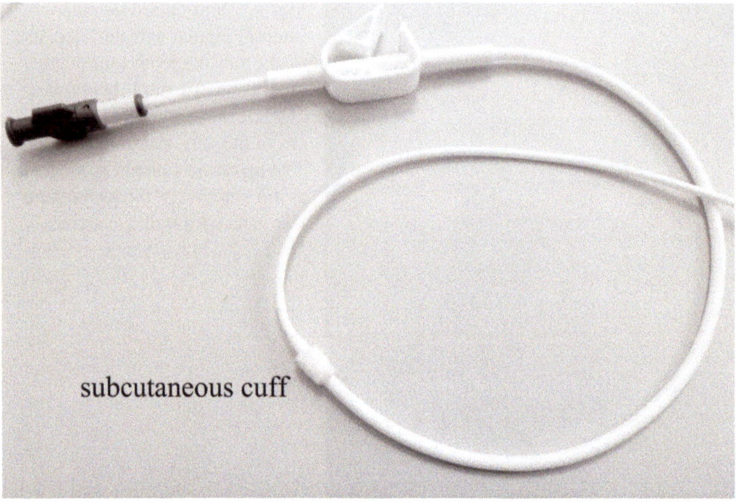

Fig. 3.2 Hickman-Broviac cuffed catheter

3.3.3 Peripherally Inserted Central Venous Catheters (PICCs)

Peripheral insertion of PICCs via the basilic or the cephalic vein abolishes the risk of hemorrhage and pneumothorax associated with subclavian access. PICCs are available with single, dual and triple lumen. They can be inserted at the bedside by specially trained nurses. The risk of BSI associated with PICCs is around 1.1 per 1000 catheter days [11].

3.3.4 Special Features

3.3.4.1 Groshong Catheters

The tip of Groshong catheters is not open-ended but contains a valve which prevents back bleeding and air embolism (Fig. 3.3). This system is also available on PICCs and implantable ports. The incidence of obstruction caused by clot formation in the catheter may be reduced with the use of a Groshong, but this has not proven its efficacy. As most reports and clinical trials dealing with other types of distally valved catheters have pointed out, inability to draw blood samples (withdrawal occlusion) is a major concern in their clinical use. In Biffi's study the use of a Groshong catheter was not superior to a traditional, open-ended device in terms of early and late complications of the implant and its use [14].

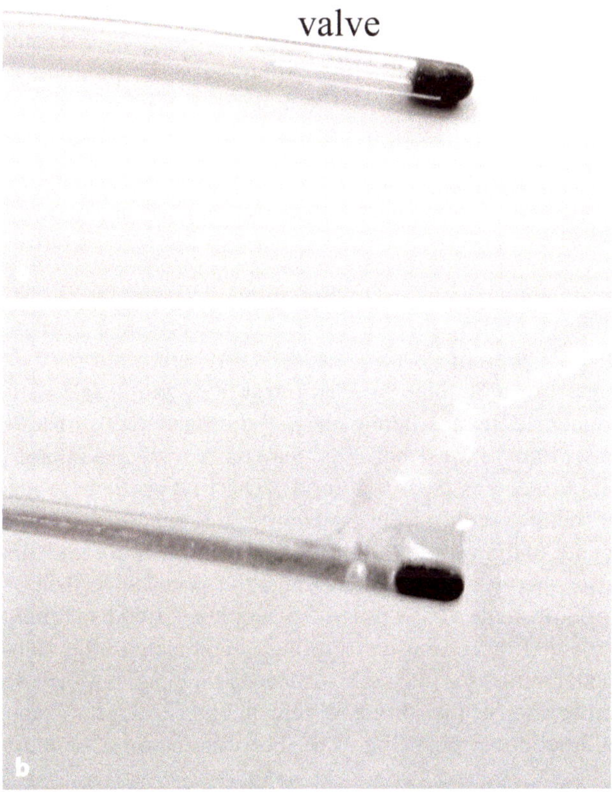

Fig. 3.3 **a** Groshong catheter tip. No pressure is applied and the valve is closed. **b** Groshong catheter tip. The pressure opens the valve and the fluid is injected

3.3.4.2 Power Catheters

Modifications on power catheters allow the radiologist to utilize them for contrast media injection during computer tomography scans in clinical routine with high infusion rates of up to 5 mL/s. This particular feature is available only on some PICCs and ports, and not on tunneled CVCs.

3.3.5 Catheter Tip Position

All recent studies have shown that the position of the tip of central venous devices is a significant factor for predicting catheter dysfunction and catheter-related venous thrombosis. When the tip is located in the last third of the superior vena cava or the right atrium, the rate of venous thrombosis is between 3% and 5%, compared with 42-46% when the tip lies in the proximal third of the vena cava or in the brachiocephalic veins [5, 6]. The most recent recommendations of the American College of Chest Physicians and of a French multidisciplinary working group in 2008 are that the optimal tip position for central venous catheters and ports should be the distal third of the superior vena cava or the proximal right atrium (Fig. 3.1) [15, 16]. The latter position does not conform to manufacturer and Food and Drug Administration guidelines, although no complications have been observed in long-term silicone central venous lines, the tip of which lies in the right atrium.

3.4 Implanted Ports

Ports are totally implanted venous devices. The first implanted ports were tested in 1982 with the Infuse-A-Port™, then in 1983 with the classical Port-A-Cath™ (Fig. 3.4) [17-19]. At present Port-a-Cath™ or PAC are often used as a generic term! Ports consist of a titanium or plastic reservoir with a self-sealing silicone septum connected to a silicone or polyurethane radio-opaque catheter (Fig. 3.5). This septum allows 1000-2000 punctures with special non-coring needles called Huber needles (see Chapter 4). The first ports were initially square-shaped and heavy, while recent ports are light, spherical or profiled, adapted to the age and to the weight of adult, children and infant patients (Fig. 3.5). The connection between the catheter and the port can either be sealed during manufacture or made at the time of placement. Blood sampling is possible with ports provided that extensive flushing is completed after sampling. Plastic ports are better suited for magnetic resonance imaging, but they do not allow radiologic interpretation of the correct placement of a needle, for example in the case of a malfunctioning port (Fig. 3.6). For this reason a titanium

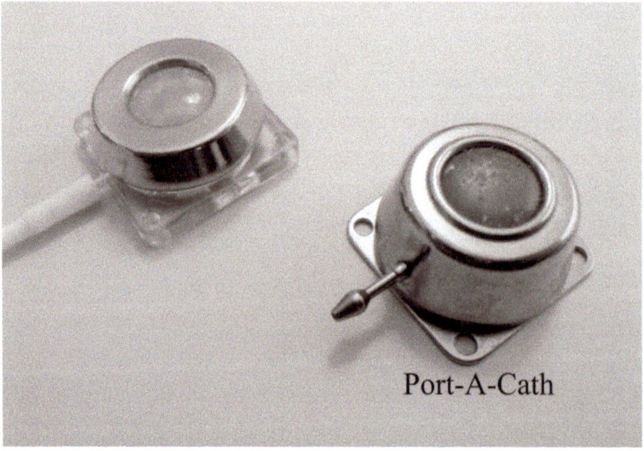

Fig. 3.4 First ports, square-shaped, including original Port-A-Cath™

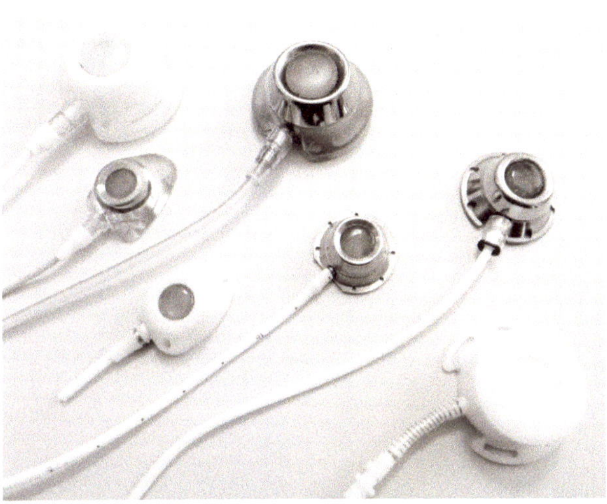

Fig. 3.5 Adult and pediatric ports made in titanium, plastic with titanium or only plastic

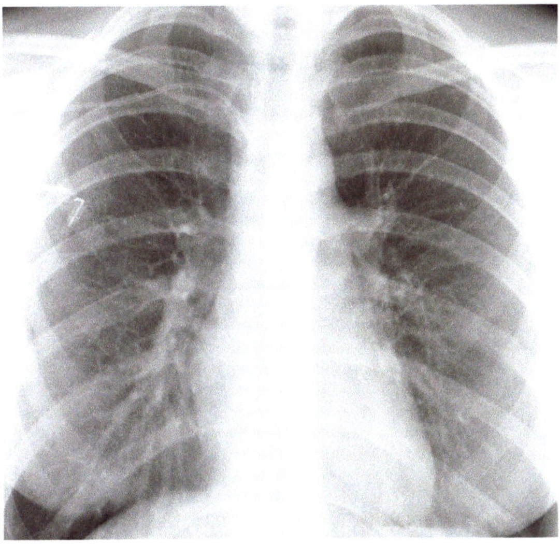

Fig. 3.6 Chest radiograph of a malfunctioning plastic port. The correct placement of the Huber needle is difficult to assert

reservoir should be preferred to a plastic reservoir. Most ports are now authorized for high pressure injection of contrast agent with a maximum pressure of 300 PSI and flow rates of up to 5 mL/s [20]. Ports are available with open-ended tips as well as Groshong tips.

The best indication of ports is long-term intermittent access, for example sequential chemotherapy for solid tumors, rather than continuous or intensive access. Ports allow the patient to take showers and to perform normal activities, sports and swimming. Usually patient acceptance is excellent compared with external catheters. The risk of BSI associated with ports is very low, around 0.2 per 1000 catheter days [11].

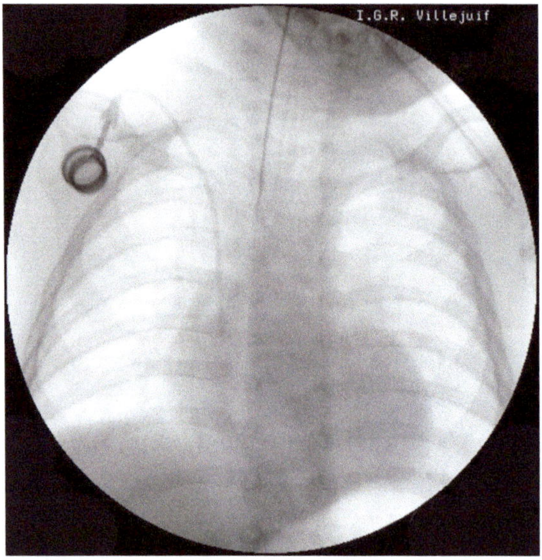

Fig. 3.7 Chest pediatric port in a 5-month-old baby

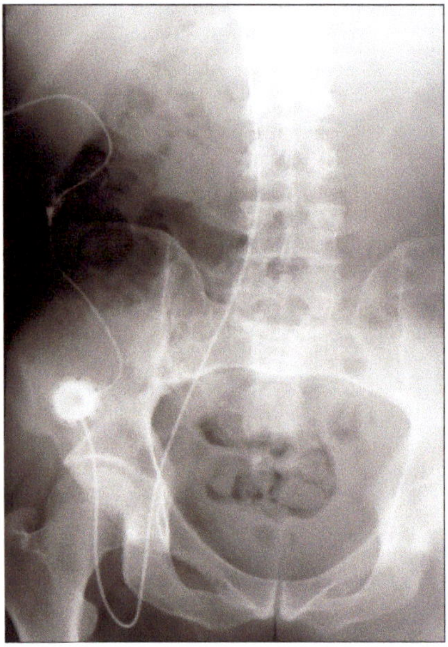

Fig. 3.8 Abdominal port with femoral venous access in a patient with lung cancer and mediastinal invasion

Implantation of ports is performed by different specialists in the operating room or in the interventional radiology suite, under local anesthesia, sedation or general anesthesia for children and infants. Ports are implanted in the subcutaneous tissue, usually on the chest wall (Fig. 3.7), sometimes on the upper arm, the lower limb below the groin or the abdominal wall in cases of contraindication of superior vena cava access (Fig. 3.8).

References

1. Galloway S, Bodenham A (2004) Long-term central venous access. Br J Anaesth 92:722-734
2. Sansivero GE (2010) Features and selection of vascular access devices. Semin Oncol Nurs 26:88-101
3. O'Grady NP, Alexander M, Dellinger EP et al (2002) Guidelines for the prevention of intravascular catheter-related infections. Centers for Disease Control and Prevention. MMWR Recomm Rep 51:1-29
4. Mermel LA, Parenteau S, Tow SM (1995) The risk of midline catheterization in hospitalized patients. A prospective study. Ann Intern Med 123:841-844
5. Luciani A, Clement O, Halimi P et al (2001) Catheter-related upper extremity deep venous thrombosis in cancer patients: a prospective study based on Doppler US. Radiology 220:655-660
6. Cadman A, Lawrance JA, Fitzsimmons L et al (2004) To clot or not to clot? That is the question in central venous catheters. Clin Radiol 59:349-355
7. Caers J, Fontaine C, Vinh-Hung V et al (2005) Catheter tip position as a risk factor for thrombosis associated with the use of subcutaneous infusion ports. Support Care Cancer 13:325-331
8. Keohane PP, Jones BJ, Attrill H et al (1983) Effect of catheter tunnelling and a nutrition nurse on catheter sepsis during parenteral nutrition. A controlled trial. Lancet 2:1388-1390
9. Timsit JF, Sebille V, Farkas JC et al (1996) Effect of subcutaneous tunneling on internal jugular catheter-related sepsis in critically ill patients: a prospective randomized multicenter study. JAMA 276:1416-1420
10. Timsit JF, Bruneel F, Cheval C et al (1999) Use of tunneled femoral catheters to prevent catheter-related infection. A randomized, controlled trial. Ann Intern Med 130:729-735
11. Maki DG, Kluger DM, Crnich CJ (2006) The risk of bloodstream infection in adults with different intravascular devices: a systematic review of 200 published prospective studies. Mayo Clin Proc 81:1159-1171
12. Broviac JW, Cole JJ, Scribner BH (1973) A silicone rubber atrial catheter for prolonged parenteral alimentation. Surg Gynecol Obstet 136:602-606
13. Hickman RO, Buckner CD, Clift RA et al (1979) A modified right atrial catheter for access to the venous system in marrow transplant recipients. Surg Gynecol Obstet 148:871-875
14. Biffi R, De Braud F, Orsi F et al (2001) A randomized, prospective trial of central venous ports connected to standard open-ended or Groshong catheters in adult oncology patients. Cancer 92:1204-1212
15. Geerts WH, Bergqvist D, Pineo GF et al (2008) Prevention of venous thromboembolism: American College of Chest Physicians Evidence-Based Clinical Practice Guidelines (8th Edition). Chest 133:381S-453S
16. Debourdeau P, Kassab Chahmi D, Le Gal G et al (2009) 2008 SOR guidelines for the prevention and treatment of thrombosis associated with central venous catheters in patients with cancer: report from the working group. Ann Oncol 20:1459-1471
17. Niederhuber JE, Ensminger W, Gyves JW et al (1982) Totally implanted venous and arterial access system to replace external catheters in cancer treatment. Surgery 92:706-712
18. Ecoff L, Barone RM, Simons RM (1983) Implantable infusion port (Port-A-Cath). NITA 6:406-408
19. Bothe A Jr, Piccione W, Ambrosino JJ et al (1984) Implantable central venous access system. Am J Surg 147:565-569
20. Wieners G, Redlich U, Dudeck O et al (2009) [First experiences with intravenous port systems authorized for high pressure injection of contrast agent in multiphasic computed tomography]. Rofo 181:664-668

Huber Needle: Different Types, Uses, Prevention of Accidents

4

José Luis Fougo

Abstract

This chapter deals with the nature of Huber needles, its different types and applications and the systems recently developed to permit their use without the risk of puncture.

Keywords

Punctures • Extravasations • Coring • Non-coring needles • Huber • Rebound

Totally implantable venous access devices (TIVADs) consist of two components: the catheter itself and the port. The port (or chamber, or reservoir) serves as a way to connect the catheter to the outside. To achieve this goal, the port is composed of a rubber membrane which can be subject to numerous punctures. It should be recalled that the main use of these devices is for chemotherapy perfusions and that extravasations of chemotherapy perfusate are unacceptable.

In recent years, TIVADs have been adapted to different purposes. Ports have been developed for epidural prolonged and repeated administration of analgesics and for the adjustable gastric bands used for the surgical treatment of morbid obesity, among other things.

A port is accessed by using a needle which punctures the skin and the rubber (silicone) membrane. Multiple punctures by ordinary coring needles can damage the silicone membrane and cause loss of substance. In the event of chemotherapy administration, there will be an increased risk of cytostatic extravasation and skin and soft tissue injury.

J.L. Fougo (✉)
Breast Centre and Department of General Surgery,
Hospital de São João,
Porto, Portugal
e-mail: joseluisfougo@gmail.com

I. Di Carlo, R. Biffi (eds.), *Totally Implantable Venous Access Devices*,

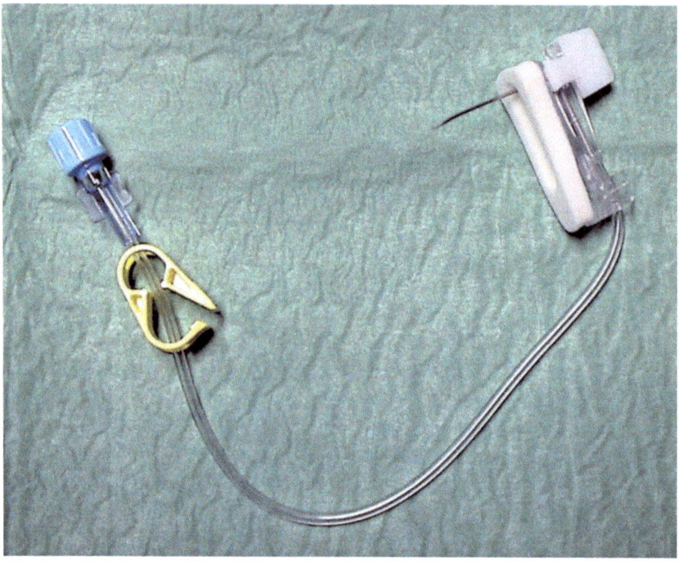

Fig. 4.1 Huber needle

Huber needles are non-coring needles especially designed for port puncture (Fig. 4.1). Ordinary needles have a bevel at the tip, and they may make a kind of biopsy of the silicone septum. Huber needles instead have a lateral hole which precludes the biopsy effect (Fig. 4.2 a, b).

A recently published paper described a study designed to compare the effect of multiple port puncture using standard coring needles with Huber non-coring needles under high perfusion pressure in the setting of adjustable gastric bands [1]. The authors stated that the use of standard needles to access the ports does not create the circumstances where fluid will leak from a cored septum. Surprisingly, they concluded that there is no more risk of damaging the septum with an ordinary needle than with a Huber needle. This finding must be tested in the context of chemotherapy and until now the use of the Huber needle is strongly recommended for port safety.

There are different types of Huber needles. They can vary in shape, length, diameter, bevel design and mechanism of protection against the exposure to blood.

Professionals may find commercially available simple, straight needles or 90º needles. Needle length varies from 12 to 37 mm. Needle diameter varies from 19 to 22 Gauge.

The choice of the needle varies with patient biotype, port height, port location in the body, the reason for the puncture and the product to be infused. For example:

- an overweight patient will need a +25 mm length needle;
- a thin patient with a low profile port will need a 15 mm length needle;
- sometimes we are confronted with ports placed well within the breast: these chambers may need a long (30 mm) needle as well;

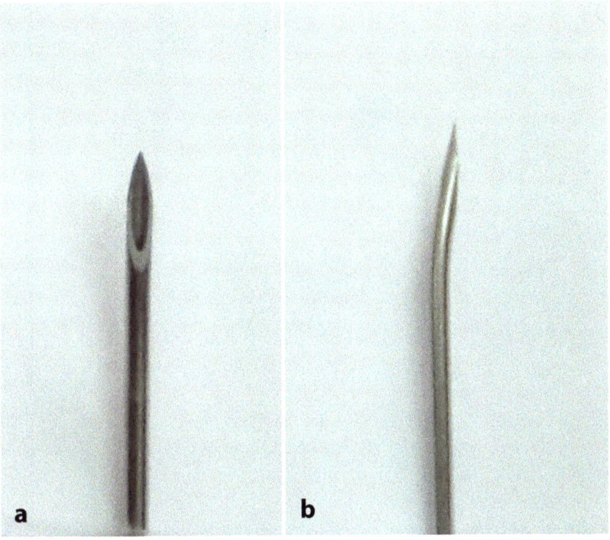

Fig. 4.2 a Huber needle special hole. b Structure of the needle manufactured to prevent damage to the port membrane

- ordinary chemotherapy preparations may be perfused through a 22 G needle;
- blood derivatives or some types of parenteral nutrition may need a larger, 19-G needle;
- in cases of a port puncture to assess TIVAD patency, or heparin flushing, a straight needle can be used;
- in cases of prolonged chemotherapy, a 90º needle that will be easily adapted to the body of the patient and to the dressings should be used.

The rebound effect/needle stick injury that results from the retrieval of Huber needles is a serious issue. To avoid this type of injury, manufacturers have been developing systems to protect healthcare professionals from needle puncture and contact with the blood. The systems are very different in conception, varying from simple tip encasement, to the coating of the entire needle and even to a method that allows the removal of the needle with just one hand, while the other hand may be used to simultaneously flush the port, thereby obtaining a positive pressure during the retrieval. This detail may obviate the need for the ordinary monthly catheter heparinization.

A recent Japanese study was designed to compare the applicability of two of these protected Huber needles (Huber Plus, C. R. Bard, Inc., New Jersey, USA vs. PolyPerf Safe, Perouse Medical, France) (Figs. 4.3, 4.4). Both devices were found to have advantages over the other, but care providers, patients and their relatives preferred the PolyPerf Safe in the overall assessment [2].

However, these products do not permit the use of a simple Huber needle, which is less expensive in relation to the more complex system. Other devices have been developed to avoid needle stick injury, including the simple device

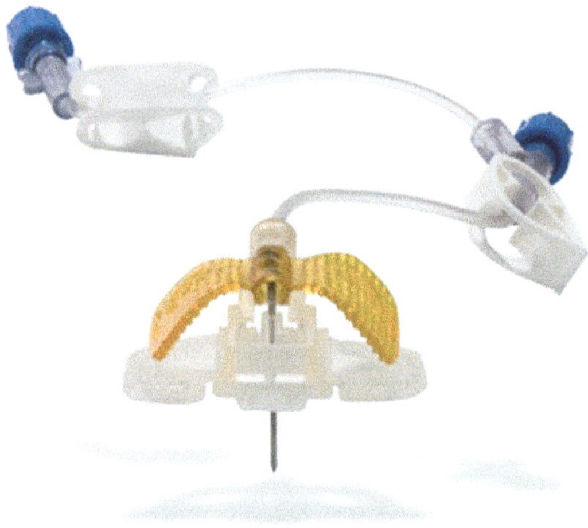

Fig. 4.3 Huber plus. Courtesy of Bard

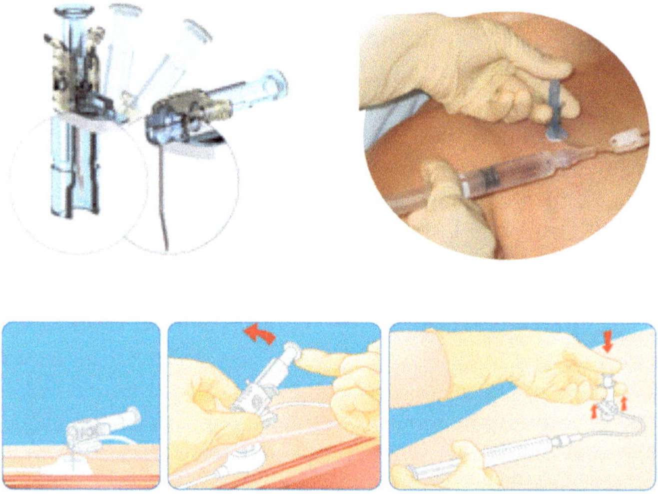

Fig. 4.4 Polyperf safe. Details of the device and how to use it, retrieving the needle while keeping positive pressure. Courtesy of Perouse Medical

depicted in Figure 4.5. This product is advantageous, in that it can be used with a normal Huber needle, thereby reducing supplementary costs. It can be adapted to each patient and protection is achieved with a safe method because both hands stay far from the needle, thus eliminating any chance of accidental puncture [3].

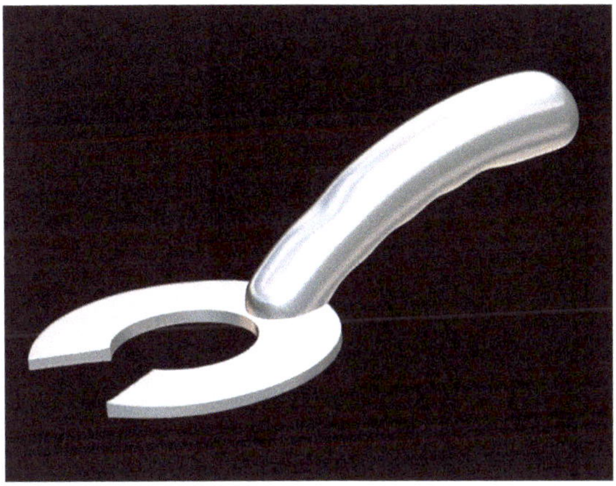

Fig. 4.5 Device for safely introducing and extracting the Huber needle and thus preventing accidental puncture

References

1. Bewsher SM, Azzi A, Wright T (2010) Use of standard hypodermic needles for accessing laparoscopic adjustable gastric band ports. Obes Surg 20:761-767
2. Shimono C, Tanaka A, Fujita A et al (2010) Comparison of port needle with safety device between Huber Plus (HP) and Poly Perf Safe (PPS). Gan To Kagaku Ryoho 37:947-951
3. www.wipo.int/pctdb/en/wo.jsp?WO=2006114801. Accessed 23 May 2011

Part II

Totally Implantable Access Devices

Clinical Indications, Preoperative Assessment, Set-up and Organizational Aspects

5

Makoto Sonobe

Abstract

A totally implantable access port is indicated for long-term, repeated administration of medications, chemotherapy agents, and blood products; parenteral nutrition; frequent collection of blood samples; and when alternative access cannot easily be achieved. These ports have several advantages over external central venous catheters, including less frequent maintenance, less risk of infection and thrombosis, and greater acceptance by patients. Before insertion of a totally implantable access port, indications for its need, how it will be used, and the overall physical condition of the patient should be considered. A minor surgical procedure is required to insert the port, although no special training is needed. The surgery should be performed in an operating room or interventional radiology unit using maximum sterile barrier precautions and sterile technique. Fluoroscopy and/or ultrasonography are needed to identify an appropriate vessel for catheter insertion and to confirm the final position of the catheter.

Keywords

Chemotherapy • Pneumothorax • Extravasation • Catheter-related infection • Catheter-related thrombosis • Non-coring needle • Ultrasonography • Fluoroscopy • Seldinger technique • Cut-down • Haemophilia

M. Sonobe (✉)
Department of Thoracic Surgery, Kyoto University Hospital,
Kyoto, Japan
e-mail: mysonobe@kuhp.kyoto-u.ac.jp

I. Di Carlo, R. Biffi (eds.), *Totally Implantable Venous Access Devices*,

5.1 Clinical Indications and Contraindications

5.1.1 Indications

Insertion of a totally implantable access port is principally indicated for intravenous infusates that cannot be administered through peripheral veins, damaged peripheral veins that can no longer accept an indwelling needle, and/or patients and treating practitioners who strongly prefer easy and safe venous access. These indications are similar to those for external central venous catheters. The advantages of a totally implantable access port over an external central venous catheter include the following: (1) less frequent catheter care; (2) lower risk of catheter-related infections and catheter-related thrombosis; (3) fewer restrictions on patient activities; and (4) less obvious and better cosmetic appearance. The disadvantages of implantable ports include: (1) need for a specialized needle (non-coring needle); (2) possible extravasation of infusate due to inadequate puncture; and (3) need for minor surgical procedure. Therefore, totally implantable access ports are used for patients who will need central venous access for an extended period of time (3 to 6 months or longer) or for patients who prefer an unobtrusive subcutaneous device [1, 2].

Cancer patients undergoing chemotherapy are good candidates for implantation because (1) there are many vesicant/irritant chemotherapy agents that can induce tissue necrosis if extravasation occurs; (2) long-term chemotherapy frequently damages peripheral veins so that peripheral access is difficult; (3) a safe and convenient venous access route is needed for long-term chemotherapy regimens; (4) blood products, fluids for volume expansion, and/or parenteral nutrition are often administered; and (5) frequent blood samples are needed for therapeutic monitoring. Therefore, patients with hematologic malignancies undergoing intensive chemotherapy and/or bone-marrow transplantation, and patients with solid tumors undergoing long-term continuous or intermittent chemotherapy (colorectal cancer and cancers of the breast, ovary, lung, etc.) are good candidates for implantation [1, 3–6].

In patients without cancer, intravenous nutrition for long-term care and repeated administration of blood products for hemophilia or other hematologic diseases are good indications for totally implantable venous access ports (Table 5.1).

5.1.2 Contraindications

There are no absolute contraindications for insertion of totally implantable access ports. Relative contraindications for patients include the following: (1) anticoagulant agents or abnormal hemostatic function (risk of bleeding); (2) bacteremia or active infection that can lead to bacteremia, such as pneumonia, pyelonephritis, or cholangitis (risk of early catheter/port-site infection) [3]; (3) the healthy lung is ipsilateral to the puncture site (risk of life-threatening

Table 5.1 Clinical indications and contraindications for totally implantable access port

Indications
Cancer patients in long-term care
• Chemotherapy agents cannot be given peripherally
• Damaged peripheral veins cannot accommodate indwelling needle
• Peripheral veins cannot tolerate vesicants/irritants
• Repeated fluid and/or blood-product administration
• Repeated blood tests for monitoring
Intravenous nutrition for long-term care
Repeated blood-product administration for hematologic diseases
Contraindications (relative)
Bleeding tendency
Bacteremia or infection with potential for bacteremia
Healthiest lung ipsilateral to insertion site
Abnormal venous return

pneumothorax); (4) abnormalities in venous return, such as superior vena cava syndrome or thrombus at the planned insertion site; and (5) allergy to materials used in implantable devices (e.g. silicone rubber, titanium) (Table 5.1).

5.2 Preoperative Assessments

Medical oncologists, surgeons / interventional radiologists, and nurses caring for a given patient should confer with each other about the indications for a totally implantable access port. Attention should first be paid to types of medication to be infused; expected duration of treatment; expected prognosis, especially in oncology patients; and patient ability to maintain the port. Evaluations should then be undertaken for the presence of coagulopathy, infection, superior vena cava obstruction, and heart and lung disease. These evaluations necessitate a medical history, physical examination, blood tests, including complete blood count and coagulation studies, and chest X-rays. Finally, the insertion site and implantation approach should be selected. Ultrasonography is useful for confirming venous return and ruling out thrombus at the planned insertion site.

Whenever possible, serious abnormalities in hemostatic function should be corrected by infusion of blood products, and ongoing infections should be treated. However, other clinical concerns may not allow these corrections. There is no need to stop anticoagulants (e.g. warfarin) or antiplatelet agents (e.g. aspirin) before implantation surgery. In addition, the patient should be adequately hydrated for easy access to the internal jugular vein and subclavian vein.

Identification of the healthy lung is important. For example, if the right lung is healthy and the left lung is diseased or absent (e.g. pleural effusion, presence of multiple cancer lesions, history of left lung resection, etc.), it is important to avoid using the right side for insertion and implantation. In this situation, right-sided pneumothorax could be life-threatening. An approach through the left internal jugular / subclavian vein or through a peripheral vein (arm or forearm) is a safer choice. Tumors in the neck or upper mediastinum or an open wound may also require changing the insertion site / approach.

5.3 Set-up and Organization

5.3.1 Hardware

For surgical implantation, the following three considerations are important: (1) adherence to sterile technique and maximum barrier precautions, (2) appropriate selection of insertion and implantation site, and (3) proper positioning of the catheter tip. Therefore, surgery should be performed in an operating room or interventional radiology unit. Essential equipment includes an ultrasound machine to determine the existence, direction, and size of the target vessels, and a fluoroscopy system to confirm positioning of the guidewire and catheter tip. C-arm fluoroscopic X-ray equipment is useful.

5.3.2 Instruments and Supplies for Implantation Surgery

Many hospitals have presterilized, packaged catheter-insertion instrument trays. The tray used at Kyoto University Hospital is shown in Figure 5.1. Several disposable instruments are also used. The following instruments are important: a scalpel with a size 11 or 15 blade; several dissecting instruments such as curved Kelly clamps or mosquito forceps; tweezers; needle holder; scissors; wound retractors; 10-mL or 20-mL syringes; small-gauge needle (size 22 or 23) for anesthetic infiltration; electrocautery unit; and surgical drapes. Sutures can be provided according to the preference of the surgeon (the author prefers 4-0 absorbable monofilament sutures). Heparinized saline solutions (10 IU/mL to fill the catheter and port, and 100 IU/ml to flush after implantation), 1% lidocaine for local anesthesia, and contrast medium for venography (if needed) are prepared for the procedure.

5.3.3 Port System

A package containing a commercially available totally implantable access port system is prepared. The package usually includes the catheter, port, guidewire, non-coring needle, vessel dilator, and catheter introducer with split-sheath mechanism (Fig. 5.2). Several commercially available packages

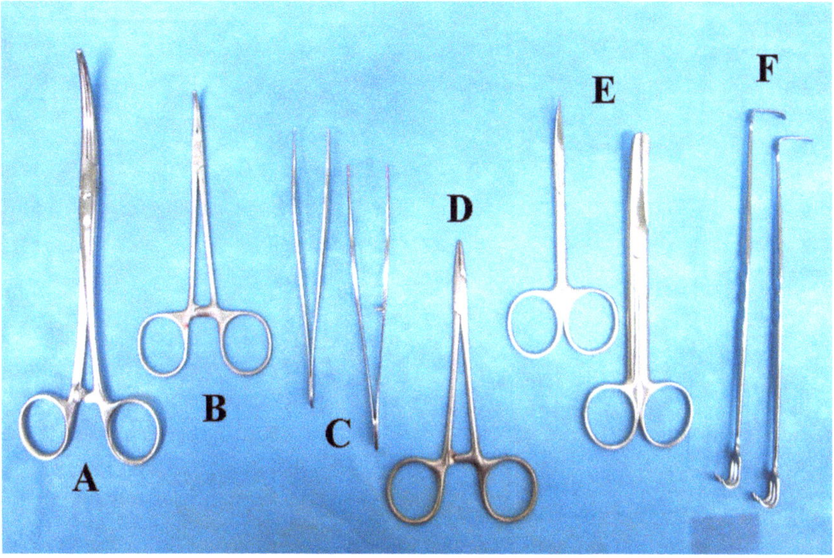

Fig. 5.1 Catheter-insertion instrument tray used at Kyoto University Hospital. Important instruments include curved Kelly clamps [A] and mosquito forceps [B] for dissection, tweezers [C], needle holder [D], scissors [E], and wound retractors [F]

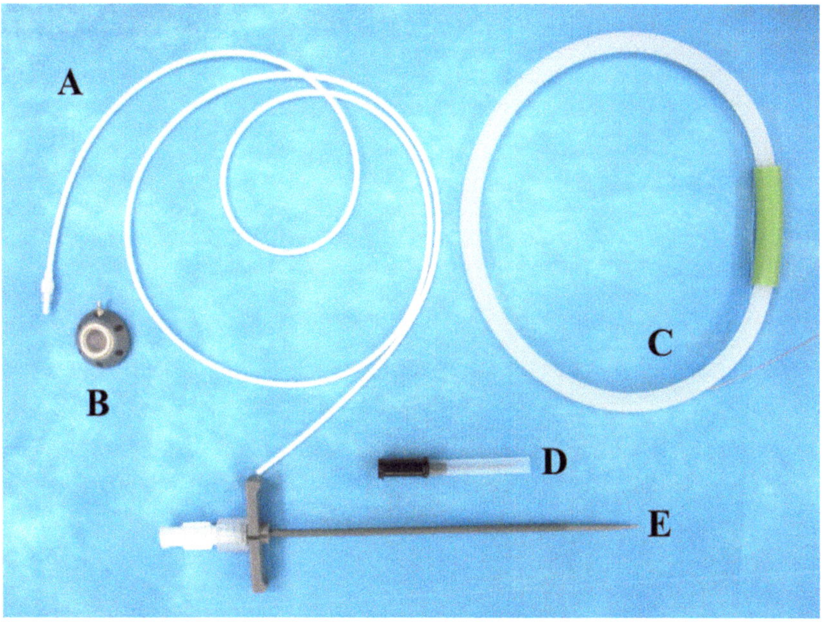

Fig. 5.2 Example of port system (Titanium Vital-Port System Mini, IP-S5116; Cook Vascular Incorporated, Vandergrift, PA, USA). Catheter [A], port [B], guidewire [C], non-coring needle [D], vessel dilator and catheter introducer with split-sheath mechanism [E], and other instruments (not shown) are packaged

include a special cannula for catheter insertion. Surgeons should confirm that they are able to correctly use this equipment before surgery.

5.3.4 Other Considerations

Implantation surgery requires at least one or two surgeons or interventional radiologists, one X-ray technician to operate the fluoroscopy system, and one surgical nurse. Surgical procedures include vascular access to the central vein, subcutaneous tunneling, and subcutaneous dissection to make a pocket for the port. These procedures require no special training for surgeons. Because changes in the approach or insertion and implantation site may be needed during the procedure, surgeons should be familiar with several alternative methods and approaches such as the Seldinger and cutdown techniques, and peripheral insertion of a central venous catheter [3, 7–10].

References

1. Vescia S, Baumgärtner AK, Jacobs VR et al (2008) Management of venous port systems in oncology: a review of current evidence. Ann Oncol 19:9-15
2. Kurul S, Saip P, Aydin T (2002) Totally implantable venous-access ports: local problems and extravasation injury. Lancet Oncol 3:684-692
3. Sonobe M, Chen F, Fujinaga T et al (2009) Use of totally implantable central venous access port via the basilic vein in patients with thoracic malignancies. Int J Clin Oncol 14:208-212
4. Schwarz RE, Groeger JS, Coit DG (1997) Subcutaneously implanted central venous access devices in cancer patients: a prospective analysis. Cancer 79:1635-1640
5. Kock HJ, Pietsch M, Krause U et al (1998) Implantable vascular access systems: experience in 1500 patients with totally implanted central venous port systems. World J Surg 22:12-16
6. Kreis H, Loehhberg CR, Lux MP et al (2007) Patients' attitudes to totally implantable venous access port systems for gynecological or breast malignancies. Eur J Surg Oncol 33:39-43
7. Di Carlo I, Barbagallo F, Toro A et al (2005) External jugular vein cutdown approach, as a useful alternative, supports the choice of the cephalic vein for totally implantable access device placement. Ann Surg Oncol 12:570-573
8. Chang HM, Hsieh CB, Hsieh HF et al (2006) An alternative technique for totally implantable central venous access devices. A retrospective study of 1311 cases. EJSO 32:90-93
9. Seiler CM, Frohlich BE, Dorsam UJ et al (2006) Surgical technique for totally implantable access ports (TIAP) needs improvement: A multivariate analysis of 400 patients. J Surg Oncol 93:24-29
10. Goltz JP, Scholl A, Ritter CO et al (2010) Peripherally placed totally implantable venous-access port systems of the forearm: clinical experience in 763 consecutive patients. Cardiovasc Intervent Radiol 33:1159-1167

Choice of Venous Sites. Surgical Implant/Technique

6

Isidoro Di Carlo and Adriana Toro

Abstract

Totally implantable venous access devices (TIVADs) can be positioned using a surgical or percutaneous technique. The surgical technique using the cephalic vein is the only approach able to avoid immediate fatal complications. Many different venous sites using the surgical technique have been described, including the external jugular vein, the internal jugular vein, the axillary vein, the saphenous vein, the gonadal vein and the inferior vena cava. The cephalic vein is generally used because it is easy to identify, but when it is unavailable due to hypoplasia or fibrosis, an external jugular vein cutdown approach can be useful. The internal jugular vein is used in patients when the cephalic vein or external jugular vein are unsuitable because of multiple previous lines, recent line-related infection, chemotherapy or thrombosis or in patients having tissue compromised by previous surgery, metastases, open wounds or previous radiation on the anterior chest wall. If the cephalic vein is not useful and the external jugular veins are unavailable, the axillary vein may be preferred especially in overweight subjects. When the superior central venous routes are not available, the most common technique used to obtain central venous access to the inferior vena cava is the inguinal approach using the saphenous vein or the gonadal vein.

Keywords

Cephalic vein • External jugular vein • Internal jugular vein • Axillary vein • Saphenous vein • Gonadal vein • Inferior vein cava

I. Di Carlo (✉)
Department of Surgical Sciences, Organ Transplantation and Advanced Technologies,
University of Catania, Cannizzaro Hospital,
Catania, Italy
e-mail: idicarlo@unict.it

I. Di Carlo, R. Biffi (eds.), *Totally Implantable Venous Access Devices,*

6.1 Introduction

The first placement of a totally implantable venous access device (TIVAD) was performed in 1982 at the MD Anderson Cancer Centre in Houston by John Niederhuber, using the cephalic vein and a surgical technique [1]. After that time the technique spread throughout the world and has been used above all by surgeons. Following on from the first description of the use of the cephalic vein to insert a TIVAD, many other different venous sites using surgical technique have been described, including the external jugular vein (EJV), the internal jugular vein (IJV), the axillary vein, the azygos vein, the superior vena cava, the right atrium, the femoral vein, the saphenous vein, the inferior epigastric vein, the gonadal vein, the lumbar vein and the inferior vena cava [2-6]. With the increasing request for TIVAD placement, surgeons were unable to meet demand. Consequently in 1992 a TIVAD was successfully implanted in an angiographic unit by using a radiologically guided technique [7]. Since then the percutaneous technique has spread throughout the world and in association with an increasing request for different clinical conditions, different specialists have begun to perform this procedure [8-10]. As a result, the surgical technique is less frequently used and the percutaneous approach has become the most utilized. However, with the increase in percutaneous procedures we have seen a concomitant rise in immediate post-procedural life-threatening complications, such as pneumothorax and/or hemopneumothorax, in part related to operator inexperience and in part to the technical limitations of the percutaneous approach itself [11]. This is why surgical cutdown, due to its safety, remains the only approach able to avoid possible immediate fatal complication. The aim of this chapter is to describe the surgical technique in the placement of a TIVAD in the most commonly used veins.

6.2 Patient Preparation

When assessing any patient for vascular access a thorough history and physical examination should be performed. Important historical items include previous catheter insertions and complications associated with them. Multiple previous lines should suggest potential venous scarring or thrombosis. In addition, a history of previous operations or radiation therapy in the vicinity of the vein should be sought. This is important if one is to be aware of potential anatomical deformities of the vein due to radiation injury or the presence of a large mediastinal tumor. The patient's overall health status and coagulation history are also important.

A physical examination can disclose *sequelae* of venous compromise, such as limb swelling, cyanosis, or the presence of subcutaneous venous collaterals.

Ultrasound (US) color Doppler is safe, noninvasive, and is the optimal preoperative study for vein patency. Lastly, a minimum of 1500 WBC are requested and coagulation status should be carefully evaluated.

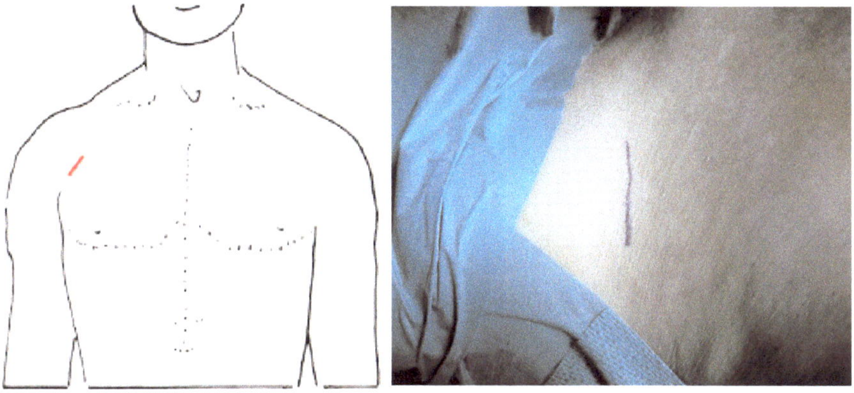

Fig. 6.1 Marked incision line in the right deltopectoral groove for the skin incision (schema and photo). Non dominant arm is preferred but both may be used

6.3 Cephalic Vein

The patient is positioned on the table in a five degree reverse Trendelenburg position. The non dominant arm is preferred. The neck, chest, and shoulder of the patient are surgically disinfected and draped in the customary sterile manner.

Usually 10 mL of 2% mepivacaine hydrochloride is sufficient to perform the entire procedure, depending on the sensitivity of each patient [12]. Local anesthesia is infiltrated in a sterile fashion into skin and subcutaneous layer and the skin in incised 4 cm inferolaterally to the clavicle into the deltopectoral region. The subcutaneous tissue is dissected down to the fascia overlying the junction of the deltoid muscle then the pectoralis major muscle, thus identifying the deltopectoral groove (Fig. 6.1). A self-retaining retractor should be used to perform the entire procedure.

The cephalic vein is located along the deltopectoral groove (Fig. 6.2). Except for the very thin patient, a good landmark for identifying the cephalic vein is the fat around the vein located under the fascia between the deltoid and the pectoral muscles. This fat is yellow ochre and is a different color from the brighter subcutaneous fat.

The cephalic vein is circumferentially dissected out for approximately 2-3 cm and ligated distally and encircled proximally with a 3-0 absorbable suture (Fig. 6.3).

The vein is transected ventrally and dilated using microsurgical forceps or a plastic hook usually furnished by the manufacturer with some TIVADs. After the catheter has been flushed with heparin-saline solution, it is introduced with gentle traction of the ligated vein to facilitate insertion of catheter (Fig. 6.4 a, b).

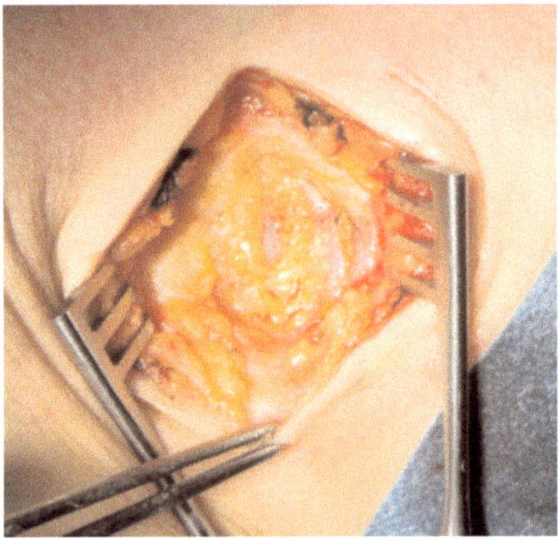

Fig. 6.2 Cephalic vein in the deltopectoral groove. The color of fat in the deltopectoral groove is yellow ochre in relation to the subcutaneous fat

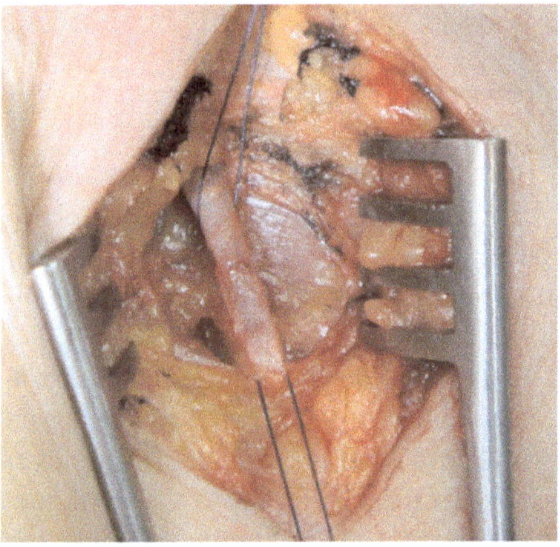

Fig. 6.3 Cephalic vein prepared for venotomy

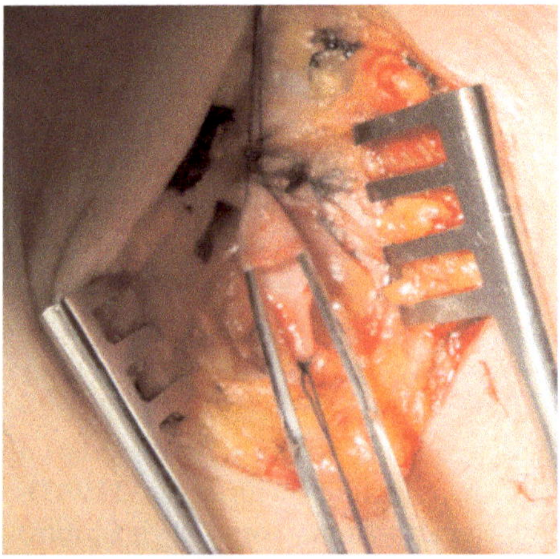

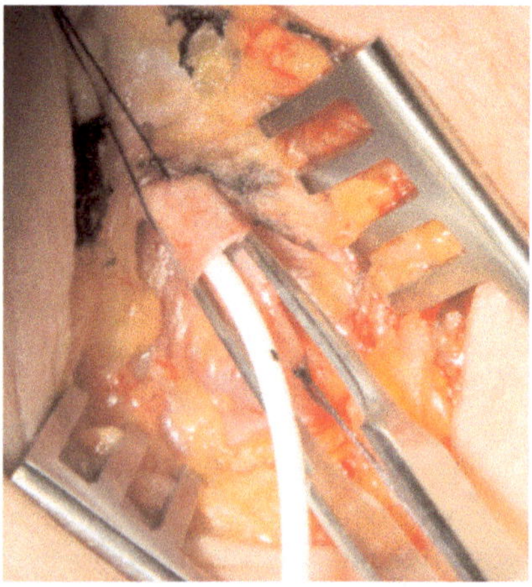

Fig. 6.4 a The vein is transected ventrally and microsurgery forceps are used to enlarge the vein. **b** The catheter is inserted and advanced into the vein. The proximal suture is tractioned to avoid venous back-bleeding

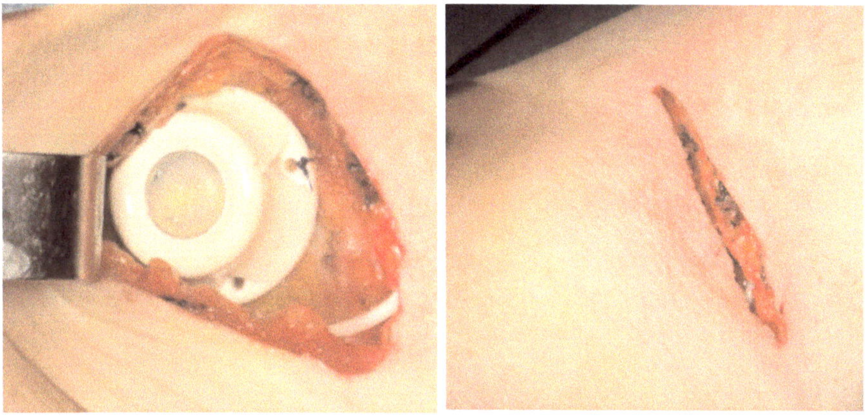

Fig. 6.5 a Port chamber is sutured to the fascia. b When the skin is released the port should not be visible in the middle of the incision

Back-bleeding from the proximal end of the cephalic vein is controlled by applying traction to the proximally placed 3-0 absorbable suture. The catheter is inserted through venotomy and advanced into the subclavian vein and innominate vein as far as the superior vena cava, so that the tip of the catheter lies just proximal to the right atrium. Correct catheter tip positioning may be controlled by using different methods such as fluoroscopy, electrography, Cath-finder®, or previous measurement of the catheter. After correct positioning of the catheter, the proximal absorbable suture around the proximal end of the cephalic vein and the catheter inside is tied down in a non constricting fashion in order to prevent back-bleeding and catheter migration. Difficulties in insertion of the catheter into the subclavian vein sometimes occur. In these patients the catheter is cut to the appropriate length based on surface landmarks, and a 40 cm J guidewire is inserted into the cephalic vein through the catheter gently. Guidewire positioning in the superior vena cava is confirmed by fluoroscopic guidance. After the catheter has been correctly positioned, the guidewire is withdrawn and the catheter is secured with a ligature around the vein proximally and connected to the port chamber.

Using the same incision, a subcutaneous pocket is prepared on the pectoral fascia. During this procedure the dissection of the subcutaneous fat from the fascia of the muscle pectoralis major should be performed very carefully to avoid bleeding and particular care should be used for hemostasis to avoid post operative hematoma of the pocket. Port chamber size should be adopted in relation to the thickness of the subcutaneous fat. In the very thin patient a pediatric port may be used to avoid the risk of skin necrosis. In contrast, for a severely overweight patient it is convenient to eliminate the fat tissue in order to leave in place a maximum depth of 2 cm of subcutaneous fat between the skin and the port [12]. If this procedure is performed, hemostasis should be very meticulous. This condition permits the Huber needle to be left stable in place, thus avoiding the risk of instability and extravasation with their related complications. The port chamber is sutured to the fascia of the pectoral muscle with at least three single nonabsorbable sutures to avoid port rotation. If the port has been correctly positioned it should not be visible through the incision line when the retractor has been removed (Fig. 6.5 a, b).

The patency of the catheter lumen is tested by aspirating blood and by flushing the lumen with a diluted heparin solution via percutaneous puncture. The subcutaneous fat can be sutured by continuous suture and intradermal suture may be used to suture the skin. No antibiotic is needes to implant a TIVAD [13] and this procedure may be performed in an out-patient department or in a surgical clinic. This reflects the cost of the procedure and the different reimbursements in each country.

6.4 External Jugular Vein

In cases where the cephalic vein cannot be visualized, or where it is hypoplastic or fibrotic because of previous chemotherapy, an EJV cutdown approach can be used [14]. Before surgery, the course of the EJV is marked on the skin using a dermographic pen, while the patient maintains the skin taught. The Trendelenburg position is not necessary. The EJV should be marked before each cephalic vein TIVAD implant, due to the possibility of failure of each procedure. In this way the EJV may be easily found. The patient's entire chest and neck are prepared and draped in a sterile fashion. Under local anesthesia a transversal 1.5 cm skin incision is performed 2 cm above the clavicle, requiring a shorter tunnel later. The EJV is dissected out and surrounded by two separate 3-0 absorbable sutures. The distal suture is tied and the EJV is partially transected transverse to the vessel midline while light traction is applied to the proximal suture.

A catheter is inserted into the EJV with the assistance of microsurgery forceps used to enlarge the vascular lumen (Fig. 6.6). Under fluoroscopic control, the catheter is driven as far as the superior vena cava where the tip of the catheter is positioned.

Once correctly positioned, the catheter is secured to the EJV using the proximal suture. If the catheter is inserted primarily in the EJV, the skin in incised 4 cm in the Morhenheim fossa and a subcutaneous pocket is prepared on the pectoral fascia. In contrast if the EJV has been used due to failure of cephalic vein insertion, the pocket is prepared as described for the cephalic vein. The catheter is then tunneled from the supraclavicular incision to the prepared pocket using a smooth instrument. Some of these tunnelers are furnished by the manufacturers. However, should these not be available in the operating room, simple smooth forceps such as Bengolea may be used to create a subcutaneous tunnel. The remainder of the procedure is then the same as described for the cephalic vein. Special care should be given to the catheter exiting the EJV. The curve directing the catheter towards the pocket has to be as large as possible to prevent kinking of the catheter and all its related complications.

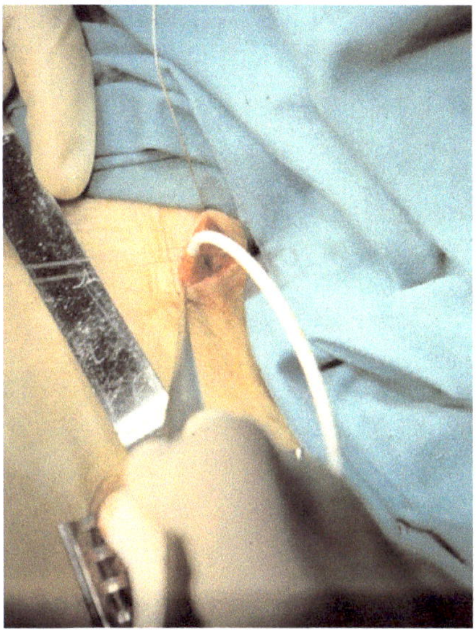

Fig. 6.6 Catheter inserted into the external jugular vein

6.5 Internal Jugular Vein

This access is used in patients when the cephalic or EJV are unsuitable because of multiple previous lines, recent line-related infection, chemotherapy or thrombosis. In addition this approach is useful in patients having tissue compromised by previous surgery, metastases, open wounds or previous radiation on the anterior chest wall. This vein can be used as first intention surgery or as a failure of cephalic or external jugular or both veins.

The procedure may be performed using local or general anesthesia, the choice depends on the clinical conditions of the patient. The patient is positioned supine with the head slightly elevated. The patient's head is turned at a 45° angle to the contralateral side. This position allows definition of the two heads of the sternocleidomastoid muscle. The skin over the sternocleidomastoid muscle needs to be marked and the area must draped in the customary sterile manner.

The skin incision is made longitudinally in the midcervical region approximately 2 to 3 cm above the clavicle. The necessary length of the incision varies but can range from 3 to 5 cm. Electrocautery is used to divide the platysma and the midcervical fascia. The sternocleidomastoid muscle is identified and the clavicular head is retracted laterally. The sternal head may be retracted medially or partially divided if needed for exposure. If the IJV is difficult to identify, palpation of the carotid artery pulse located medially to the vein and observation for the deep blue color of the vein can be used to guide the dissection. Once the vein is identified, care is taken while isolating a segment of vein.

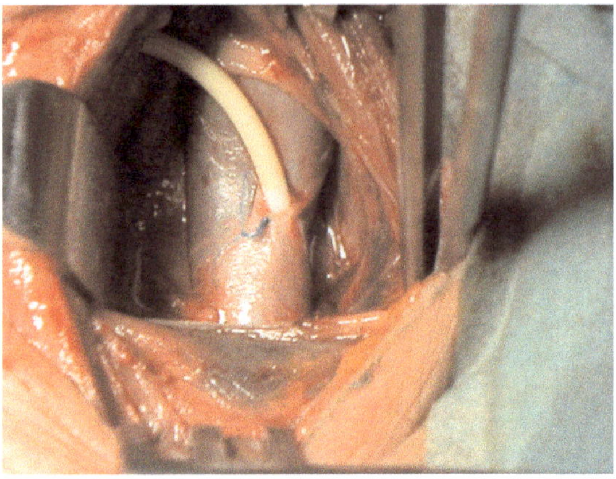

Fig. 6.7 Catheter threaded into the internal jugular vein

Initially a right-angle dissector is placed around the vein allowing an elastic vascular tape to be passed. This tape is then used for gentle retraction of the vein while the remainder of the venous segment is cleared on all sides of the adventitial tissue with sharp dissection. The midportion of the vein generally has no branches, which allows safe and easy isolation. A 4-0 or 5-0 Prolene® is placed in a purse-string suture. The suture is placed on the anterior surface of the vein in the center of the wound to allow ease of threading. It is best to allow a generous area (approximately 1 cm) inside the purse-string so that the vein wall will be insinuated between the catheter and the suture. This protects the purse-string from tearing the vein. After having positioned a Satinsky clamp above and below, a small venotomy is then made in the center of the purse-string. The assistant then enlarges the venotomy by forceps and the catheter is introduced into the vein. At this moment the Satinsky is released, the purse-string suture is tractioned and the catheter is advanced until the vena cava. After the position of the catheter is checked the purse-string suture is definitively ligated (Fig. 6.7).

A subcutaneous pocket is prepared and the procedure to complete the operation is the same used for the EJV.

6.6 Axillary Vein

If the cephalic vein is not useful and the EJVs are not utilizable the axillary vein may be preferred in thin patients. In contrast the dissection of the neck for the IJV is easier than the axillary vein in overweight subjects [15]. If the cephalic vein is unavailable or unsuitable for use, the pectoralis major and the deltoid muscles are retracted, the clavipectoral fascia is incised and the pectoralis minor muscle is divided. This surgical maneuver provides an approach to the axillary vein or its branches (Fig. 6.8).

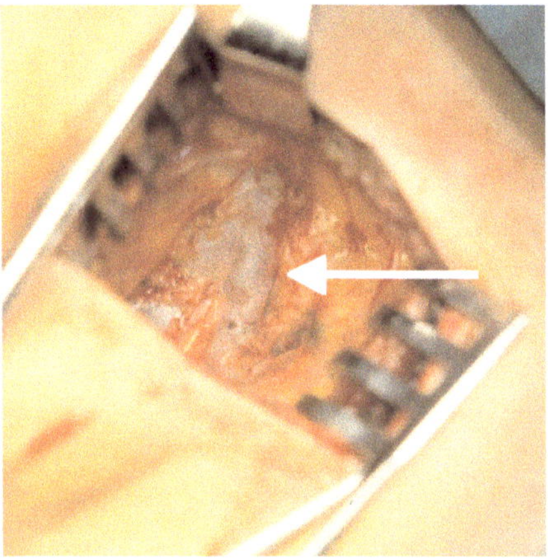

Fig. 6.8 Axillary vein (*arrow*)

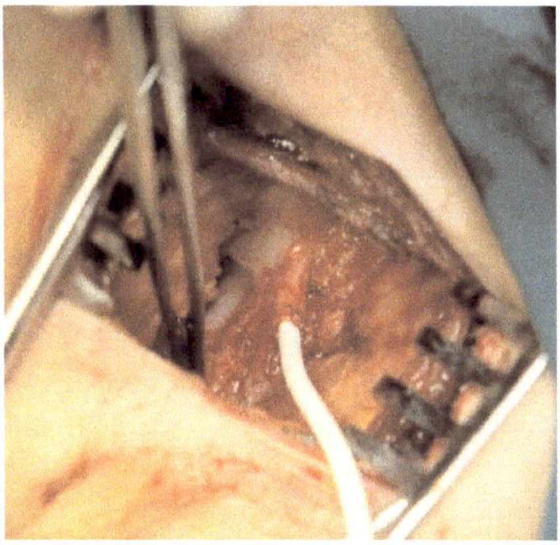

Fig. 6.9 Catheter tip is introduced in the axillary vein

A purse-string suture is placed on the superior wall of the vein, and the vein is then clamped. Using a Satinsky clamp a small venotomy is made in the centre of the purse-string and the catheter tip is introduced through the purse-string site and positioned in the superior vena cava (Fig. 6.9).

Correct catheter positioning is controlled via one of the methods previously described. The purse-string suture is ligated and the catheter is connected to a port located in the subcutaneous pocket anterior to the pectoralis major. Then the technique is the same as described for the cephalic vein.

6.7 Saphenous Vein

When the superior central venous routes are not available, the most commonly technique used to obtain central venous access to the inferior vena cava is

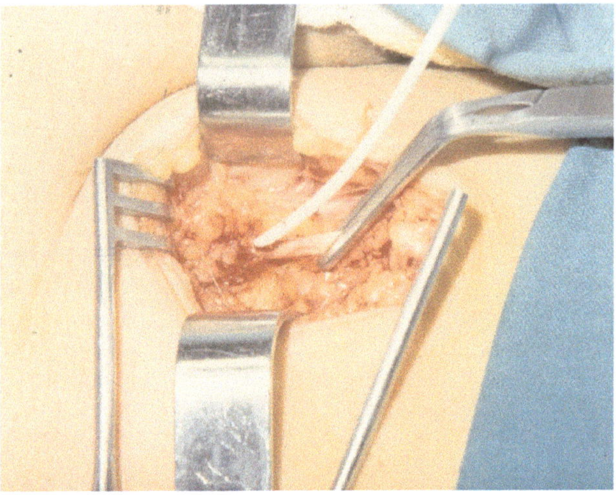

Fig. 6.10 Tip of the catheter is threaded in the saphenous vein

the inguinal approach. Relative contraindications to using the central venous system include venous thrombosis, burns of the head and neck, previous or planned radiation therapy to the neck or mediastinum, extensive cervical or thoracic trauma, oropharyngeal fistula and tracheostomy [16].

An inguinal incision is made and the saphenous vein is isolated. The saphenous vein is encircled by two nonabsorbable ties, the tie distal is ligated, and venotomy is performed, so that the tip of the catheter is introduced into the inferior vena cava through the saphenous vein. The vein can also be clamped and ligated after catheter introduction (Fig. 6.10).

Under fluoroscopic guidance, the tip of the catheter is threaded to the level of the renal veins. The catheter is secured to the saphenous vein with the absorbable ties. When using the saphenous vein access to place a TIVAD there is an elevated risk of contamination and subsequent infection in the inguinal region. For this reason a minimum of 5-10 cm distance is used between the inguinal incision and the port pocket. Abdominal pocket is the most used site, but the absence of a solid plane such as the thorax makes the insertion of the Huber needle difficult. For this reason the wall of the leg may be considered a valid alternative site [17]. The catheter is tunneled subcutaneously and the port chamber is sutured to the fascia with three single non absorbable sutures (Fig. 6.11).

The leg may be considered a valid alternative to position the port. The catheter is connected to the port and flushed with heparin solution to confirm system patency. The inguinal incision is properly cleaned and closed in multiple layers to prevent contamination of the catheter by skin organisms in this region.

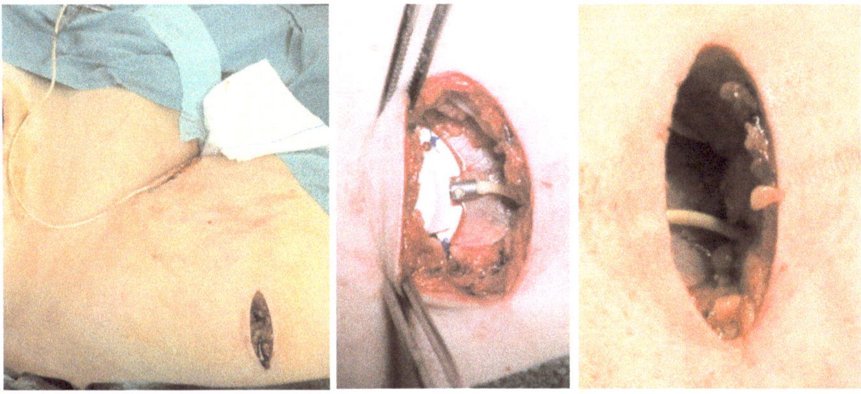

Fig. 6.11 a Alternative site of positioning of port when the saphenous vein is used. b Port chamber is sutured to the fascia. c If correctly implanted, when the retractor is released the port should not be visible from the midline incision

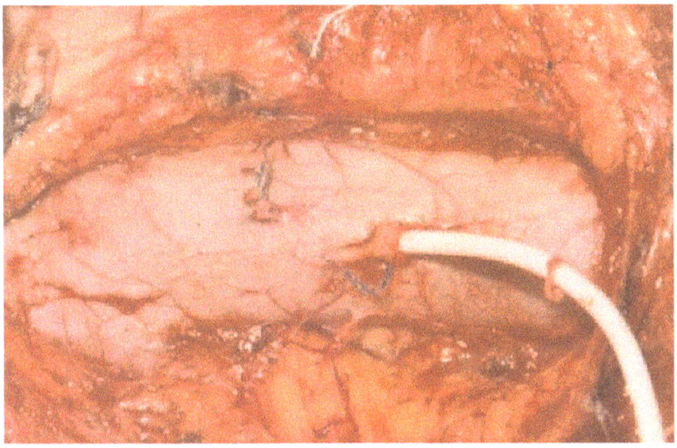

Fig. 6.12 Catheter in the gonadal vein. From [18] with permission

6.8 Gonadal Vein

This approach is rarely used but it can be useful in patients having undergone abdominal surgery.

The right gonadal vein is preferable to the left because of its direct takeoff from the inferior vena cava. The catheter is inserted under general anesthesia. The right gonadal vein is exposed by Kocherizing the duodenum and then dissected 2-3 cm from the vena cava. The vein is ligated in its distal part and clamped in its proximal part. Following the venotomy the tip of the catheter is introduced and positioned in the superior vena cava before its confluence into the right atrium.

After the fluoroscopic control the catheter is secured with two ligatures, and connected with the implantable device lodged in a right prethoracic subcutaneous pouch [18]. The vena cava can also be used at the confluence of the gonadal vein (Fig. 6.12).

References

1. Niederhuber JE, Ensminger W, Gyves JW et al (1982) Totally implanted venous and arterial access system to replace external catheters in cancer treatment. Surgery 92:706-712
2. Malt RA, Kempster M (1983) Direct azygos vein and superior vena cava cannulation for parenteral nutrition. JPEN 7:580-581
3. Maher JW (1983) A technique for the positioning of permanent central venous catheters in patients with thrombosis of the superior vena cava. Surg Gynecol Obstet 156:659-660
4. Starkhammar H, Bengtsson M (1985) Totally implanted device for venous access. Experience in tumour patients. Acta Radiol Oncol 24:173-176
5. Boddie AW Jr (1989) Translumbar catheterization of the inferior vena cava for long-term angioaccess. Surg Gynecol Obstet 168:55-56
6. Williard W, Coit D, Lucas A, Groeger JS (1991) Long-term vascular access via the inferior vena cava. J Surg Oncol 46:162-166
7. Morris SL, Jaques PF, Mauro MA (1992) Radiology-assisted placement of implantable subcutaneous infusion ports for long-term venous access. Radiology 184:149-151
8. Laurenzi L, Fimiani C, Faglieri N et al (1996) Complications with fully implantable venous access systems in oncologic patients. Tumori 82:232-236
9. Munro FD, Gillett PM, Wratten JC et al (1999) Totally implantable central venous access devices for paediatric oncology patients. Med Pediatr Oncol 33:377-381
10. Lorch H, Zwaan M, Kagel C, Weiss HD (2001) Central venous access ports placed by interventional radiologists: experience with 125 consecutive patients. Cardiovasc Intervent Radiol 24:180-184
11. Di Carlo I, Pulvirenti E, Mannino M, Toro A (2010) Increased use of percutaneous technique for totally implantable venous access devices. Is it real progress? A 27-year comprehensive review on early complications. Ann Surg Oncol 17:1649-1656
12. Di Carlo I, Cordio S, Privitera G et al (2001) Totally implantable venous access devices implanted surgically. A retrospective study on early and late complications. Arch Surg 136:1050-1053
13. Di Carlo I, Toro A, Pulvirenti E et al (2011) Could antibiotic prophylaxis be necessary to implant totally implantable venous access devices? Randomized prospective study. Surg Oncol 20:20-25
14. Di Carlo I, Barbagallo F, Toro A et al (2005) External jugular vein cutdown approach as an useful alternative support the choice of the cephalic vein for the totally implantable access device placement. Ann Surg Oncol 12:570-573
15. Di Carlo I, Puleo S (2001) A new technique for totally implantable venous access device (TIVAD) insertion. Surgery 129:768-769
16. Chen SY, Lin CH, Chang HM et al (2008) A safe and effective method to implant a totally implantable access port in patients with synchronous bilateral mastectomies: modified femoral vein approach. J Surg Oncol 98:197-199
17. Toro A, Sofia M, Sparatore F et al (2005) Assessment of patient's comfort and functioning of a totally implantable venous system placed in the safenous vein. G Chir 26:282-285
18. Di Carlo I, Lombardo R, Russello D, Puleo S (2000) Totally implantable venous access device inserted during major abdominal operations for cancer. A new technique. Hepatogastroenterology 47:907-908

Choice of Venous Sites. Percutaneous Implant/Technique/ US Guidance

7

Roberto Biffi

Abstract

The percutaneous approach to the subclavian or internal jugular vein is currently the most popular procedure for placing central venous catheters in the superior vena cava, both for short- and long-term use. There is compelling evidence that ultrasound (US)-guided venipuncture (with realtime ultrasonography) is associated with a substantial benefit, and US support is therefore strongly recommended (Grade A) for all central venous catheter insertions. Concerns have been raised with respect to training, as the novel techniques should be incorporated into the US courses that are currently being set up for radiologists, anesthesiologists, and surgeons. Moreover, the landmark method would remain important for emergencies when US equipment and/or expertise might not be immediately available. A recent randomized trial concluded that central venous insertion modality and sites had no impact on either early or late complication rates when performed by experienced operators, but US-guided insertion showed the lowest proportion of failures. While many RCTs have clearly shown that US guidance is superior to the landmark technique - at least in terms of immediate outcome - for internal jugular vein cannulation in a variety of clinical settings, doubts still persist for the subclavian insertion site. A very recent RCT in ICU patients has suggested that US-guided cannulation of the subclavian vein is superior to the landmark method in terms of average access time, number of attempts, frequency of artery puncture, hematoma, hemothorax, pneumothorax, brachial plexus and phrenic nerve injury. More studies are needed to address long-term benefits (if any) and cost-effectiveness.

R. Biffi (✉)
Division of Abdomino Pelvic Surgery, European Institute of Oncology, Milan, Italy
e-mail: roberto.biffi@ieo.it

I. Di Carlo, R. Biffi (eds.), *Totally Implantable Venous Access Devices*,

Keywords
Central venous catheters • Percutaneous implantation • Ultrasounds • Ultrasound guidance • Internal jugular vein • Subclavian vein • Femoral vein

7.1 Choice of Venous Sites

The use of central venous access devices has become an essential component in the treatment of many medical disorders. It has been estimated that several million devices are inserted each year, facilitating many emerging therapies, including long-term chemotherapy. Stable and safe venous access is indeed of paramount importance in cancer patients, although it is difficult to estimate how many of these devices are actually used in oncology patients. However, it is reasonable to assume that the proportion is high, since most surgery, chemotherapy, and radiotherapy protocols for the management of oncologic disease require intravenous infusions, including even those for palliative care, for which a long-term device is usually the best route of administration. As a matter of fact, the need for intravenous access devices for the administration of cancer therapy has increased proportionally with the increasing number of patients diagnosed with cancer.

Long-term (>3 months) therapies require a long-term venous access device, such as a cuffed tunneled central catheter (Hickman, Broviac, Groshong) or a totally implanted port. The choice between tunneled catheters and ports depends on many factors, mainly related to patient compliance and choice, the experience of the nursing staff and the frequency of venous access required. Totally implantable access devices have been recommended only in patients who require long-term, intermittent vascular access, while a tunneled central venous catheter is preferable in patients requiring long-term frequent or continuous access. However, the evidence base underlying this recommendation is weak (Grade C).

The percutaneous approach to the subclavian or internal jugular vein is currently the most popular procedure for placing central venous catheters (CVC) in the superior vena cava, both for short- and long-term use. In selecting the most appropriate insertion site for a CVC, several factors should be considered, including patient-specific factors (e.g. pre-existing CVC, anatomic abnormalities, bleeding diathesis, some types of positive-pressure ventilation), the relative risk of mechanical complications (e.g. bleeding, pneumothorax, thrombosis), as well as the risk of infection and the feasibility of adequate nursing care of the catheter exit site. Such venous approaches were made possible in the 1970s by the development of specific tools, like the Seldinger J-wire and the peel-away introducer-dilator, formerly not available. These technological instruments offer the option to avoid open surgical vein cannulation, which at that time was necessary for the placement of the silicone and polyurethane catheters required for long-term access. The great flexibility of percutaneous cannulation, the short duration of the procedure in most situations, and the possibility of switching from a procedure that requires an operating theater to a less demanding (especially cost-wise) outpatient or even bedside procedure have made the superiority of percutaneous central vein access quite obvious. At present, indeed, good medical practice does not recommend using a venous cutdown surgical procedure as a standard method to insert catheters, even for long-term ones [1].

Percutaneous techniques have reduced significantly - or even eliminated - the need for open cutdown procedures and the associated wound-related morbidity. Nonetheless, percutaneous techniques have left the operating physician exclusively reliant upon the relationships between surface anatomic landmarks and the underlying deep anatomic structures. Blind positioning of CVCs is usually achieved by direct venipuncture of the subclavian vein (via a supraclavicular or infraclavicular approach), the internal jugular vein (high posterior approach; high anterior approach; axial approach, between the two heads of the sternoclavicular muscle; low lateral approach; etc.) or the femoral vein. Placement of a totally implantable and especially a non-tunneled CVC in the femoral vein is not recommended as routine procedure in adult patients, since this route is associated with a relevant risk of venous thrombosis, as well as a high risk of extraluminal contamination and catheter related bloodstream infections (CRBSI), due to the difficulties inherent in dressing this exit site.

Venipuncture of the internal jugular vein carries less risk of insertion-related complications than venipuncture of the subclavian vein; in particular, the low lateral approach to the internal jugular vein (or Jernigan's approach) appears to be the technique of blind venipuncture associated with the lowest risk of mechanical complications [2].

Possibility of ultrasound (US) guidance is not a selection criterion, as US-guided positioning of any type of device (short-term CVCs or ports) may be achieved by supraclavicular venipuncture of the subclavian vein, of the internal jugular vein, or of the innominate vein; by infraclavicular venipuncture of the axillary/subclavian vein; or by femoral venipuncture.

Though positioning of central venous catheters on the left side is usually associated with a higher risk of malposition than on the right side, there are no evidence-based recommendations in this regard. In addition, there may be specific clinical and anatomic conditions which enforce the use of one or the other side (poor visualization of the veins on the other side, skin invasion by cancer, post-traumatic abnormalities etc.), and the risk of malposition may be minimized by using a technique for intraoperative control of the position of the catheter tip (including fluoroscopy and EKG-based methods).

Increased difficulty in nursing the exit site of an external catheter is to be expected when the exit site is in the neck area; therefore, approaches that facilitate dressing changes are preferable, such as the infraclavicular area (subclavian or axillary venipuncture) or the area just above the clavicle (low lateral approach to the internal jugular vein; supraclavicular approach to the innominate vein or to the subclavian vein). Most of these limitations do not apply to totally implantable devices.

A review and meta-analysis [3] of nonrandomized studies, mostly carried out in intensive care unit settings and published up to year 2000, reported that there were significantly more arterial punctures with jugular than with subclavian access, but that there were significantly fewer malpositions with jugular access, with no difference in the incidence of hematoma, pneumothorax or vessel occlusion. The authors concluded that selection bias could not be ruled out. A recent randomized, multicenter trial of 750 severely ill, bed-bound adults requiring a first catheter insertion for renal replacement therapy showed that jugular venous catheterization access does not appear to reduce the risk of infection compared with femoral access, except among adults with a high body mass index, and may have a higher risk of hematoma [4]. A review of the Cochrane Database of Systematic Reviews published in 2007 did not discover any randomized trials of subclavian versus jugular venous access, concluding that more evidence on whether the subclavian or the jugular access route is optimal was required [5].

Again in an intensive care unit (ICU) environment, a recent study failed to demonstrate any advantage of the subclavian route compared to the internal jugular vein in terms of infection rate [6]. In a prospective study of 988 ICU patients, the internal jugular route and the femoral route were associated with a higher risk of local infection of the exit site, but there was no difference in terms of CRBSI. In addition, since US guidance is now considered a standard of care, it was recommended that future comparative trials should incorporate US-guided venipuncture, as well as take into account other central routes made possible by US guidance, such as the axillary or the innominate (brachiocephalic) vein.

With respect to long-term use of totally implantable ports in oncology patients, we recently investigated this issue in a randomized three-arm trial [7]. Briefly, four hundred and three patients eligible for receiving IV chemotherapy for solid tumors were randomly assigned to implantation of a single type of port (Bard Port, Bard Inc., Salt Lake City, UT), either through a percutaneous landmark access to the internal jugular, a US-guided access to the subclavian or a surgical cutdown access through the cephalic vein at the deltopectoral groove. Early and late complications were prospectively recorded until removal of the device, patient death or end of the study. Four hundred and one patients (99.9%) were assessable: 132 with the internal jugular, 136 with the subclavian and 133 with the cephalic vein access. The median follow-up was 356.5 days (range 0–1087). No differences were found for early complication rate in the three groups (internal jugular: 0% [95% confidence interval (CI) 0.0-2.7%], subclavian: 0% [95% CI 0.0-2.7%], cephalic: 1.5% [95% CI 0.1-5.3%]). US-guided subclavian insertion site had significantly lower failures (e.g. failed attempts to place the catheter in agreement with the original arm of randomization, p=0.001). Infections occurred in one, three and one patients (internal jugular, subclavian and cephalic access, respectively,

$p=0.464$), whereas venous thrombosis was observed in 15, 8 and 11 patients ($p=0.272$). We concluded that central venous insertion modality and sites had no impact on either early or late complication rates when performed by experienced operators, but US-guided subclavian insertion showed the lowest proportion of failures. This report presents the first randomized evidence on this topic; our results illustrate that central venous access insertion site does not influence early or late occurrence of complications of venous ports connected to a standard open ended catheter implanted in an experienced environment. 2D-US guidance to subclavian vein catheterization had significantly less failures compared with landmark access to internal jugular vein or cutdown surgical access to cephalic vein at the deltopectoral groove. Cost, patient quality of life (QoL) and procedure compliance could be additional critical issues in deciding which insertion site should be used and these are currently under investigation. Indeed, in the same patient population we investigated QoL and psychological distress at regular intervals by means of EORTC QLQ-C30 and HADS (hospital anxiety and depression scale) questionnaires, using univariate and multivariate repeated measure linear mixed models. A *post hoc* analysis investigated the impact of type of administered chemotherapy (adjuvant vs. palliative). We found that mean-score changes for the items of the EORTC QLQ-C30 scales were significantly associated with type of administered chemotherapy only ($p<0.001$), and not with implantation site. Frequency distribution of patients with depression and anxiety score greater than 10 at HADS was not significantly different, with respect either to type of administered chemotherapy or TIVAD implantation site. The conclusion was that central venous insertion sites had no impact on patient QoL and psychological distress. Patients undergoing palliative therapies showed worse EORTC QLQ-C30 scales [8]. While awaiting further evidence, skilled operators may therefore rely on their experience and on proper assessment of clinical setting and patient characteristics when choosing the most appropriate venous access site for long-term drug administration. A regular use of US guidance is able to minimize implant failures and shifting to other veins, even in an experienced environment.

7.2 Techniques of Percutaneous Implant

Central venous catheter (CVC) insertion represents a risk of pneumothorax and major bleeding, infection and CVC-related vein thrombosis. Mechanical complications of CVC insertion without US guidance, such as arterial puncture and pneumothorax, are seen in up to 21% of attempts, and up to 35% of insertion attempts are not successful. Central venous cannulation can be an unsafe procedure: the National Confidential Enquiry into perioperative deaths has reported one death resulting from a procedure-induced pneumothorax. Recognition of risk factors for difficult catheterization is essential, and all patients should be evaluated for conditions that might increase the difficulty of

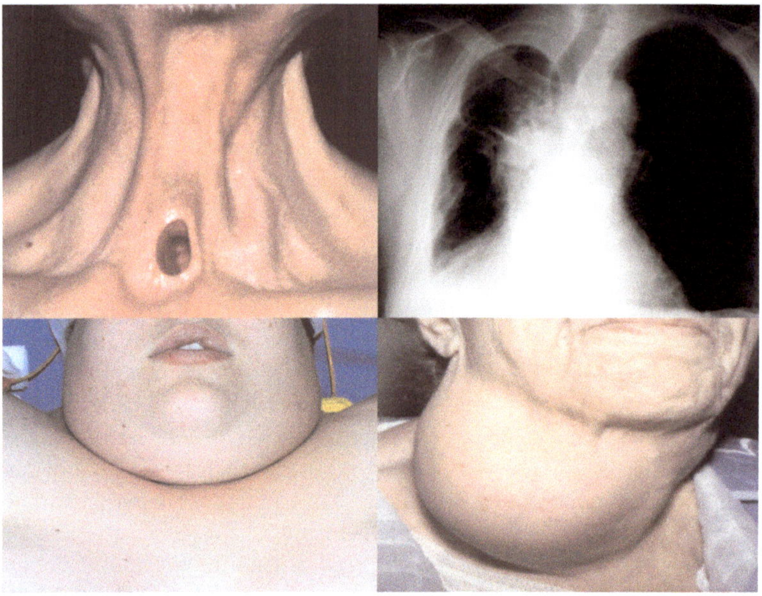

Fig. 7.1 Examples of predictable difficult cases for central venous cannulation

catheter insertion, such as skeletal deformity, presence of scars, obesity, or previous surgery at insertion site (Fig. 7.1). The preferential use of the internal jugular vein for the percutaneous "blind" (based on anatomic landmarks) approach for central venous cannulation is not able to eliminate the risk of pneumothorax, especially when anatomic abnormalities, dehydration, inexperience or disease-related alterations may force the operator to resort to subclavian venipuncture after failed attempts.

Before introducing techniques of percutaneous implant, it should be underlined that respect of sterility is of paramount importance in both the percutaneous and surgical implant of a long-term central venous access. Prospective trials suggest that the risk of CRBSI may be reduced by using maximal sterile barriers, including a sterile gown and sterile gloves for the operator, and a large sterile drape for the insertion of central venous access devices. Full-barrier precautions during CVC insertion are recommended by most guidelines, and this practice has been adopted by most 'bundles' of evidence-based interventions aiming to reduce CRBSI in multicenter prospective trials. Proper education and specific training of the staff is universally recommended as one of the most important and evidence-based strategies for reducing the risk of catheter-related infections (Grade A). There is good evidence demonstrating that the risk of infection declines following the standardization of aseptic care and increases when the maintenance of intravascular catheters is undertaken by inexperienced healthcare workers. In addition, it has been proven that relatively simple education programs focused on training healthcare workers to adhere to local evidence based protocols may decrease the risk to patients of

CRBSI. In a very important multicenter prospective study carried out in 108 ICUs, Provonost et al. [9] showed that the adoption of a bundle of a small number of evidence-based interventions (hand washing; full-barrier precautions during the insertion of central venous catheters; skin antisepsis with chlorhexidine; avoiding the femoral site if possible; removing unnecessary catheters as soon as possible) was highly effective in producing a clinically relevant (up to 66%) and persistent reduction in the incidence of CRBSI.

7.2.1 Internal Jugular Vein

Basically, there are three percutaneous approaches to the internal jugular vein, i.e. anterior, central, and posterior. The essential surface anatomy is comprised of the borders of Sedillot's triangle, the sternal head of the sternocleidomastoid muscle medially, the clavicular head of the sternocleidomastoid laterally, and the superior border of the medial third of the clavicle inferiorly. The central *axial* method is the most favored; cannulation begins with cutaneous puncture at the superior apex of this triangle. The needle and syringe are angled 45° off a coronal plane, and the needle is advanced in a sagittal plane.

The internal jugular vein lies immediately posterior to the apex of Sedillot's triangle with a frequency of 97% on the right and 79% on the left, and is thus relatively superficial in location. The internal jugular vein will be accessed at a needle depth of 1.0–1.5 cm beneath the cutaneous surface in most patients. If the vein is not accessed at this superficial level, one should consider that the advancing needle may have opposed the anterior and posterior walls of the internal jugular vein, collapsing the lumen, and allowing the transluminal passage of the needle out of the vein through its posterior wall. Consequently, slowly withdrawing the needle is recommended if it has been advanced 2.0–2.5 cm below the cutaneous surface without successful cannulation of the vein. If this maneuver is unsuccessful, the needle should be advanced from the cutaneous puncture site with a slightly lateral trajectory to puncture the vein posterior to the clavicular head of the sternocleidomastoid. The occurrence of carotid arterial puncture is due to the close relationship between the internal jugular vein and the carotid artery, so understanding this relationship is crucial to avoid this complication. The internal jugular vein generally lies anterolateral to the carotid artery. However, the vein may also lie directly anterior to the artery, predisposing to arterial puncture. Chandrasekaran found this relationship in 26% on the right and 20% on the left side in young healthy volunteers [10].

The effects of head rotation, carotid artery palpation, and Trendelenburg position on internal jugular vein diameter have been studied. Contralateral rotation of the head brings the sternocleidomastoid muscle into an anterior position over the internal jugular vein impeding cannulation, especially from the anterior approach. Contralateral rotation beyond 40° increases the anterior-posterior overlap of the internal jugular vein with the carotid artery, increasing the risk of arterial puncture. Carotid artery palpation diminishes internal jugular vein diameter. Trendelenburg position reliably increases internal jugular vein diameter. Consequently, Trendelenburg position should be employed whenever feasible, the carotid artery should not be palpated during venipuncture, and the head should be rotated to the contralateral side only so far as to provide access to the neck [11].

Due to the need to tunnel the catheter to the infraclavicular region to reach the port's chamber, the author's preferred approach for internal jugular cannulation in the long-term setting is the posterior-inferior (low lateral) route, according to the Jernigan method [12]. The needle is placed at the posterior border of the sternocleidomastoid muscle, at a point 1 cm above the border of the clavicle and is advanced toward the ipsilateral sternoclavicular joint.

It is important to recognize that the deep courses of the left and right internal jugular veins are not bilaterally symmetric. The right internal jugular vein follows a direct course inferior to the superior vena cava. The left internal jugular vein runs to the right after it joins the left subclavian vein to become the innominate vein, and the innominate vein subsequently runs inferiorly as it joins the superior vena cava. The angle at the junction of the left internal jugular vein and innominate vein can create difficulties when passing catheters through introducer sheaths. Given the more consistent presence of the right internal jugular vein immediately deep to the apex of Sedillot's triangle, and the nonlinear course from the left internal jugular vein to the superior vena cava, right internal jugular vein cannulation is preferred whenever feasible. Furthermore, total complications have been found more frequently after left versus right internal jugular cannulation.

7.2.2 Subclavian Vein

The subclavian vein offers an alternative to the internal jugular vein for central venous access. An infraclavicular approach to the subclavian vein is preferred by the author. The operator stands on the side to be cannulated. The patient should be placed in the Trendelenburg position to maximize venous filling and minimize the risk of air embolus; the head and neck position should be neutral. The appropriate course for the needle passes immediately beneath the junction of the medial one-third and lateral two-thirds of the clavicle. This junction, i.e. the *break* of the clavicle, is the point at which the anterior convexity of the medial clavicle transitions into an anterior concavity laterally. The appropriate point for cutaneous puncture lies 1–2 cm inferior and lateral to the clavicular transition point. A cutaneous puncture site closer to the clavicle creates difficulty maneuvering the needle beneath the clavicle. More medial cannulation may be impeded by calcification of the costoclavicular ligament. As the needle is advanced, it must remain absolutely parallel to the floor; if the needle is directed posteriorly to negotiate the clavicle, the risk of pneumothorax is greatly increased. As the needle is advanced from the cutaneous puncture site to a point beneath the clavicular transition point, its tip should be aimed just above the tip of the operator's nondominant index finger placed in the sternal notch. The needle is advanced along this course passing through the subclavius muscle until the subclavian vein is accessed.

The subclavian vein can also be cannulated using a supraclavicular approach, which is preferred by some authors. The essential landmark for the supraclavicular approach is the junction of the lateral border of the clavicular head of the sternocleidomastoid with the clavicle. The point of cutaneous puncture lies 1 cm superior and 1 cm lateral to this junction. The junction of the sternocleidomastoid with the clavicle defines the claviculosternomastoid angle. The cannulating needle tip is angled posteriorly 5°–15° off a coronal plane and advanced along a line that bisects the claviculosternomastoid angle. This will lead to subclavian venipuncture between the clavicle and the anterior scalene muscle. US visualization of the subclavian vein can confirm patency or identify thrombosis. However, the anatomic position of the subclavian vein between the clavicle and first rib complicates real-time US localization during venipuncture. US localization without real-time US guidance does not improve success of subclavian venipuncture attempts, nor does it decrease complication rates. However, the axillary vein and artery can be easily visualized with US more laterally on the chest wall anterior to the lateral clavicle. Here, the axillary vein can be recognized as a compressible structure lying anterior to the noncompressible, pulsating axillary artery. US-guided cannulation of the axillary vein may prove to be a safer technique than blind subclavian cannulation, especially for those operators without extensive experience with the latter approach. Blind approaches to the axillary vein have been described, but there is no reason to pursue these if US is available.

7.2.3 Femoral Vein

At present it is commonly believed that the femoral approach should never be considered as a primary choice for short and especially long-term central venous access, for the reasons previously explained. Therefore, the femoral vein is now considered the third choice for catheterization and is used only when subclavian and internal jugular approaches are not feasible. Femoral cannulation may indeed be favored during emergent resuscitation, when procedures such as endotracheal intubation and cardiac compressions limit safe concurrent access to the internal jugular vein and subclavian vein.

Femoral venipuncture is performed in the anterior superior thigh, just below the level of the inguinal ligament. This ligament runs from the pubic tubercle medially to the anterior superior iliac spine laterally. The femoral artery generally bisects the inguinal ligament. The femoral vein lies immediately medial to the femoral artery. Cutaneous puncture is performed approximately 1 cm medial to the point of maximal pulsation of the femoral artery. It is critical to ensure that the puncture of the vein occurs below the level of the inguinal ligament, i.e. meaning the skin insertion point should be slightly inferior on the thigh. Puncture above the inguinal ligament is in fact a puncture of the external iliac vein, which quickly becomes a deep retroperitoneal structure making it difficult to place pressure on the insertion site if bleeding occurs. Each femoral vein provides equally efficacious access and can be employed. As with venipuncture of the internal jugular and axillary/subclavian veins, venipuncture of the femoral vein can be facilitated by realtime US localization. The US probe can be placed in a sterile sheath and be used in realtime to visualize the puncture site. The femoral vein will be a typically larger caliber, compressible structure anteromedial to the femoral artery, which appears as a noncompressible and pulsatile vessel.

7.3 Technique and Role of US Guidance

Realtime sonography provides a means to safely direct the cannulating needle toward the internal jugular, axillary/subclavian, and femoral veins while avoiding puncture of the accompanying arteries and other organs. According to this technique, a US probe is used to locate the vein, and the introducer needle is guided through the skin and into the vessel (Figs. 7.2-7.4). US does not obviate the need for anatomic knowledge, so surface anatomic landmarks remain necessary for orientation of both cannulating needles and the US probe itself. Given the superficial location of the central veins at the sites of venipuncture, a high frequency probe of 7.5 mHz creates optimal images. US equipment can be easily used within a sterile field. Needle guides which orient the needle within the field of view along the path of the US beam can facilitate venipuncture in some conditions, but they are not favored by many operators (including the author of this chapter), as they require complete maneuverability of the needle.

Two main techniques have been described for US-guided central venous cannulation: the in-plane (IP) and out-of-plane (OOP) technique (Fig. 7.5). The IP technique is performed with the needle along the long axis of the US probe, whereas the OOP technique is performed with the needle along the short axis of the US probe. In the IP method the needle is placed in line with, and parallel to the transducer and US beam. Both the full length of the needle shaft and tip are visualized. Conversely, in the OOP technique the needle crosses the US probe and is visualized as a single spot. Most experts (including the Author of this chapter) favor the first technique, which is considered safer and more effective in obtaining the cannulation of the vein as a "single-shot" procedure. The author routinely uses realtime US guidance for internal jugular vein cannulation. The issues created by the close proximity of the carotid artery to the internal jugular vein are most efficaciously dealt with by US localization of the carotid artery and internal jugular vein in realtime during venipuncture. US imaging visually differentiates the internal jugular vein and common carotid artery, facilitates venipuncture rather than arterial puncture, guards against

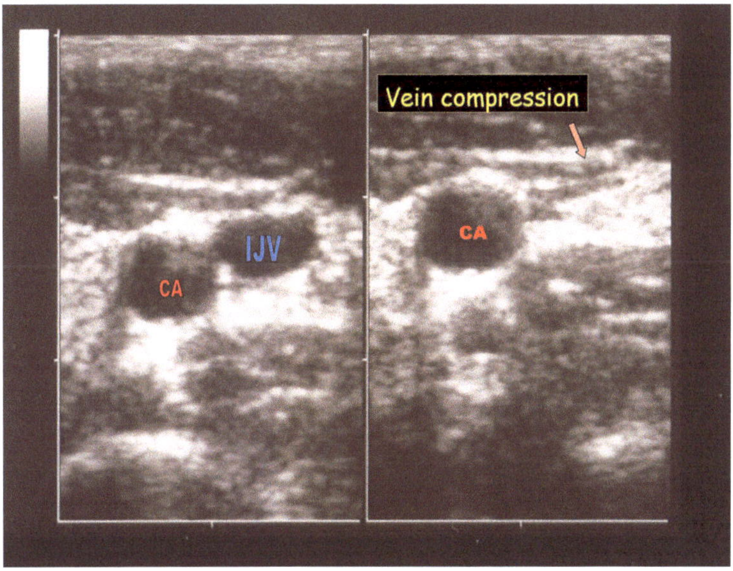

Fig. 7.2 Transverse US scan appearance of carotid artery and internal jugular vein. Compressibility makes the identification of the vein easier. Gentle pressure applied to the US probe will completely flatten the diameter of the internal jugular vein while leaving the diameter of the carotid artery unchanged. *CA*, carotid artery; *IJV*, internal jugular vein

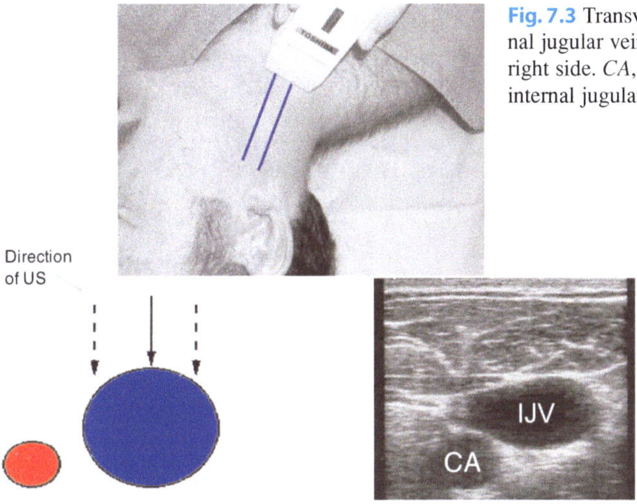

Fig. 7.3 Transverse US scan of internal jugular vein and carotid artery – right side. *CA*, carotid artery; *IJV*, internal jugular vein

through-and-through puncture of the internal jugular vein, and prevents deep passage of a needle into deep cervical and thoracic structures.

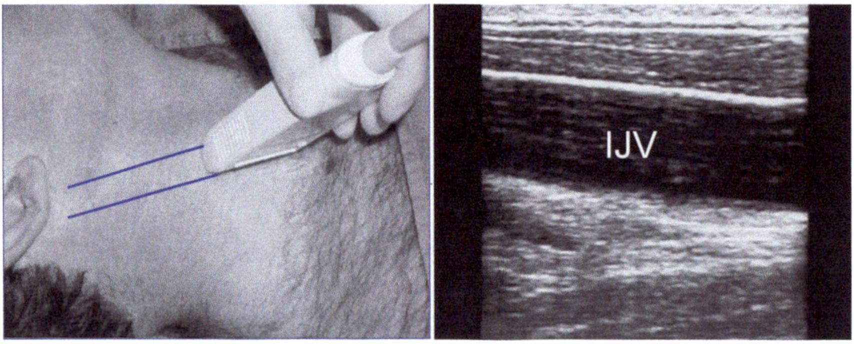

Fig. 7.4 Longitudinal US scan of internal jugular vein – right side. *IJV*, internal jugular vein

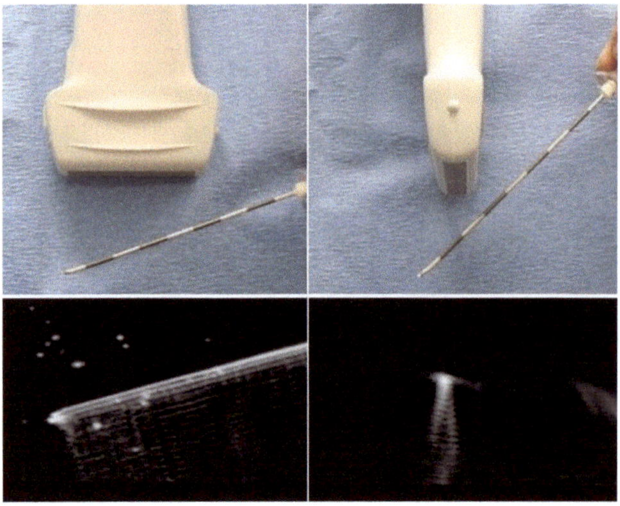

Fig. 7.5 Position of the needle in the "in-plane" (*left*) and "out-of-plane" (*right*) techniques. *IP*, in plane; *OOP*, out of plane

There is compelling evidence that US-guided venipuncture (with realtime ultrasonography) is associated with a substantial benefit, and US support is therefore strongly recommended (Grade A) for all CVC insertion. US guidance has been evaluated in randomized controlled trials (RCTs), which have been pooled in 3 meta-analyses [13-15]. In a 1996 meta-analysis of eight RCTs, US-guidance was characterized by a lower rate of failure and complications and by a higher rate of success at the first attempt if compared to the landmark technique. In 2001, the Stanford Evidence Based Practice Center at the UCSF published the results of the project 'Making Health Care Safer: A critical analysis of patient safety practices', identifying US-guidance for CVC placement as one of eleven evidence-based clinical tools which should be enforced in clinical practice.

The UK National Institute for Clinical Excellence made the following recommendations in 2002:

- 2D-imaging US guidance should be the preferred method when a CVC is inserted into the internal jugular vein of adults and children in "elective situations";
- 2D-imaging US guidance should be considered in most clinical situations where CVC insertion is necessary, regardless of the situation (elective or emergency procedure);
- Everyone who uses 2D-imaging US guidance to insert CVCs should be appropriately trained so that they can use the technique competently.

The implementation of UK National Institute for Clinical Excellence guidelines has been associated with a significant reduction in complication rates in a UK tertiary referral center. Similar recommendations, based on the published data of RCT meta-analyses, have been made by several scientific societies. Most recently, the Association for Vascular Access drafted a position statement on the use of realtime imaging for placement of central vascular access devices (available at www.avainfo.org) advocating the use of US guidance for all non emergent central vascular access procedures, including percutaneously inserted central catheters. Other prospective studies, some of which were RCTs, have addressed this issue in a number of settings, such as the intensive care unit, emergency room, oncology, pediatrics and dialysis, leading to the conclusion that US guidance improves the success rate of vein cannulation, reducing the number of attempts, complications, and failures. Finally, a randomized study of US-guided versus blind catheterization of the internal jugular vein in critical care patients showed that US-guidance was also associated with a decrease in catheter-related infections [16].

Concerns have been expressed with respect to training, as the novel techniques should be incorporated into the US courses that are currently being set up for radiologists, anesthesiologists, and surgeons. Moreover, the landmark method would remain important for emergencies when US equipment and/or expertise might not be immediately available. Cost analysis is certainly a key issue. Calculations should be precise and also include costs for US devices and operator training. Calvert et al. [15] compared the economics of using 2D-US locating devices and more traditional landmark methods for central venous cannulation. They concluded that the cost of using US for central venous cannulation was less than 10 pounds sterling (corresponding to about 20 USD) per procedure, and that the introduction of 2D US for central venous cannulation would save the UK National Health Service money (£2,000 for every 1,000 procedures). However, some criticism has surrounded the incidence of arterial puncture that the authors used in their analysis. Based on experience and published data, a 12% incidence of arterial puncture using the landmark approach was judged almost an order of magnitude too high. Using a significantly lower and more realistic arterial puncture incidence reduces the cost of the landmark technique and may change the cost-effectiveness calculation to the point where the choice of US may no longer be dominant, meaning that while US is more effective, it also costs more. Lastly, since the reference is internal jugular vein cannulation in the operating theater, the question of whether the results can be extrapolated to other central venous cannulations performed outside that setting was not addressed. While many RCTs have clearly shown that US guidance is superior to the landmark technique - at least in terms of immediate outcome - for internal jugular vein cannulation in a variety of clinical settings, doubts still persist for the subclavian insertion site. US guidance for subclavian venous catheterization has yielded inconsistent results in a small number of trials [17, 18]; limited evidence favored 2D US guidance for subclavian vein procedures in adults (relative risk 0.14; 95% confidence interval, 0.04 to 0.57). An indirect comparison of relative risks suggested that 2D ultrasonography would be more successful than Doppler guidance for subclavian vein procedures in adults (relative risk 0.09; 95% CI, 0.02-0.38). A very recent RCT in ICU patients [19] has suggested that US-guided cannulation of the subclavian vein is superior to the landmark method in terms of average access time, number of attempts, frequency of artery puncture, hematoma, hemothorax , pneumothorax, brachial plexus and phrenic nerve injury. More studies are needed to address long-term benefits and cost-effectiveness.

References

1. Centers for Disease Control (2002) Guidelines for the prevention of intravascular catheter-related infections. MMWR Morb Mortal Wkly Rep 51:1–36
2. Pittiruti M, Malerba M, Carriero C et al (2000) Which is the easiest and safest technique for central venous access? A retrospective survey of more than 5,400 cases. J Vasc Access 1:100–107
3. Reusch S, Walder B, Tramer MR (2002) Complications of central venous catheters: internal jugular versus subclavian access—a systematic review. Crit Care Med 30:454–460
4. Parienti JJ, Thirion M, Mégarbane B et al (2008) Femoral vs jugular venous catheterization and risk of nosocomial events in adults requiring acute renal replacement therapy: a randomized controlled trial. JAMA 299:2413–2422
5. Hamilton HC, Foxcroft DR (2007) Central venous access sites for the prevention of venous thrombosis, stenosis and infection in patients requiring long-term intravenous therapy. Cochrane Database Syst Rev 3:CD004084
6. Deshpande KS, Hatem C, Ulrich HL et al (2005) The incidence of infectious complications of central venous catheters at the subclavian, internal jugular, and femoral sites in an intensive care unit population. Crit Care Med 33:3-20
7. Biffi R, Orsi F, Pozzi S et al (2009) Best choice of central venous insertion site for the prevention of catheter-related complications in adult patients who need cancer therapy: a randomized trial. Ann Oncol 20:935-940
8. Biffi R, Orsi F, Pozzi S et al (2010) No impact of central venous insertion site on oncology patients' quality of life and psychological distress. A randomized three-arm trial. Support Care Cancer [Epub ahead of print] doi:10.1007/s00520-010-0984-9
9. Pronovost P, Needham D, Berenholtz S et al (2006) An intervention to decrease catheter-related bloodstream infections in the ICU. N Engl J Med 355:2725–2732
10. Chandrasekaran S, Chandrasekaran VP (2010) Anatomical variations of the internal jugular vein in relation to common carotid artery in lesser supra clavicular fossa – a colour doppler study. Int J Basic Med Sci 1. Available at: http://www.ijbms.com/anatomy/supra-clavicular-fossa

11. Marcus HE, Bonkat E, Dagtekin O et al (2010) The impact of Trendelenburg position and positive end-expiratory pressure on the internal jugular cross-sectional area. Anesth Analg 111:432–436
12. Jernigan WR, Gardner WC, Mahr MM, Milburn JL (1971) The internal jugular vein for access to the central venous system. JAMA 218:97-98
13. Randolph AG, Cook DJ, Gonzales CA, Pribble CG (1996) Ultrasound guidance for placement of central venous catheters: a meta-analysis of the literature. Crit Care Med 24:2053–2058
14. Hind D, Calvert N, McWilliams R et al (2003) Ultrasonic locating devices for central venous cannulation: meta-analysis. BMJ 327:361-367
15. Calvert N, Hind D, McWilliams R et al (2004) Ultrasound for central venous cannulation: economic evaluation of cost-effectiveness. Anaesthesia 59:1116–1120
16. Karakitsos D, Labropoulos N, De Groot E et al (2006) Real-time ultrasound-guided catheterisation of the internal jugular vein: a prospective comparison with the landmark technique in critical care patients. Crit Care 10:R162
17. Lefrant JY, Cuvillon P, Bénézet JF et al (1998) Pulsed Doppler ultrasonography guidance for catheterization of the subclavian vein: a randomized study. Anesthesiology 88:1195–1201
18. Bold RJ, Winchester DJ, Madary AR et al (1998) Prospective, randomized trial of Doppler-assisted subclavian vein catheterization. Arch Surg 133:1089–1093
19. Fragou M, Gravvanis A, Dimitriou V et al (2011) Real-time ultrasound-guided subclavian vein cannulation versus the landmark method in critical care patients: A prospective randomized study. Crit Care Med [Epub ahead of print] doi:10.1097/CCM.0b013e318218a1ae

8

Modified Seldinger Technique for Open Central Venous Cannulation for Totally Implantable Access Device

Phillip Knebel, Roland Hennes, Markus K. Diener, Christoph M. Seiler and Markus W. Büchler

Abstract

Open cannulation of the cephalic vein and percutaneous puncture of the subclavian or internal jugular vein are the two main approaches for totally implantable venous access device (TIVAD) implantation. The mean primary success rate of the open cannulation techniques with 80% is low compared to nearly 100% of percutaneous puncture. Therefore a rescue strategy after failed open cutdown of the cephalic vein is needed. The modified Seldinger technique can close this gap. It is a combination of open cutdown and the Seldinger technique using a guide wire, dilator and peel-away sheath through the dissected cephalic vein. The PORTAS 1 and PORTAS 2 trial could show an increase of successfully implantated TIVAD through open cutdown with the modified Seldinger technique as rescue strategy. In this chapter the modified Seldinger technique is explained and shown in detail.

Keywords

Modified Seldinger technique • TIVAD implantation • Open cannulation technique • TIVAD • Port • Indwelling catheter

8.1 Introduction

The two main approaches for totally implantable venous access device (TIVAD) placement are insertion into the cephalic vein through an open can-

P. Knebel (✉)
Department of General Visceral and Transplantation Surgery,
University of Heidelberg,
Heidelberg, Germany
e-mail: phillip.knebel@med.uni-heidelberg.de

I. Di Carlo, R. Biffi (eds.), *Totally Implantable Venous Access Devices*,

nulation technique (OCT) by a surgeon or the percutaneous puncture (PP) of the subclavian or jugular vein by a surgeon or interventional radiologist, facilitated by contrast agent, ultrasound or using the anatomical landmark technique as described in the previous chapters. While common complications, such as kinking or dislocation of the catheter, subcutaneous hematoma, surgical site infection, and nerve palsy, are observed regardless of the technique, specific and serious risks are only associated with puncture of the subclavian vein, such as 'pinch off' phenomena and pneumothorax or hemothorax. The latter complications in particular require further treatment, including placement of a pleural drainage and, often, admission to hospital [1–3].

The median primary success rates for the OCT range from 71% to 94%, and from 90% to 99% for PP of a central vein in various retrospective studies and a few single center randomized controlled trials [4–19]. A retrospective multivariate analysis of 400 patients who received a primary TIVAD implantation through OCT identified two main reasons for failure of the open cutdown technique: either an undersized vessel or the inability to introduce the catheter through the cephalic vein into the subclavian vein [4].

In four single center randomized controlled trials examining both techniques, similar overall complication rates were observed. However, in none of these trials a pneumothorax / hemothorax occurred in the group in which OCT was successful [19–22]. For PP the rate of pneumothorax / hemothorax is reported to be up to 4.3% as secondary endpoint in various retrospective, prospective and randomized clinical trials [3, 4, 19, 21, 23, 24]. The pneumothorax / hemothorax rate of the percutaneous puncture of central veins for other indications than TIVAD placement ranges from 0.5 to even 12% [21].

The modified Seldinger technique is a combination of open cannulation of the cephalic vein and the Seldinger technique. The aim of this rescue technique is to avoid a percutaneous puncture of the subclavian vein and the risk of pneumothorax / hemothorax after a failed OCT. Therefore, a guidewire and, if necessary, a dilator and peel away sheath is introduced into the dissected cephalic vein to overcome a narrow or strongly curved vessel. This technique was first described by Coit et al. [25] in 1988 and successfully applied in a randomized controlled trial in 2006 [19].

8.2 Results of Randomized Controlled Trials Applying the Modified Seldinger Technique

The PORTAS 1 trial compared the primary success rates of OCT (classical venae sectio) of the cephalic vein versus the modified Seldinger technique of the same vessel. A total of 164 patients (82 per group) were enrolled in the trial between 2006 and 2007.

Although the primary success rates of OCT in 66 patients (81%) and modified Seldinger technique in 69 patients (84%) were not significantly different

(p=0.686), the combination of open cannulation as a first line strategy with the modified Seldinger technique as a second line/rescue strategy if open cannulation fails showed an increase in the success rate to 94% [19]. Therefore, it was possible to avoid percutaneous puncture of the subclavian vein with the risk for pneumothorax/hemothorax in an additional 13% of patients. Only 4 patients out of 82 required a percutaneous puncture for successful TIVAD placement. The median duration of TIVAD implantation did not differ significantly with 35 min (range 10–140 min) in the modified Seldinger group and 36 min (range 10–203 min) in the open cutdown group (p=0.87). Even the peri- and postoperative complication rates showed no significant difference. A multivariate analysis revealed that the educational level of the participating surgeons, patient body mass index, Karnowsky index and age did not have a significant impact on the primary endpoint.

In the PORTAS 2 trial we compared the primary success rates of OCT (modified Seldinger technique was allowed as rescue strategy) of the cephalic vein with percutaneous puncture of the subclavian vein in an expertise-based randomization setting [26]. The open cutdown technique was applied by surgeons and the percutaneous puncture was performed by interventional radiologists using contrast agent (roadmap technique). A total of 102 patients (51 per group) were included between March and August 2008. The open cutdown technique with the modified Seldinger technique as rescue strategy was successful in 48 patients (94%) and percutaneous puncture of the subclavian vein in 49 patients (96%) [22]. Therefore, the safety and efficacy of the modified Seldinger technique could be confirmed in two randomized controlled trials.

8.3 How We Do it: Modified Seldinger Technique

The standard procedure for TIVAD implantation in our department is OCT of the cephalic vein. For this purpose, all patients are positioned on the operation table in a five degree reverse Trendelenburg position. The neck, chest and shoulders of the patients are prepared and draped in customary sterile manner. Antibiotic prophylaxis is only given to patients with risk for endocarditis according to the local standards.

If the open cutdown method fails, the modified Seldinger technique is used as a rescue strategy. Only after an unsuccessful attempt of the modified Seldinger technique the puncture of the subclavian vein will be used as third line strategy.

Indication for Modified Seldinger Technique

Failed open cutdown of the cephalic vein.

Materials

Guidewire, dilator and peel-away sheath from a percutaneous puncture set.

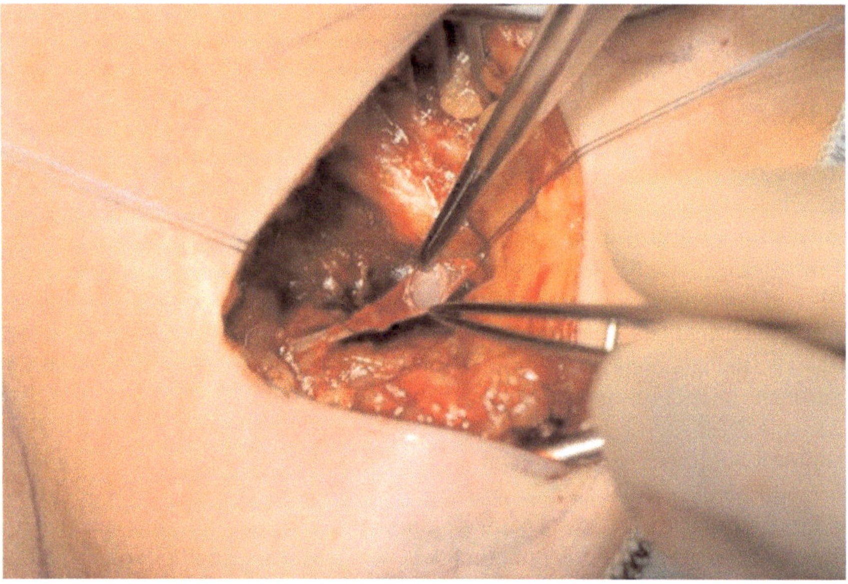

Fig. 8.1 Transverse venotomy of the cephalic vein

Procedure

Step 1: The cephalic vein is dissected, ligated distally and encircled proximally with a 3/0 absorbable suture, after which a transverse venotomy is performed (Fig. 8.1).

Step 2: The guidewire, featuring a J-shaped tip, is introduced through the dissected cephalic vein right into the brachiocephalic vein under fluoroscopy guidance. The J-shaped tip has the advantage that it may be inserted without greater difficulties even when the entrance of the subclavian vein is orthogonal to the cephalic vein. Furthermore, the guidewire can easily pass possible obstructions or stenoses of the cephalic or subclavian vein (Fig. 8.2).

Step 3: After correct placement of the guidewire in the brachiocephalic vein a dilator and peel-away sheath is passed over the guidewire (Figs. 8.3, 8.4). Alternatively, in the absence of a stenosis of the cephalic vein it may be possible to pass the TIVAD catheter directly over the guidewire without using the dilator and peel-away sheath.

Step 4: The guidewire and dilator are removed (Fig. 8.5) and the TIVAD catheter is easily inserted through the peel-away sheath (Fig. 8.6).

Step 5: After insertion of the TIVAD catheter the peel-away sheath can be removed. The correct position of the TIVAD catheter tip is checked by fluoroscopy and corrected if necessary (Fig. 8.7).

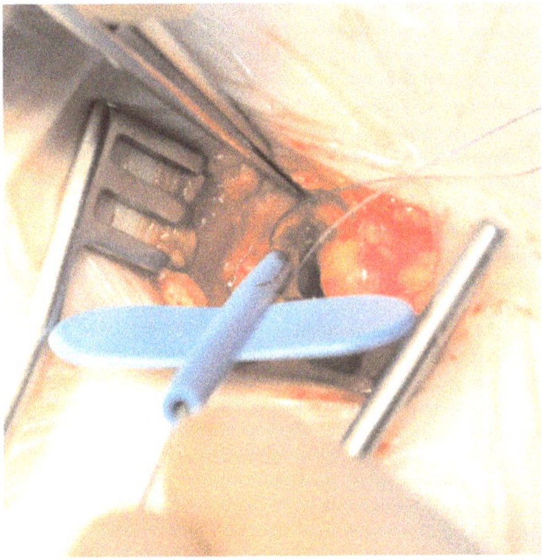

Fig. 8.2 Introducing the guidewire in the dissected cephalic vein

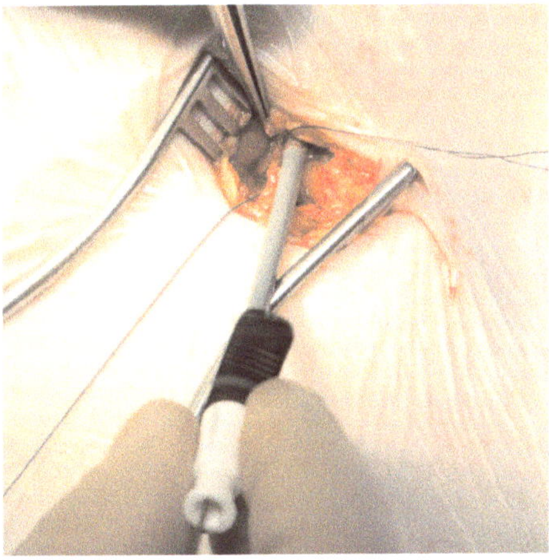

Fig. 8.3 Introducing the dilator and peel away sheath

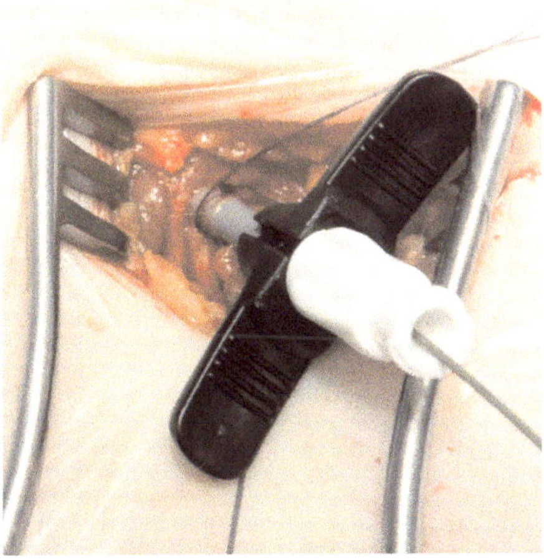

Fig. 8.4 Introduced dilator and peel away sheath

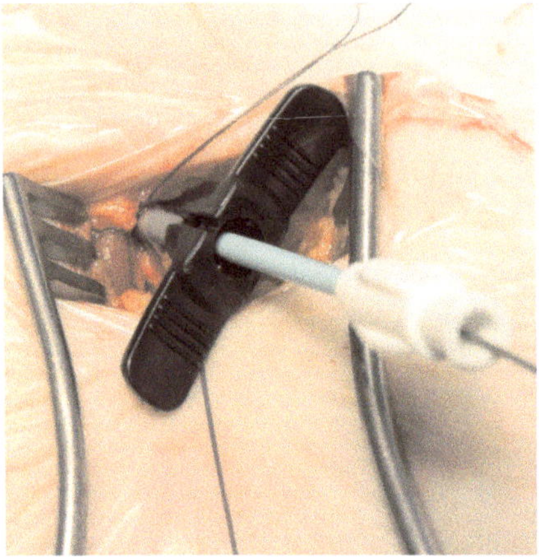

Fig. 8.5 Removal of the guidewire and dilator

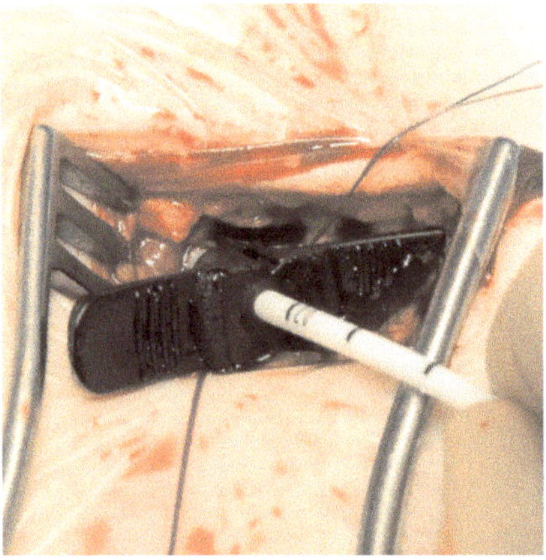

Fig. 8.6 Introducing the TIVAD catheter

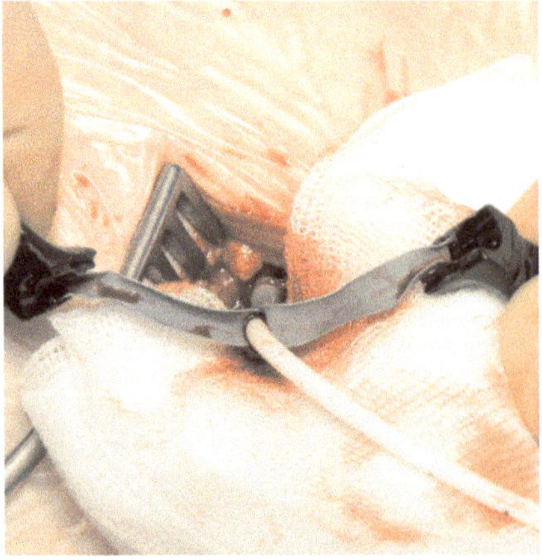

Fig. 8.7 Removal of the peel-away sheath

8.4 Conclusions

The modified Seldinger technique should be used as a second line rescue strategy after failed open cannulation of the cephalic vein. This easy technique can be applied successfully to avoid a percutaneous puncture of the subclavian vein with the risk of a pneumothorax or hemothorax.

References

1. Fischer L, Knebel P, Schroder S et al (2008) Reasons for explantation of totally implantable access ports: a multivariate analysis of 385 consecutive patients. Ann Surg Oncol 15:1124-1129
2. Kluge A, Stroh H, Wagner D, Rauber K (1998) [The fluoroscopy-guided implantation of subcutaneous venous ports: the complications and long-term results]. Rofo 169:63-67
3. Biffi R, Pozzi S, Cenciarelli S et al (2001) Treatment of pneumothorax as a complication of long-term central venous port placement in oncology patients. An observational study. J Vasc Access 2:129-136
4. Seiler CM, Frohlich BE, Dorsam UJ et al (2006) Surgical technique for totally implantable access ports (TIVAD) needs improvement: a multivariate analysis of 400 patients. J Surg Oncol 93:24-29
5. Di Carlo I, Cordio S, La Greca G et al (2001) Totally implantable venous access devices implanted surgically: a retrospective study on early and late complications. Arch Surg 136:1050-1053
6. Le Saout J, Vallee B, Person H et al (1983) [Anatomical basis for the surgical use of the cephalic vein (V. Cephalica). 74 anatomical dissections. 189 surgical dissections]. J Chir (Paris) 120:131-134
7. Davis SJ, Thompson JS, Edney JA (1984) Insertion of Hickman catheters. A comparison of cutdown and percutaneous techniques. Am Surg 50:673-676
8. Chuter T, Starker PM (1988) Placement of Hickman-Broviac catheters in the cephalic vein. Surg Gynecol Obstet 166:163-164
9. Au FC (1989) The anatomy of the cephalic vein. Am Surg 55:638-639
10. Perry EP, Nash JR, Klidjian AM (1990) Direct cephalic vein cannulation for safe subclavian access. J R Coll Surg Edinb 35:218-220
11. Torramade JR, Cienfuegos JA, Hernandez JL et al (1993) The complications of central venous access systems: a study of 218 patients. Eur J Surg 159:323-327
12. Gallichio MH, Kahn D, Lempert N, Conti DJ (1994) Placement of a double lumen silastic catheter for hemodialysis access through the cephalic vein. J Am Coll Surg 178:171-172
13. Povoski SP (2000) A prospective analysis of the cephalic vein cutdown approach for chronic indwelling central venous access in 100 consecutive cancer patients. Ann Surg Oncol 7:496-502
14. Shetty PC, Mody MK, Kastan DJ et al (1997) Outcome of 350 implanted chest ports placed by interventional radiologists. J Vasc Interv Radiol 8:991-995
15. Simpson KR, Hovsepian DM, Picus D (1997) Interventional radiologic placement of chest wall ports: results and complications in 161 consecutive placements. J Vasc Interv Radiol 8:189-195
16. Lyon RD, Griggs KA, Johnson AM, Olsen JR (1999) Long-term follow-up of upper extremity implanted venous access devices in oncology patients. J Vasc Interv Radiol 10:463-471
17. Lorch H, Zwaan M, Kagel C, Weiss HD (2001) Central venous access ports placed by interventional radiologists: experience with 125 consecutive patients. Cardiovasc Intervent Radiol 24:180-184

18. Di Carlo I, Barbagallo F, Toro A et al (2005) External jugular vein cutdown approach, as a useful alternative, supports the choice of the cephalic vein for totally implantable access device placement. Ann Surg Oncol 12:570-573
19. Knebel P, Fischer L, Huesing J et al (2009) Randomized clinical trial of a modified Seldinger technique for open central venous cannulation for implantable access devices. Br J Surg 96:159-165
20. Nocito A, Wildi S, Rufibach K et al (2009) Randomized clinical trial comparing venous cutdown with the Seldinger technique for placement of implantable venous access ports. Br J Surg 96:1129-1134
21. Biffi R, Orsi F, Pozzi S et al (2009) Best choice of central venous insertion site for the prevention of catheter-related complications in adult patients who need cancer therapy: a randomized trial. Ann Oncol 20:935-940
22. Knebel P, Lopez-Benitez R, Fischer L et al (2011) Insertion of Totally Implantable Venous Access Devices: An Expertise-Based, Randomized, Controlled Trial (NCT00600444). Ann Surg 253:1111-1117
23. Sznajder JI, Zveibil FR, Bitterman H et al (1986) Central vein catheterization. Failure and complication rates by three percutaneous approaches. Arch Intern Med 146:259-261
24. Vandoni RE, Guerra A, Sanna P et al (2009) Randomised comparison of complications from three different permanent central venous access systems. Swiss Med Wkly 139:313-316
25. Coit DG, Turnbull AD (1988) A safe technique for the placement of implantable vascular access devices in patients with thrombocytopenia. Surg Gynecol Obstet 167:429-431
26. Knebel P, Fischer L, Cremonese E et al (2008) Protocol of an expertise based randomized trial comparing surgical venae sectio versus radiological puncture of vena subclavia for insertion of totally implantable access port in oncological patients (PORTAS 2 Trial: NCT 006600444). Trials 9:60

Optimal Catheter Tip Position: Radiologic Criteria and Clinical Relevance

9

Marguerite Stas and Johan Coolen

Abstract

Correct location of the central catheter extremity attached to totally implantable ports is mandatory in order to avoid complications and to maintain functionality. But there is still a debate about the definition of the optimal position. Obviously, sites such as the very cranial segment of the vena cava superior or the caudal part of the right atrium are to be avoided. The golden middle-way is located between these extreme locations, at the junction between the lower portion of the superior vena cava and the upper right atrium. However, even if a consensus can be reached regarding this peculiar site, description of correlations between anatomical boundaries of veins and visible radiological landmarks varies in function of the chosen imaging method. This chapter will address the issues of correct catheter tip position with regard to complications and performance and provide some insight about correlations between various venous segments and surrounding bony structures.

Keywords

Correct location • Central catheter extremity • Totally implantable ports • Complications • Functionality • Junction • Anatomical boundaries of veins • Radiological landmarks • Imaging

M. Stas (✉)
Surgical Oncology, UZ Leuven,
Leuven, Belgium
e-mail: marguerite.stas@uzleuven.be

I. Di Carlo, R. Biffi, *Totally Implantable Venous Access Devices*,

"Catheter tip position emerged as the dominant independent prognostic factor for reduced device-specific duration or complication-free device-specific duration, but not the case volume of the surgeon."
Schwarz RE et al. (2000) Ann Surg Oncol 7:441-449

9.1 Introduction

For totally implantable vascular access devices (TIVAD) which have to remain in situ and function well for months or years, the precise position of the central extremity of the catheter tip is of paramount importance both for avoiding complications and maintaining functionality. However, the optimal position of the catheter tip is still a matter of debate [1,2]. Following common sense, obvious erroneous sites must be avoided, such as the feeder vessels of the superior vena cava (SVC), associated with an increased risk for venous thrombosis [3- 5] or the lower part of the right atrium (RA) where catheter tip can damage heart wall of valves and cause arrhythmias [6]. The golden middle way is located between these extreme positions, and more precisely where the SVC merges into the RA [7, 8]. It is also important to keep in mind that wherever its location, the central portion of the catheter will move inside the great vessels, following body motions [3]. The optimal site is accordingly the place where unavoidable movements of the catheter tip will not result in later catheter misplacement.

However, precise intravascular anatomical structures, such as the junction between SVC and RA, may be difficult to localise on plain film radiograph. One has to rely on radio opaque bony or cartilaginous structures in the vicinity or to inject contrast dye [2]. Patient build and conditions such as tumours or mediastinal shifting may obscure the recognition of the structures of interest. Thin catheters which contain only small amounts of barium sulphate in their wall, are not easily seen, particularly in obese patients.

Advantages and drawbacks of different control methods for catheter tip location will be discussed, ranging from plain chest radiographs to MRI scans and more invasive echo-endoscopy methods.

9.2 Catheter Tip Location and Its Relation to Complications

Two main aspects regarding the optimal location for central venous catheter tips are still matter of discussion: the definition of the optimal site, with regard to potential complications and to functional aspects, and the definition of the best assessment technique of this position. In fact, all *long-term* venous access devices aiming at more than 2-3 weeks indwelling time, are to some extent exposed to the same hazards regarding catheter tip position, irrespective of the vein accessed or the type of device: percutaneously inserted central catheters (PICCs), (non-) tunneled catheters or port catheters. For this reason, some data found in series addressing other types of catheters are applicable to TIVADs as well.

9.2.1 Evolution of the Definition for Optimal Tip Location, With Regard to Atrial and Venous Thrombosis

Initially, FDA recommendations [9] and NAVAN statements [10] were driven by complications in described patients with catheter tips located in the right atrium. Atrial perforation with a polyethylene catheter was already reported in1968, followed by atrial thrombus formation - with eventual pulmonary embolism - and cardiac tamponade, both in adults and children [6], with exceptional cases of fatal outcome. The development of soft silicone catheters limited this risk [1], and the device developed by Broviac for parenteral nutrition was qualified as "atrial" catheter.

In adherence with the FDA recommendations, tips of *central* catheters shifted to anywhere outside the RA [11], or even into the brachio-cephalic veins [12]. However, catheter tips in these peripheral locations are associated with a significant incidence of catheter as well as venous thrombosis [4, 5] and ensuing stenosis that will impair subsequent insertions.

Thrombotic complications were emphasized in a retrospective series of Cadman et al. [4] who showed the relation between tip location and venous thrombosis in 428 tunneled central venous catheters, with a follow-up of 23,040 line days. Venous thrombosis was diagnosed using venography, linograms and ultrasound (US). All cases of thrombosis were ipsilateral to the catheter tip, so if a line was inserted in the right subclavian vein and its tip malplaced in the contralateral left subclavian vein, then thrombus formation was found in the left subclavian vein. In multivariate analysis, the only significant risk factor for venous thrombosis was catheter tip location: 2.6% if the tip is located distally in the SVC, 5.3% in the middle third and in 41.7% in the cranial third of the SVC or its inlet veins. Furthermore, none of the 54 catheters with their tip located in the RA showed signs of thrombosis or caused complications [4].

9.2.2 Evolution of the Definition for Optimal Tip Location, With Regard to Functional Performance

The main purpose of TIVADs is safe administration, over a prolonged period of time, of infusates that may be harmful to the veins when injected peripherally. Before drug delivery, it is thus mandatory to assess catheter integrity and proper intravascular tip location, which are usually confirmed by ease of injection and blood aspiration. Furthermore, in contrast to patients in the operating room or intensive care units who have short term venous catheters for infusion and arterial lines for blood sampling, patients with TIVADs are supposed to receive medication injection and undergo blood sampling through the same system. However, difficult or impossible blood aspiration while injection is easy, is the most frequent hindrance reported in the literature focusing on functional aspects of TIVADs: it is responsible for 85% of malfunctions in radiological series, and 25 % when all types of malfunctions are taken into consideration [13].

Table 9.1 Relationship between catheter tip position and risk for venous thrombosis and functional problems. Caers et al. Supportive Care in Cancer 2005

Location of catheter tip	Number of patients	Venous thrombosis	Functional problems
Brachiocephalic vein	31	45.2%	6.5%
SVC cranial 1/3	42	19%	16.7%
SVC mid 1/3	142	4.2%	1.4%
SVC caudal 1/3	66	1.5%	0%
RA or inferior Vena Cava	18	5.6%	5.6%

SVC, superior vena cava; *RA*, right atrium.

There are in fact several causes either in isolation or combination which can lead to functional problems. Thrombus and sleeve formation around the catheter tip, which abuts the vessel wall [14], can act as a valve system and jeopardize aspiration, while the injection of fluids is still possible and safe; mechanical obstruction of the devices by precipitates, catheter kinking or narrowing ("pinch-off" problem) will impair fluid movements in both directions. Catheter tips that abut the vein wall also bring high doses of medication to a small surface area and can cause traumatic venous thrombosis and endothelial vein wall damage. Moreover, blood aspiration is supposed to be impaired by suction of the vein wall when a negative pressure is exerted on the catheter lumen. In this context, a clear link between catheter tip position and aspiration function is established.

A retrospective series of Caers et al. [5] showed a significant correlation between location of TIVAD tips outside the lower third of the SVC and both thrombotic complications and functional problems. Other significant factors were insertion from the left side, female gender and the presence of lung tumour (Table 9.1).

Another retrospective study followed by a randomized series by the same authors, addressed the thrombotic risk of long arm-catheters with peripherally located tip *vs* a central vein terminus. When compared to catheters ending in the SVC, tips inserted both inadvertently and on purpose in the axillary-subclavian-innominate veins were associated with more venous thrombosis (60% *vs* 21%). Catheters associated with thrombosis were also more likely to become infected ($R=0.48$, $p< .02$). Moreover, central tip catheters had an improved survival ($p<0.02$) [7]. From an ethical point of view, this randomized study is impossible to repeat nowadays.

Evidence was also gained through observation of haemodialysis catheters: tip location in the right atrium allows better flow rates, in both directions, without an increase in thrombus formation nor damage to the atrial wall. Consequently, guide-lines from the National Kidney Foundation: Dialysis Outcomes Quality Initiatives [15] advised inserting catheter tips in the right atrium.

The European Society for Clinical Nutrition and Metabolism (ESPEN) guidelines address the long-term delivery of hyperosmolar parenteral nutrition solutions. On the basis of grade A level of evidence, they recommended inserting central catheter tips in the lower third of the vena cava superior, at the atriocaval junction, or in the upper portion of the right atrium [8].

9.3 Catheter Tip Location: Anatomical Landmarks Imaging Techniques

When a "central" catheters is inserted in a vein and is able to follow the bloodstream towards the right atrium, most catheter tips will *spontaneously* reach this target, but not all.

A prospective data collection was initiated in1984 concerning location of the tip of 1,000 consecutive TIVAD catheters placed by surgical cut-down technique. Immediately after inserting a suitable catheter length in order to reach the upper atriocaval junction, perioperative fluoroscopy control of catheter tip location was performed. More than 20% were found in another location than the aimed landing zone. Catheter tips inserted through cephalic veins could be found in arm, internal jugular or subclavian veins of the same or opposite side. Inserted through the external and internal jugular veins, tips could go to ipsilateral and contralateral subclavian veins, to the internal thoracic, and azygos veins or into the internal jugular veins. From all insertion sites, catheters were able to curl back into brachiocephalic veins or SVC, without reaching the right atrium. Absence of length marks on these soft silicone catheters led to deep insertions as well. Under real-time imaging, correction attempts were always undertaken in order to place the catheter tips at the aimed location, before release for use.

Non-optimal locations of catheters inserted according to the sole anatomical landmarks were confirmed in another series on TIVADs which reported only 16 of 30 tips in a satisfactory position [16]. Similar results were found in a series on tunneled catheters where only 57 % of the tips were found inside the distal SVC or right atrium on postoperative chest radiograph [4]. Moreover, a series on 843 consecutively placed PICCs in children, without fluoroscopic guidance, required thereafter catheter manipulations in up to 85.8% cases in order to reach the distal third of the SVC [17].

In contrast, Ku et al. [18] found only 9 malpositions in their retrospective study on 1,070 TIVADs implanted through percutaneous subclavian vein puncture by a single specialist: 3 catheters twinned at the innominate vein, one at the left subclavian vein; right subclavian puncture brought 3 catheters into the left innominate vein and 2 in the right internal jugular vein. Failure to cannulate the subclavian vein (63 cases) or to advance the catheter further than the subclavian vein (20 cases) were excluded from the analysis. Nevertheless, the risk of malposition was considered low enough to waive the need for perioperative control [18].

Consensus could not be reached about the necessity of assessing catheter tip position during the insertion procedure, advocating mainly the need for cumbersome maneuvers and the high costs of radiological equipments [18].

9.4 Control Techniques for Catheter Tip Position

9.4.1 Imaging Techniques

9.4.1.1 Plain Chest Radiograph Post Insertion

Advantages

The chest radiograph after the procedure remains an important medicolegal document to assess central catheter tip location, irrespective of the insertion technique or device used for perioperative tip location control [1, 9, 18, 19]. Performed within a few hours after catheterization, a chest radiography may also rule out the presence of a small pneumothorax that can occur following *blind* percutaneous vein puncture, since small lesions are not immediately visible.

Disadvantages/Concerns

The value of plain chest radiographs is limited by the fact that imaging is performed after completion of TIVAD insertion: in case of malposition, a new intervention will be necessary in order to bring the catheter tip in the correct location. This second procedure is a waste of time, delaying catheter relief for administering the planned intravenous therapy.

This type of imaging is also discouraged in pregnant women (radiation risk to the fetus) and patients with ataxia telangiectasia (high susceptibility for tissue damage induced by ionizing radiation).

Moreover, the relationship between the visible central catheter extremity on the image and its precise location with respect to surrounding structures is often imprecise and subject to inter-observer variability [2]. Rapid movements of the catheter tip inside the vessel can also lead to misinterpretation of tip position on chest radiographs [1]. This is even more the case in small children with enlarged thymus and in patients affected by large malignant pleural effusions, lung or mediastinal tumors, heart failure, kyphosis, scoliosis, following pneumonectomy etc... Indeed, the location of the catheter tip relies on visible bony structures that are located out of the coronal plane of the SVC. For this reason variations of the direction of the incident X-ray beam on the patient and X-ray film planes will modify the final image, due to the parallax effect [2]. *Bed-side* pictures by portable devices allow only some gross evaluation due to the difficulty in standardizing all these elements. Moreover, poor contrast between the catheter and surrounding structures prevented proper tip assessment in up to 15% of cases [5]. Digital chest radiographs taken in standardized upright position of the patient may improve the reading accuracy.

SVC Boundaries

Optimal radiographic landmarks related to the different segments of the SVC are still a matter of debate as well, for veins are difficult to visualize on plain radiographs without contrast dye opacification. However, several notable radiological structures or images have been described with regard to their relationship with the mediastinal *soft tissue* elements.

The right SVC forms the **right border of the upper mediastinal shadow** and has a straight cranio-caudal course, projecting parallel to the right border of the spine, except in patients with severe scoliosis, and mediastinal shift due to large pleural effusion or total pneumonectomy. In rare cases, patients present a left-sided SVC, without *situs inversus*: this vein is not clearly visible on plain radiographs and needs specific imaging with contrast dye, CT or MRI.

The **upper border of the SVC** has been associated with the inferior border of the clavicles [20] and with the angle between the right main bronchus and the trachea [3]. Concerning the latter, MRI images revealed that the SVC begins above the tracheobronchial angle (median 1.5 cm, range 0.1-3.8 cm in adults) [21].

Distally, the "**cavoatrial junction**" was identified by the characteristic widening of the right mediastinal border at this point [19] or by the intersection of the right heart border with the contour of the SVC [3]. The inflection point resulting from the junction between the SVC and the RA was also found projecting 2 cm caudal from the place where the lower border of the right main bronchus crosses the SVC. However, more precise imaging with CT revealed that the upper border of the inflection was formed by the right atrial appendage and not the RA in 56% patients; the superior cavoatrial junction was located anterior to the T5-T6 intervertebral disk ± 0.75 vertebral body units, at a mean distance of 1.6 cm ± 1.1 cm below the right heart border, at 2.9 cm ± 1.3 cm below the right stem bronchus, and 4.0 ± 1.0 below the carina, corresponding to 2.0 ± 0.4 vertebral body units. Fortunately, the association between the length of the SVC and the vertebral body height remains constant in the same subject [22].

Relying on MRI studies, Aslamy et al. [21] were also able to show that the superior heart border belonged to the left atrium in 38% of patients, and was located at a median distance of 1 cm above the superior edge of the right atrium. The place where the SVC merges in the RA is thus located 1 cm caudally. These authors also found that the SVC ended at a median distance of 4.9 cm (range, 2.9-6.8 cm) beneath the trachea-bronchial angle [21].

Targeting the Upper Cavoatrial Junction

Even when the lower extremity of the SVC / cavoatrial junction is chosen as the optimal position on chest radiograph, authors of different series have provided different recommendations. The catheter tip has to been seen in the space between the fifth and sixth thoracic vertebrae [20], or lie between the sixth and eight vertebrae [19], or come into the cardiac silhouette [21], or land 2 cm caudal from the lower border of the right main bronchus, reach 2 vertebral bodies beneath the carina in adolescents and young adults [22] or one and a half vertebral bodies beneath the carina in children. According to anatomical landmarks, the crista terminalis was also correlated with a point projecting 5 cm below the manubriosternal junction [16].

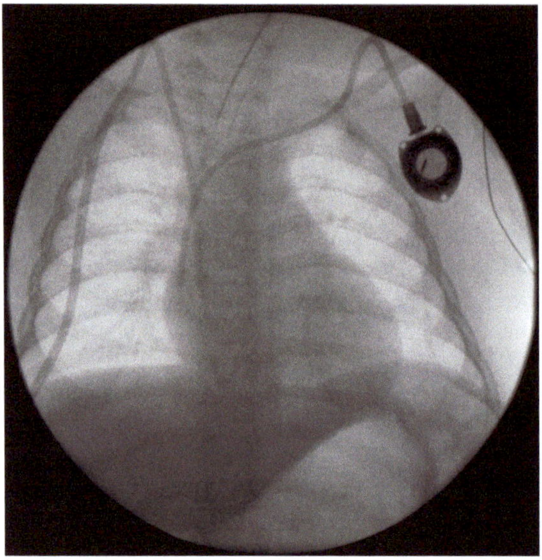

Fig. 9.1 Child with port inserted through the left external jugular vein (catheter abutting the right border of the SVC) and double lumen tunneled catheter through the right external jugular vein (catheter abutting on the left border of the SVC)

More pragmatically, to avoid having a catheter tip in contact with the vessel wall, it must be located a distance beyond the last bend before reaching the upper part of the SVC *such that the axes of the intracaval portion of the catheter and vein are aligned*. This aim was considered more difficult to achieve with catheters inserted from the left side, due to the angle between the left brachiocephalic vein and the VCS [3]. However, irrespective of the insertion side, catheters of appropriate length were found to lean on the opposite wall of the SVC (Fig. 9.1).

Effect of Patient Motion on the Location of the Catheter Tip After Insertion
Another concern is the significant change in the SVC length between the supine position of the patient during catheter insertion and the upright position requested for the control chest radiograph. These changes are even more pronounced in patients having a procedure in Trendelenburg position, which is quite popular for percutaneous venous punctures.

The effective lengthening of the SVC in upright position after placement will lead to a relative *shortening* of the catheter due to upwards migration. A compensation for this migration at the time of placement will maintain control over the final catheter position [3].

One can also take advantage of the motion of the diaphragm during the respiratory cycle to position the catheter. In inspiration, the diaphragm moves caudal wards, resulting in an elongation of the mediastinum and the catheter tip is able to *move* 2-cm upwards on average in adults. Accordingly, Schutz et al. [3] recommended performing the control radiograph while the patient takes a deep breath.

Heavy coughing or vomiting as well as Valsalva maneuvers may provoke a displacement of the catheter into peripheral veins, in particular if the catheters were initially too short. Last but not least, children are growing but their catheter is not. A systematic control imaging is requested in order to track progressive slipping of the catheter away from its initial location in the SVC in order to replace the device before complications occur.

9.4.1.2 Fluoroscopy During the Procedure

Advantages of Fluoroscopy

Central catheter positioning under fluoroscopic visualisation is a very attractive method since it can display the actual position of the catheter tip and show eventual misplacement. Moreover, the amount of radiation delivered to the patients remains limited if reduced dose pulsed fluoroscopy is used (median 54 mGy, range 1 to 921 mGy) [23]. Another advantage of fluoroscopy is the possibility of injecting contrast dye through the catheter [2, 12] in order to depict more precisely difficult venous crossroads which need to be passed through, providing that the patient is not allergic to intravenous contrast or suffering renal failure. Visualization of catheter tip movements due to respiratory and cardiac motions provides a better idea of its actual location than static perioperative images. The possibility to rotate the C-arm of the fluoroscopy device with 90°, in order to create a profile view in addition to the antero-posterior view [1], can be interesting when malposition is suspected in the thoracic or azygos veins. Moreover, a catheter tip in the right ventricle may end up in a horizontal course and show ample tip movements [12].

Limits of Fluoroscopy

The difficulties listed for the reading of plain radiographs are also encountered on perioperative fluoroscopic images and loss of precision is possible as well. Indeed, the inflection between the SVC and the heart border is not always clear. Other landmarks, as the fifth or sixth intervertebral space may be difficult to spot on the limited anatomic area shown on the screen and inclination of the X-ray beam may amplify parallax effects. Some malpositions are missed at a first glance because of the lower quality of images obtained in the operating room, when compared to static digital radiographs or to images provided by sophisticated angiography suite equipments. This is the case for catheters which curl back into the SVC in the sagittal plane, and catheters located in the internal thoracic vein (Fig. 9.2) or azygos vein, which project closely to or behind the SVC on anteroposterior views. These rare events could be avoided by taking systematically lateral views, although this is not a part of current practice. Moreover, during complex treatment courses, patients will need multiple radiological investigations and although each investigation delivers only a small amount of radiation, these doses are cumulative in time: stochastic effects, principally secondary cancer due to low doses exposures, are thus not fully excluded [23].

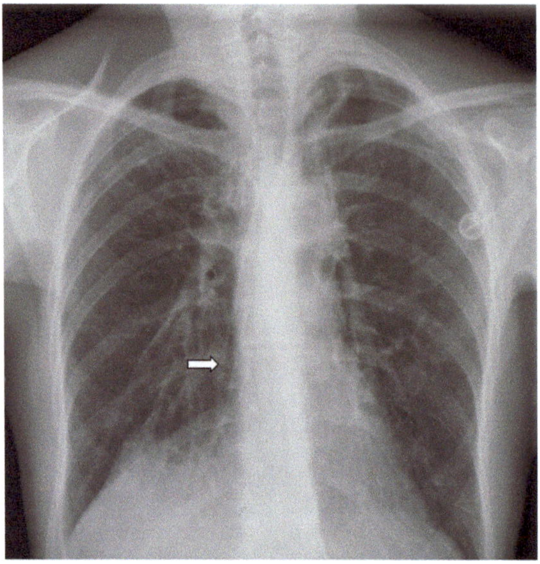

Fig. 9.2 Catheter tip in right mammary vein. Catheter position was considered correct on fluoroscopy. White arrow directed on the central extremity of the catheter projecting outside the superior vena cava

9.4.1.3 Other Imaging Techniques

Marcy et al. [24] used angiography through opacification of peripheral veins for image-guided puncture prior to placement of arm ports. They reported impossible peripheral vein access for dye injection in 2% of cases, failure of brachial vein puncture in 4%, and procedure related death in 0.4% of cases [24]. If dye injection can be achieved, it provides an excellent visualization of central veins, where stenosis is suspected. However, high quality images may only be obtained in fully equipped radiology suites; and known allergy to iodinated contrasts, renal failure and pregnancy are important contraindications.

Contrast enhanced computer tomography is also able to accurately depict blood vessels and additionally the surrounding anatomic structures. It provides relevant information in patients with a history of numerous accesses, when a new catheter is requested but TIVAD insertion under computed tomography guidance is currently not feasible.

Practical considerations and costs restrict the use of magnetic resonance imaging as well, where available, for diagnostic purposes. Moreover, patients wearing a cardiac pace-maker have to be excluded.

US guidance in general is an accurate and safe technique for localization of superficial veins, prior to puncture, providing the absence of subcutaneous emphysema, but visualization of central veins is not possible. On trans-thoracic ultrasonography, only the heart and intra-cardiac catheter tips are visible. However, performing a simultaneous injection of normal saline can cause additional turbulences and improve the detection rate of catheter tips [25]. Trans Esophageal Echography (TEE) is a refined technique able to accurately depict the heart and the important landmark formed by the crista terminalis, at the junction between the SVC and the RA, and was advocated as the standard control technique against which all other techniques have to be compared [16, 26]. However, the upper part of the SVC and its tributary veins may not be visualized since these structures are located too far from the esophagus, with air in between. Moreover the insertion of an esophageal tube is definitely less pleasant than other imaging techniques for patients having a TIVAD implanted under local anesthesia.

Different electromagnetic guidance systems have been developed to localize central catheters through the tracing of an sensor inserted in their lumen (Cathfinder®, Pharmacia; Navigator®, Navilyst; CathTrack®, Bard Inc). These systems provide a visual and audible signal to indicate the position of the sensor when a hand-held probe is placed on the skin above this sensor. The search for the typical signal is performed when the catheter tip is taught to be located in the SVC, and this allows adjustments in craniocaudal position in order to fit with pre-determined anatomic landmarks. However, in case of difficulty in threading the catheter in the SVC, fluoroscopic assistance is needed [27]. A newer device (VasoNovaTM Vascular Positioning SystemTM, Teleflex) has combined this guidance with ultrasound, with great facility of use and good precision providing that the catheter is already located in the SVC.

9.5 Conclusions

Many issues are still debated concerning long-term central venous accesses: optimal technique of insertion; optimal location of catheter tip; need and timing for correct position assessment before relieving patients for intravenous treatment.

Among the available control techniques, the postoperative chest X-ray is an easy to obtain, valuable medico-legal document, but its interpretation can lack precision. Real-time fluorosocopy allows visualization of the catheter and is a very useful tool when perioperative correction of eventual malposition is needed. However, concerns about SVC landmarks on plain radiographs can be magnified on routine radioscopic images, such as those obtained in operating rooms. Intravenous contrast dye injection or through the catheter provides better visualization of the catheter and the vessels, essentially in difficult cases. But these products are costly and routine use is limited by patient conditions. Intravascular guidance using CT or MRI is emerging but till now limited to intracardiac ablation of ectopic pace-maker sites. Transesophageal endoscopy is very reliable but quite uncomfortable for the patient, when performing TIVAD insertion under local anesthesia such as in current practice. Magnetic navigation systems were more able to raise than maintain enthusiasm of users in the past.

Complications and malfunctions associated with incorrect catheter tip position, outside the very distal portion of the SVC or the upper part of the RA, are well documented. This should prompt all users to place central catheter tips at this site, and to check its position during the insertion procedure.

References

1. Vesely TM (2003) Central Venous Catheter Tip Position: A Continuing Controversy. J Vasc Interv Radiol 14:527-534
2. Nakazawa N (2010) Challenges in the Accurate Identification of the Ideal Catheter Tip Location. JAVA 15:196-200
3. Schutz JCL, Patel AA, Clark TWI et al (2004) Relationship between Chest Port Catheter Tip Position and Port Malfunction after Interventional Radiologic Placement. J Vasc Interv Radiol 15:581-587
4. Cadman A, Lawrance JA, Fitzsimmons L et al (2004) To clot or not to clot? That is the question in central venous catheters. Clin Radiol 59:349-355
5. Caers J, Fontaine C, Vinh-Hung V et al (2005) Catheter tip position as a risk factor for thrombosis associated with the use of subcutaneous infusion ports. Support Care Cancer 13:325-331
6. Korones DN, Buzzard CJ, Asselin BL, Harris JP (1996) Right atrial thrombi in children with cancer and indwelling catheters. J Pediatr 128:841-846
7. Kearns PJ, Coleman S, Wehner JH (1996) Complications of long-arm-catheters: A randomized trial of central vs peripheral tip location. JPEN 20:20-24
8. Pittiruti M, Hamilton H, Biffi R et al (2009) ESPEN guidelines on parenteral nutrition: central venous catheters (access, care, diagnosis and therapy of complications) Clinical Nutrition 28:365-377
9. Food and Drug Administration Task Force (1989) Precautions necessary with central venous catheters. FDA Drug Bulletin 15-16
10. National Association of Vascular Access Networks (1998) NAVAN Position Statement. J Vasc Access Devices 3:8-10
11. McGee WT, Ackerman BL, Rouben LR et al (1993) Accurate placement of central venous catheters: A prospective randomized, multicenter trial. Crit Care Med 21:1118-1123
12. Barnacle A, Arthurs O, Roebuck D, Hiorns M (2008) Malfunctioning central venous catheters in children: a diagnostic approach. Pediatr Radiol 38:363-378
13. Goossens GA, Stas M, Moons P (2011) Management of functional complications of totally implantable venous access devices by an advanced practice nursing team: 5 years of clinical experience, submitted
14. Xiang DZ, Verbeken EK, Van Lommel ATL, Stas M, De Wever I (1998) Composition and formation of the sleeve enveloping a central venous catheter. J Vasc Surg 28:260-271
15. National Kidney Foundation (2001) K/DOQI Clinical Practice Guidelines for Vascular Access. Am J Kidney Dis 37(Suppl 1):S137-S181
16. Chu K-S, Hsu J-H, Wang S-S et al (2004) Accurate central venous Port-A-Catheter placement: Intravenous electrocardiography and surface landmark techniques compared by using transesophageal echocardiography. Aesth Analg 98:910-914
17. Fricke BL, Racadio JM, Duckworth T et al (2005) Placement of peripherally inserted central catheters without fluoroscopy in children: Initial catheter tip position. Radiology 234:887-892
18. Ku YH, Kuo PH, Tsai YF et al (2009) Port-A-Cath implantation using percutaneous puncture without guidance. Ann Surg Oncol 16:729-734
19. Peres PW (1990) Positioning central venous catheters – a prospective study. Aneasth Intens Care 8:536-539
20. Greenall MJ, Blewitt RW, McMahon MJ (1975) Cardiac tamponade and central venous catheters. BMJ 2:595-597
21. Aslamy Z, Dewald CL, Heffner JE (1998) MRI of central venous anatomy. Implications for central venous catheter insertion. Chest 114:820-826
22. Baskin KM, Jimenez RM, Cahill AM et al (2008) Cavoatrial junction and central venous anatomy: Implications for central venous access tip position. J Vasc Interv Radiol 19:359-365
23. Storm ES, Miller DL, Hoover LJ et al (2006) Radiation Doses from Venous Access Procedures. Radiology 238:1044-1050

24. Marcy PY, Magné N, Castadot P et al (2007) Is radiologic placement of an arm port mandatory in oncology patients?: an analysis of a large bi-institutional experience. Cancer 110:2331-2338
25. Radke J, Lange LP, Bartels A, Brunsch C (1990) Control of the placement of a central venous catheter using Doppler ultrasound. Aneasthesist 39:283-287
26. Schummer W, Schummer C, Schelenz C et al (2004) Central venous catheters – the inability of 'intra-atrial ECG' to prove adequate positioning. Br J Anaesth 93:193-198
27. Popp MB, Dobrilovic N, Matern W et al (2005) Accuracy of implanted port placement with the use of the electromagnetic CathTrack ® catheter locator system. The Journal of Vascular Access 6:9-12

Verifying Catheter Tip Position: Fluoroscopy vs Intravasal Electrogram

10

Marguerite Stas and Rik Willems

Abstract

Taking into account the hazards of *blindly* positioning of catheter tips and the full subcutaneous implantation of ports, it is important to assess a correct catheter tip location during insertion of the device, for later corrections are cumbersome or impossible without a new procedure. Perioperative fluoroscopy was considered as the golden standard for this control as it allows to visualise the catheter in situ and to perform correcting manoeuvres when needed. This can be done under direct 2-dimentional real-time imaging, but patients and care providers are repeatedly exposed to a small amount of radiation, and false-positive results are not fully ruled out. An alternative assessment method, based on electrocardiographic principles, could be useful to determine the best location for the catheter tip and to assist precise positioning. Indeed, the shape of the intravasal electrocardiogram waves (IEG) is closely related to the place where they are captured. Tracking changes in the IEG pattern, mainly involving the *P-wave* of the ECG complex taken inside large vessels or heart allows thus to position catheter tips very accurately. For this technique, a conductive solution or a metallic guidewire can be used as guidance systems. This chapter will describe the theoretical basis of the Intravasal Electrogram and its application to perioperative central catheter positioning, and will provide a comparison with fluoroscopic performances.

Keywords

During insertion • Perioperative fluoroscopy • Changes in the IEG pattern • Conductive solution • Guidewire

M. Stas (✉)
Surgical Oncology, UZ Leuven,
Leuven, Belgium
e-mail: marguerite.stas@uzleuven.be

I. Di Carlo, R. Biffi, *Totally Implantable Venous Access Devices*,

10.1 Introduction

Series reporting on central catheter insertion techniques that rely solely on anatomical landmarks without other verification of tip position, showed a definite risk of initial catheter malposition. This is the case for all kinds of central access lines [1, 2, 3]. Assessment of catheter tip location is therefore needed, before releasing the device for use. The plain chest radiograph was counselled as control [4], immediately after the procedure. However, for totally implantable venous access devices (TIVADs), in contrast to external catheters (tunnelled and non-tunneled catheters and peripherally inserted central catheters), postoperative correction of eventual malposition is impossible without a new, costly procedure. This led to the implementation of several perioperative checking techniques, among which fluoroscopy and intravasal electrogram, whether captured through a ionic conducting solution [5, 6] or a metallic guidewire [7], are the most widely used.

Fluoroscopy is considered as the golden standard for it allows to visualise the catheter in situ and to position its tip under direct 2-dimentional real-time imaging. Patients receive only a small amount of radiation during fluoroscopy [8] but repeated exposure remains a concern for care providers. Furthermore, this method has several drawbacks, some of which were already listed in Chapter 9, and an expensive equipment is needed, which is not constantly available on all wards.

An assessment method based on electrocardiography can skirt around these problems, taking advantage of the relation between the shape of the intravasal electrocardiogram and the place where it is captured. Briefly, the first deflection displayed during the cardiac activity cycle on the surface electrocardiogram (ECG) is the P-wave, due to the depolarisation of the muscle cells of the atrial wall. It is seen as a positive deflection on the surface ECG if the electrical vector of depolarization is directed towards the measuring electrode, best depicted on the DII lead. But this atrial activity can also be measured within the heart, by the Intravasal Electrogram (IEG) technique. We will refer to this as the IEG *"P-wave"*. An intravenous electrode, that replaces the right shoulder electrode of the surface ECG, is advanced toward the right atrium (RA). Coming closer to its source, the amplitude of the IEG *"P-wave"* will increase in the lower part of the superior vena cava (SVC) and peak in the RA. Tracking the IEG *"P-wave"* changes during intravascular motion of the electrode allows thus to detect very precisely the junction between the SVC and the RA, but only in the presence of atrial contractions. Consequently, the absence of a clear P-wave on the surface ECG (for example in case of atrial fibrillation) or catheter malposition in one of the affluent veins of the SVC, precludes IEG changes and information about the intravasal electrode location may not be obtained.

Features of the IEG technique, advantages and limits of fluoroscopy and IEG for perioperative catheter tip location will be discussed.

10.2 Monitoring the Intravasal Electrogram During the Insertion Procedure

The surface electrocardiogram (ECG) concept was developed by the Dutchman Einthoven at the dawn of the 20th century: electric waves generated by the depolarization of cardiac myocytes during the heart contraction cycles can be visualized as a repetitive series of specific spikes and depressions. In 1949, Hellerstein, Pritchard and Lewis [9] adapted these principles for recording and monitoring of intracavitary potentials through a single lumen, saline filled cardiac catheter. The technique was named Intravasal Electrogram (IEG) and implemented for intra-procedural control of correct positioning of central venous lines in Europe. It was legally accepted as sole control technique for this purpose soon thereafter in Germany. The technique was also tested and proved to be both feasible and reliable for TIVAD insertion through a surgical venous cut-down technique [7] and through venous puncture [6].

10.2.1 Principles of Electrocardiography Applied to the Intravasal Electrogram

This section summarizes the basics of electrocardiography with relevance to the perioperative control of the catheter tip location, based on the work of Friedman [10], *Diagnostic Electrography and Vectography*. The rhythmic excitatory process of the heart has normally its origin in the sinoatrial (SA) node, a specialized tissue lying within the atrial musculature, near the upper cavoatrial junction. It is the normal pacemaker of the heart but the electrical forces produced by the node itself are too small to be recorded on a surface electrocardiogram. However, the P wave, representing the atrial depolarization initiated by the SA node, can be detected. From the SA node, the activation process is first transmitted to the RA, spreads thereafter to the interatrial septum and finally to the left atrium (LA), following an electrical vector directed roughly towards leads I-II of the surface ECG. Lead II will display the largest P-wave, with an amplitude of 0.5 to 2.5 mm (a deflection of 1 mm on the ECG stroke correlates with an electrical activity of 0.1 millivolt) and a duration in time of 0.07 to 0.10 s. Since the depolarization of RA and LA occur very close to each other in time and space, the resulting P wave in DII appears as one single "positive" spike, directed upwards. In other leads, the P wave shape can appear as negative or biphasic. Increased voltage or duration of the P wave is usually diagnostic of atrial abnormality, irrespective of the SA node condition. In right atrial enlargement for example, the amplitude of the P wave will increase; in left atrial enlargement, the duration of the wave is increased and two spikes may be seen, partially overlapping each other. In summary, the P-wave morphology on the surface ECG is determined by the interatrial and intra-atrial conduction patterns [11]. In atrial fibrillation, there is no synchronized atrial depolarization nor visible P-wave on the surface ECG which displays only oscillations of the baseline.

10.2.2 Intravasal Electrogram

10.2.2.1 Principle of IEG

The sinus node function is assessed electrocardiographically by analyzing the frequency and pattern of atrial depolarization, namely the P-wave morphology, frequency and regularity [11]. Using specially designed bipolar intravascular steerable catheters for cardiac pacing, atrial activitiy can also be recorded in atrial fibrillation or junctional rhythms [11]. These catheters were further developed for the ablation of atrial arrhythmia and cannot be compared to the blind, less sensitive unipolar recording devices used for perioperative IEG. Due to its low electrical activity, evaluation of sinus node automaticity and conduction is therefore usually performed indirectly by assessing atrial activity. The intravasal electrogram takes advantage of a unipolar intravascular catheter, able to guide the proper location its tip. Advancing into the SCV towards the RA, this electrode will record typical changes in the IEG pattern. Coming closer to the RA, the amplitude of the electrical atrial activity will rise progressively, due to the proximity of the catheter to the atrial tissue and to its allignement with the vector of the atrial activation. Moreover, the intracardiac atrial electrogram is superimposed on top of the P wave of the surface ECG with this technique of recording [12]. The amplitude of the QRS complex will increase as well, but in a lesser proportion, and the maximal amplitude of the atrial activity captured inside the RA may even surpass the height of the ventricular activity. The amplitude of this large *atrial* deflection (IEG *"P-wave"*)

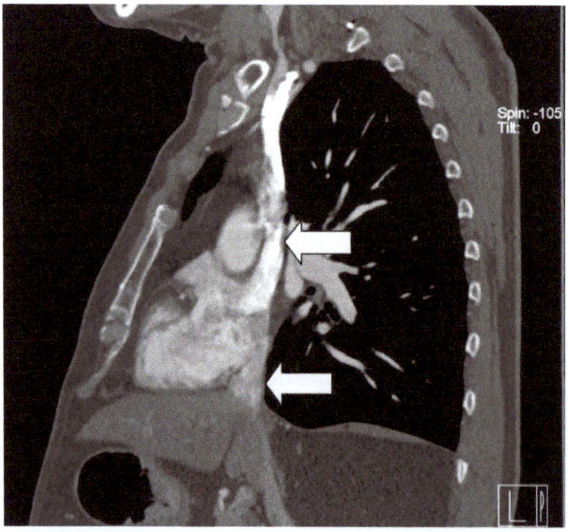

Fig. 10.1 Sagittal CT view of the chest. Note the alignment of the superior vena cava (SVC) and inferior vena cava (IVC) indicated with white arrows containing legend

will remain comparable as long as the recording electrode is located in the RA, at the epicenter of the atrial electrical activity. Indeed the increase in amplitude is inversely related to the square of the source distance [13]. When the electrode leaves the RA, whether down to the inferior vena cava (IVC) or up to the SVC, the *IEG "P-wave"* amplitude will decrease, back to the size of the P-wave displayed on the *surface* ECG. The shape of the atrial electrical activity recorded in the RA is essentially a positive spike. Biphasic waves are only seen in 20% to 48 % cases [7, 14] and multiple extra-systoles induced by this technique are infrequent. Due to the anatomical location of the RA anterior to the plane of the SVC prolonged by the IVC (Fig. 10.1), straight intravasal guidewire electrodes – and catheters – are prone to descend in the IVC rather than to curl into the RA and induce extra systoles by triggering the atrial wall [14] or tricuspid valve.

10.2.2.2 Conducting Devices

Both metallic guidewires exceeding the length of the catheter (included in the port tray of the Celsite® ports, BBraun [7, 15] and Districath®, Districlass) and ionic solutions to be injected with a separate syringe (Alphacard®, BBraun – Vygocard®, Vygon – Johans® ECG adapter, Arrow International [16, 17]) can serve as electrodes, providing a connection with the ECG monitor. Note that guidewires fully covered by insulating Teflon are not suitable. Different ionic conducting solutions can be used, such as normal saline [16], 5.85% NaCl [5], 10% saline [13], 0.8mEq/mL $NaHCO_3$ [6]. Some authors reported more arrhythmias with the guidewire technique than with a catheter filled with a saline solution [18]. Based on more than 10 years of experience in routine use of IEG for positioning over 1000 catheters yearly, we found a stable IEG pattern when using a metallic guidewire and very few cases of arrhythmias induced by this device. On the contrary, several cycles of saline flush alternating with rest periods were needed in order to detect the maximal *P-wave*. Indeed, the time span during which the ECG curve remains stable after flushing is short and the saline injection itself causes disturbing baseline shifting and artifacts, precluding visualization of the typical waves.

10.2.3 Practical Set-up for Perioperative IEG

10.2.3.1 General Set-up in Surgical Exposure and US Guided Approach

Patients are installed in supine position on a table allowing fluoroscopic rescue, if needed. Three standard surface ECG electrodes are placed on the skin and connected to a classical 3-leads ECG monitor: the *negative* electrode is located behind the right shoulder, the *neutral* behind the left shoulder and the *positive* at the apex of the heart (Fig. 10.2, ECG set-up). In full aseptic conditions, the vein is accessed, whether by surgical cutdown or by US guided puncture.

For the surgical technique, cutdown of the cephalic, external or internal jugular veins is usually performed under local anesthesia in adults and gener-

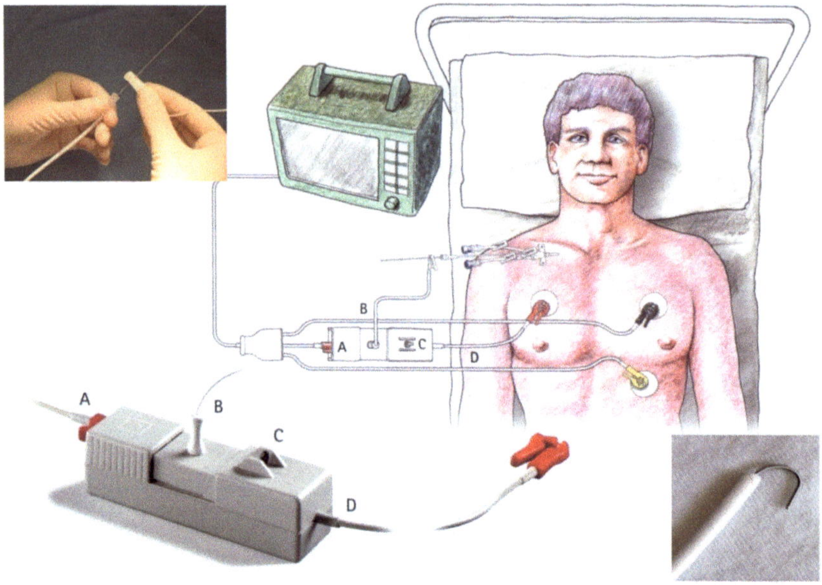

Fig. 10.2 Set-up for perioperative IEG (A) Switch box with connection to ECG monitor – (B) insertion site of sterile cable to be attached to the intravasal guidewire for IEG (replaces the right-shoulder ECG lead) – (C) switch converting *surface* ECG to IEG mode – (D) cable to external ECG pad on right shoulder. *IEG* Intravasal electrogram (with permission of Prof. Dr. Motsch, Heidelberg - Germany and BBraun)

al anesthesia in children. After exposing the vein, the catheter is gently advanced for 10 cm, until it reaches a large vessel. The metallic guidewire is then inserted in the catheter, in order to present only the J-tip extremity to the bloodstream. The opposite extremity of the guidewire comes out the other end of the catheter and is clamped by a sterile conducting cable. This allows the right shoulder electrode to be replaced by the guidewire tip and to transmit the intracardiac electrical activity to the monitoring device, through a switchbox (Certodyn® BBraun) or directly (Sapiens®, Bard, exclusively developed for PICC catheters – Nautilus®, Romedex). The median portion of the guidewire remains isolated from the surrounding tissues or blood by the catheter itself. Indeed, non-insulated guidewires will transfer the electrical activity to the surrounding tissues instead of transmitting this signal to the monitor. Continuous recording of IEG can start. Coming in the caudal portion of the SVC, the amplitude of the IEG *"P-wave"* captured by the intra-vascular electrode will increase and reach a maximum level when entering the RA at the junction between the SVC and the RA (Fig. 10.3). Catheter tips are best left 2 cm deeper in caudal direction, anticipating for the expected upwards migration when patients move back to the upright position [19, 6]. An alternative is to search for the begin of the area with the maximal IEG *"P-wave"* amplitude in deep

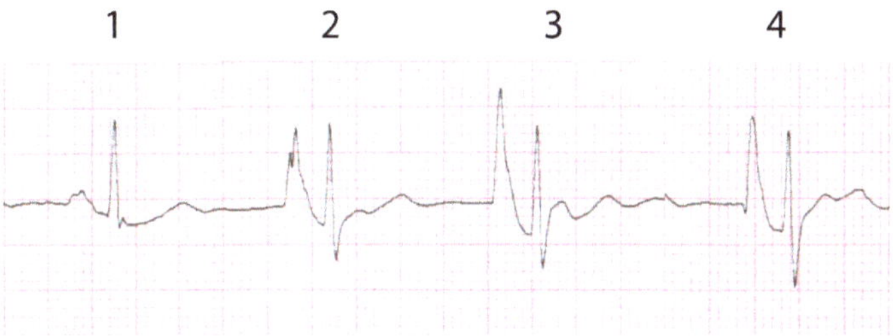

Fig. 10.3 Typical IEG patterns with regard to the P-wave: 1, in proximal part of superior vena cava; 2, lower SVC; 3, junction SVC-Right atrium; 4, caudal in RA, with minimal negative deflection preceding the high P-wave. Note the changes of the QRS when reaching the RA

inspiration and to position the catheter tip at that site, following the same principles as for the intra-procedural fluoroscopic technique [20].

If the tall IEG "*P-wave*" does not appear in the DII derivation on the monitor after inserting the appropriate length of catheter, a misplacement is to be suspected. The catheter can be withdrawn a short distance and then advanced again [5] after changing the patient's position. Simple maneuvers such as turning the head and neck towards the shoulder on the insertion side may be helpful. If not, fluoroscopic assistance is requested.

Once the catheter tip is positioned correctly, the guidewire is removed and the catheter flushed vigorously in order to remove all the blood sucked up into the catheter lumen during guidewire withdrawal. The catheter can be trimmed at the appropriated length and connected to the port.

Using the modified Seldinger technique for percutaneous puncture of the internal jugular or subclavian vein under US guidance, the IEG can be helpful as well to assess the correct direction of the guidewire before entering the vein with a large-bore dilator and peel-away sheet. After puncture of the vein, the guidewire is advanced for 15-20 cm, the needle is removed and the dilator advanced over the guidewire until the resistance of the vein wall is felt. At that moment, the guidewire is isolated from the skin surface and can serve as intravasal electrode by switching the ECG to the IEG mode. An increase in the *P-wave* (and QRS) amplitude appears - although less pronounced than the *atrial* P obtained through an insulated guide - when the caudal part of the SVC or the RA are reached, indicating that the dilator may be advanced further in the vessel without harm. However, for searching the precise location of the SVC-RA junction, it is better to reinserted the guidewire into the catheter as mentioned above.

10.2.3.2 False positive and false negative findings

Absence of clear IEG "*P-wave*", despite correct catheter tip position, may be seen when the monitor is not set in DII mode, in the event of technical failure or absence of formal atrial contractions, such as in patients with cardiac pacemakers. In cases of atrial fibrillation, there is no P-wave, but inserting the

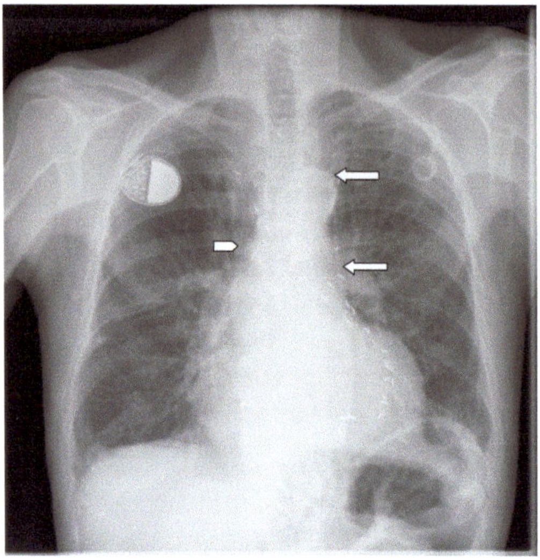

Fig. 10.4 Port catheter in left-sided SVC (*white arrows*) and pacemaker lead inserted through the right-sided SVC (*arrowhead*)

catheter further into the right ventricle is able to display large ventricular complexes in some patients. False-negative findings are not harmful but require rescue by direct imaging technique. In turn, some true-negative IEG's can be misinterpreted by fluoroscopy, such as catheters entering the internal thoracic (see Chapter 9) or azygos vein, or curling back in the SVC in the sagittal plane.

False positive results were reported following accidental or intended arterial punctures, bringing catheters in the ascending aorta: IEG was similar to the pattern found in the SVC [13]. Catheters located in the coronary sinus or epicardial veins, or entering the left atrium through an open foramen ovale will display an IEG *"P-wave"* as well. Finally, venous access from the left can bring catheter tips in a left-sided SVC (Fig. 10.4), a rare but known condition. A tall biphasic IEG *"P-wave"* will appear after insertion of a much shorter catheter length when compared to the expected length for that site, based on anatomical landmarks.

The intravasal IEG principle for location of the tip of central catheters is not device-specific, but some considerations may limit its use. Indeed, if the *Instructions For Use* provided with a particular device do not mention the possibility of using ECG/IEG guidance, this will be considered an *off label* use and any adverse event occurring during placement – even if obviously unrelated to IEG recording – will fall under the sole responsibility of the user.

10.3 Comparison of Fluoroscopy with IEG

Comparison of perioperative fluoroscopy with IEG in terms of success rate and accuracy is scarce. Information has to be collected indirectly, through series comparing IEG with anatomical landmarks, perioperative TEE or ultrasound, or postoperative radiographs, in supine or erect position.

Furthermore, variability across different authors determining the ideal IEG "*P wave*" shape is as evident as the variability of the ideal landing zone definition, when using radiological landmarks. Series aiming essentially to position the catheter tip outside the RA, in compliance with the FDA recommendations [13, 16, 21, 22] achieved this aim in over 95% cases by pulling the catheter back after obtaining the tallest IEG "*P-wave*". Others preferred to insert the catheters at the cavoatrial junction [7,6,14] and leave the tips at the tallest IEG "P" level, or deeper (Table 10.1).

In a pilot study, perioperative fluoroscopy was compared with IEG during insertion of TIVAD catheters. First, a good radiologic correlation was found between the place where the SVC is transected by the right heart border and a point projecting 2 cm distal from the right main bronchus. Second, these sites correlated with the begin of the area where the "*P-wave*" displayed its maximal amplitude on IEG. All patients had a standing chest radiograph after the procedure: 88% of catheter tips were found within a range of 2 cm of the radiological targets but 12% of the catheters were 3-5 cm too short. There were no adverse events [7]. At that time, correction for catheter tip migration due to body motions was not yet implemented. These results allowed us to define typical patterns of IEG "*P-waves*", specific for particular intravascular sites and to design the next study.

A randomized controlled trial addressed the precision of the IEG method when compared to perioperative fluoroscopy, for catheters reaching directly the SVC without additional radiologic rescue. Over 1,000 implantable ports were placed, whether under fluoroscopic guidance or with IEG. More than 20 residents and staff members of one surgical department inserted the devices. All patients received a digital upright chest radiograph after the procedure, with anterior and lateral views. Images were read by one radiologist blinded for the preoperative catheter tip control technique. Position of the catheter tip was recorded with regard to the 2 radiological landmarks tested in the pilot study. Statistical analysis showed a non-inferiority of the IEG technique, which was the main end-point of our study (manuscript in progress).

Following this trial, the IEG technique was implemented in 2002 as upfront approach in all our patients, except those with a cardiac pace-maker and in accesses through the IVC. In over 90% cases, the junction of the SVC and RA could be localized with this technique, using a metallic guidewire. In case of smooth progression of the catheter into the vein, without visualization of the typical IEG "P-wave", correcting maneuvers were attempted after changing the patient's position. If catheter threading into the SVC remained impossible, fluoroscopic assistance was requested, with the use of Teflon covered guidewires and contrast dye injection when needed. In case of unexpected stenosis revealed by perioperative imaging, insertion of the catheter was postponed until full imaging of central veins was obtained in order to chose the most appropriate access site.

Table 10.1 Definition of optimal anatomical site and corresponding P-wave shape on Intravasal Electrogram for catheter tip location

Author	Study	Set-up	Reference	Anatomical target	IEG	Conclusion
Radke 1990	Obs	Doppler US + IEG	Post-op XR	Right Sternal border where Doppler sound was most distinct	Atrial P -1 cm	Correct position if no time lag between injection and perception of turbulences
McGee 1993	RCT	IEG vs LM	Post-op supine XR	Outside the heart	Tallest P wave -3 cm	IEG 100 % correct – LM 44 % correct
Stas 2001	Obs	IEG + fluoroscopy	Post-op erect XR antero-posterior + lateral	SVC-RA junction or 2 cm under RMB	Begin tallest P-wave zone	Best correlation: IEG tallest P and fluoroscopy 2 cm under RMB
Chu 2004	RCT	IEG vs LM	Per-op TEE: 1 cm of CT + Post-op XR	CT	Tallest P before biphasic P	IEG 100 % correct – LM 53% correct
Schummer 2004	Prosp	IEG	TEE & open heart surgery	CT, outside RA	Site of 1st increase in P wave	All out of RA
Popp 2005	Obs	Electromagnetic + per-op fluorosocpy	Post-op erect XR antero-posterior + lateral	Center 3d IC space (right sterna border)	-	Fluoroscopic rescue in 2/27 cases
Jeon 2006	Obs	IEG	TEE	SVC-RA = superior edge CT	Tallest P wave	Biphasic P = to deep in RA
Gebhard 2007	RCT	IEG vs LM	Post-op supine XR	SVC	Pull back to normal P – 2 cm	IEG 96% correct – LM 76% correct
Lee 2009	RCT	IEG vs LM	Post-op XR	Carina	Where atrial P returned normal	IEG 95% correct – LM 96% correct
Gavecelt 2010*	Prosp	IEG	Post-op XR	Lower 1/3 SVC-upper RA	Tallest P wave	Overall accuracy 95.4%

Obs, observational study; *RCT*, randomized controlled trial; *Prosp*, prospective study; *US*, ultrasound; *IEG*, Intravasal electrogram; *LM*, anatomical landmark; *Post-op XR*, postoperative chest radiograph; *TEE*, perioperative transesophageal echography; *CT*, crista terminalis; *SVC*, superior vena cava; *RA*, Roght Atrium; *RMB*, lower border of right main bronchus; *IC*, inter-costal;
* article in press in JAVA.

Our data were confirmed by a recent multicentric study of the Italian GAVeCeLT group that was able to demonstrate a success rate of more than 90 % with IEG for the correct insertion of port catheters [18].

10.4 Conclusions

The advantages and limitations of imaging techniques for control of central venous catheter tip position were discussed in the previous chapter. The intravasal electrogram technique, developed in the present section, constitutes a good alternative: it is safe, easy to learn and to use in daily practice, accurate, precise, fast and cheap. The typical *IEG "P-wave"*, which is seen during intravasal catheter progression, is related to the contraction of both right and left atrium and remains at a maximal level as long as the catheter tip is located within the right atrium. It decreases only when the catheter is leaving the atrium towards the SVC or IVC and extrasystoles are rare. With the available J-tip guidewire – and even more with the use of conducting saline solutions – the low electrical activity emitted by the sinus node itself, which is located at the level of the crista terminalis, can certainly not be captured.

Using the intravasal IEG perioperatively, post procedural control chest radiograph is no longer necessary, providing that the risk of pneumothorax is totally ruled out by the chosen insertion technique. This is the case for surgical cutdown procedures and peripherally inserted central catheters.

However, IEG use is less suitable in patients with heart rhythm abnormalities or cardiac pacemakers. Any difficulty to position the catheter at the junction SVC-RA based on IEG alone (less than 10 % cases for TIVADs) should prompt at least fluoroscopic assistance. Indeed, the absence of typical P-wave changes after easy insertion of the catheter is suspicious for a malposition, and IEG alone is unable to locate the catheter tip outside the central veins or the right atrium.

Following our own observational study and randomized controlled trial, IEG became our upfront choice for perioperative control of catheter tip position in TIVAD more than 10 years ago, and is still our preferred technique, due to sustained success and enthusiasm among our residents.

Acknowledgments

The authors wish to thank S. Mulier MD, for the concept of the pilot study on IEG; J. Vijgen MD, PhD for the assistance in cardiac electrophysiology; L. De Wever MD for the reading of the chest radiographs; S. Dymarkowski MD PhD and R. Oyen MD PhD who provided the radiological images; G.A. Goossens PhDC, RN for her assistance and reviewing the manuscript. Residents and staff members of the Department of Surgical Oncology and nurses of surgical and oncological wards in UZleuven who took care of patients needing a TIVAD are acknowledge as well.

References

1. De Wever I, Stas M, Mulier S (1998) Poorten en Katheters voor langdurige I.V. therapie, Universitaire Pers, Leuven
2. Cadman A, Lawrance JA, Fitzsimmons L et al (2004) To clot or not to clot? That is the question in central venous catheters. Clin Radiol 59:349-355
3. Fricke BL, Racadio JM, Duckworth T et al (2005) Placement of Peripherally Inserted Central Catheters without fluoroscopy in Children: Initial Catheter Tip Position. Radiology 234:887-892
4. Food and Drug Administration Task Force (1989) Precautions necessary with central venous catheters. FDA Drug Bulletin 15-16
5. Neubauer AP (1995) Percutaneous central iv access in the neonate: experience with 535 silastic catheters. Acta Paediatr 84:756-760
6. Chu K-S, Hsu J-H, Wang S-S et al (2004) Accurate Central Venous Port-A-Catheter Placement: Intravenous Electrocardiography and Surface Landmark Techniques Compared by Using Transesophageal Echocardiography. Aesth Analg 98:910-914
7. Stas M, Mulier S, Pattyn P et al (2001) Peroperative intravasal electrographic control of catheter tip position in access ports placed by venous cut-down technique EJSO 27:316-320
8. Storm ES, Miller DL, Hoover LJ et al (2006) Radiation Doses from Venous Access Procedures. Radiology 238:1044-1050
9. Hellerstein HK, Pritchard WH, Lewiw RL (1949) Recording of intracavity potentials through a single lumen, saline filled cardiac catheter. Proc Soc Exp Biol Med 71:58-60
10. Friedman HH (1985) Diagnostic electrography and vectography. McGraw-Hill, New-York
11. Josephson ME, Seides SF (1979) Clinical Cardiac Electrophysiology. Techniques and Interpretations. Lea & Febiger, Philadelphia
12. Gallagher JJ, Kasell JH, Cox JL et al (1982) Techniques of intraoperative electrophysiologic mapping. Am J Cardiol 49:221-240
13. Schummer W, Schummer C, Schelenz C et al (2004) Central venous catheters – the inability of 'intra-atrial ECG' to prove adequate positioning. Br J Anaesth 93:193-198
14. Jeon Y, Ryu HG, Yoon SZ et al (2006) Transesophageal echographic evaluation of ECG-guided central venous catheter placement. Can J Anesth 53:978-983
15. Pawlik MT, Kutz N, Keyl C et al (2004) Central venous catheter placement: comparison of the intravascular guidewire and the fluid column electrocardiograms. Eur J Anaesthesiol 21(8):594-599
16. McGee WT, Ackerman BL, Rouben LR et al (1993) Accurate placement of central venous catheters: A prospective randomized, multicenter trial. Crit-Care-Med 21:1118-1123
17. Tsui BCH, Richards GJ, Van Aerde J (2005) Umbilical vein catheterization under electrocardiogram guidance. Pediatric Anesthesia 15:297–300
18. Pittiruti M, La Greca A, Scopettuolo G (2011) The electrocardiographic method for positioning the tip of central venous catheters. J Vasc Access (in press)
19. Kowalski CM, Kaufman JA, Rivitz SM et al (1997) Migration of central venous catheters: implications for initial catheter tip positioning. J Vasc Interv Radiol 8:443-447
20. Schutz JCL, Patel AA, Clark TWI et al (2004) Relationship between Chest Port Catheter Tip Position and Port Malfunction after Interventional Radiologic Placement. J Vasc Interv Radiol 15:581-587
21. Gebhard RE, Szmuk P, Pivalizza EG et al (2007) The accuracy of electrocardiogram-controlled central line placement. Anaesth Analg 104:65-70
22. Lee JH, Bahk JH, Ryu HG et al (2009) Comparison of the bedside central venous catheter placement techniques: landmark vs electrocardiogram guidance. Br J Anaesth 102:662-666

Part III

Immediate Complication: Prevention and Treatment

Pneumothorax

11

Roberto Biffi

Abstract

Percutaneous placement of central venous catheters, causing a direct lesion of the lung parenchyma, is a remarkable cause of iatrogenic pneumothorax, the incidence of which is approximately 1 to 4%. Clinical presentation, diagnosis and treatment guidelines of iatrogenic pneumothorax complicating central venous access placement are presented.

Keywords

Central venous catheters • Percutaneous implantation • Iatrogenic pneumothorax • Tube thoracostomy

11.1 Introduction

Percutaneous placement of central venous catheters, through an inadvertent, direct lesion of the lung parenchyma, is a remarkable cause of iatrogenic pneumothorax. Its incidence is approximately 1 to 4% and largely dependent on the experience of the operator, the site of venipuncture and the technique employed [1–4]. Surprisingly few papers have specifically addressed the topic of the best treatment of this condition, in contrast with the large amount of information available regarding the recognition and therapy of spontaneous pneumothorax [5]. In our own previous experience [6], 22 patients out of 1421 (1.54%) experienced a radiologically-proven pneumothorax, with the pleural space affected ranging from 5 to 70%. No cases of associated lung disease or limited cardiopulmonary reserve were detected in this clinical series. No sig-

R. Biffi (✉)
Division of Abdomino Pelvic Surgery, European Institute of Oncology, Milan, Italy
e-mail: roberto.biffi@ieo.it

I. Di Carlo, R. Biffi (eds.), *Totally Implantable Venous Access Devices*,

nificant difference were observed with regard to the side approached (right: 13; left: 9). Sixteen patients out of 22 (72.7%) with minor portions of affected pleural space received simple observation; in these patients the most common finding was an uncomplicated tachycardia (more than 100 bpm); 8 of these did not complain of any symptoms. Six patients (27.2%) underwent an additional procedure (3 tube-thoracostomies and 3 aspirations of the pleural space), claiming symptoms of chest pain and various degrees of dyspnea. Tube thoracostomy was mainly adopted at the beginning of our experience, and in patients with a severe degree of pleural involvement (55 to 70% of the pleural space), whereas aspiration has been used more recently and in patients with varying degrees of pleural space involvement, ranging from 40 to 60%. All the patients of this clinical series had a full recovery and could receive their programmed chemotherapy with a delay of 1-4 days (mean: 1.5) on the scheduled timing; no surgery was needed and no fatality occurred.

11.2 Clinical Features and Diagnosis

Clinical presentation of iatrogenic pneumothorax complicating central venous access placement in patients without a severe underlying pulmonary disease is largely dependent on the size of the pleural space involved. Individuals with a small pneumothorax (one involving less than 30 percent of the hemithorax) are usually asymptomatic and may have a normal physical examination. Tachycardia is usually the most common physical finding in this setting. In patients with a larger pneumothorax, deep chest pain, dyspnea and coughing are often present and findings on examination may include decreased movement of the chest wall, a hyperresonant percussion note, diminished fremitus, and decreased or absent breath sounds on the affected side. Moreover, a large pneumothorax results in a decrease in vital capacity, low ventilation-perfusion ratio and increased shunting, causing varying degrees of hypoxemia. When the lung function is normal (this usually occurs in spontaneous pneumothoraxes and iatrogenic ones without underlying pulmonary disease), hypercapnia does not develop. In contrast, in patients with underlying lung disease dyspnea is always present and usually severe, even in those with a small pneumothorax [7]. The physical findings are often subtle and may be masked by the underlying lung disease, particularly in patients with chronic obstructive pulmonary condition.

Tachycardia of more than 135 beats per minute, hypotension, respiratory distress or cyanosis should raise the suspicion of a tension pneumothorax. This is a life-threatening condition produced by a one-way valve mechanism and causes a progressive accumulation of air within a hemithorax, eventually compressing the vena cava and shifting the mediastinum. Immediate decompression of the pleural space is mandatory in this condition, using a large-bore needle inserted percutaneously into the second interspace at the mid-clavicular line, as studies using animal models suggest that over hypotension there is a delayed finding that immediately precedes cardiorespiratory collapse [8]. Thoracostomy tube placement can be undertaken at a nonemergent pace, so long as the patient responds to the first measure.

The diagnosis of iatrogenic pneumothorax always has to be confirmed by the identification of a thin, visceral pleural line, which is found to be displaced from the chest wall on a posterior-anterior chest radiogram, performed with the patient in an upright position. A confirmatory radiogram must be routinely obtained after implant, usually soon after the procedure or a few hours later, depending on the available facilities and on-site protocols. As there have been anecdotal reports of delayed, severe pneumothorax not visible on earlier roentgenograms, occurring hours and even days after the procedure [9, 10], particularly in oncology patients, a delayed radiogram (at least 2 hours after implant) should be preferred and a new, urgent chest X-ray should be obtained in all patients having a central venous port and developing acute respiratory symptoms. A radiogram obtained during expiration may help in identifying a small apical pneumothorax; however, the routine use of this type of radiography does not improve the diagnostic yield [11]. Radiographic evidence of a giant bulla may appear to be a pneumothorax; bullous lesions that abut the chest wall usually have a concave appearance. In patients in whom the diagnosis is not clear, computed tomography of the chest should be performed to differentiate between these two conditions [12].

11.3 Treatment

As the information in the literature regarding the treatment of iatrogenic pneumothorax complicating central venous access placement is limited, most considerations and remarks have been obtained from the literature data on the management of spontaneous pneumothorax and iatrogenic pneumothorax following percutaneous pulmonary biopsies. The treatment of iatrogenic pneumothorax centers on evacuating air from the pleural space and re-expanding the lung. Available therapeutic options include simple observation, aspiration with a catheter either with or without immediate removal of the catheter after pleural air is evacuated, and insertion of a chest tube or tube-thoracostomy. Thoracoscopy through a single insertion port into the chest, pleurodesis, video-assisted thoracoscopic surgery and thoracotomy are possible treatment modalities in spontaneous primary and secondary pneumothoraxes, but are fortunately extremely rare in the clinical setting of iatrogenic pneumothorax complicating central venous access. The selection of an approach depends on the size of the pneumothorax, the severity of symptoms, and whether there is or not a persistent air leak. Looking at our own data and contributions from the literature, a small asymptomatic pneumothorax (one involving less than 30 percent of the hemithorax) should be first approached by observation alone, with repeat chest X-ray and supplemental oxygen, which is able to accelerate by a factor of four the reabsorption of air by the pleura, which occurs at a rate of 2 percent per day in patients breathing room air [13]. Most physicians hospitalize patients with a small pneumothorax, although the treatment of patients who are likely to comply with treatment plans may be managed at home after six hours of observation and new X-ray, if such patients can obtain emergency services quickly [5].

Pneumothoraxes that are large (involving greater/equal 30 percent of the hemithorax) or progressive may be drained by simple aspiration with a thoracentesis catheter or small-bore (7 to 14 French) catheter or by the insertion of a chest tube. Simple aspiration is successful in 70 percent of patients with moderate-sized primary spontaneous pneumothorax [14], and no data can be obtained from the medical literature regarding the success rate of this treatment in iatrogenic pneumothoraxes complicating central venous catheter placement. In our series all the three cases treated with this approach achieved full recovery after 1–3 days of treatment, even when the amount of affected pleural space was relevant (up to 60%). According to clinical series of uncomplicated spontaneous pneumothorax, it may be anticipated that this method is likely to fail if the patient is more than 50 years old, or if more than 2.5 liters of air is aspirated immediately [15]. Successfully treated patients can be discharged from the hospital with follow-up within several days if a chest radiogram obtained six hours after aspiration shows resolution of the pneumothorax and if such patients can obtain emergency services quickly. If aspiration through a catheter fails to expand the lung, the catheter can be attached to a one-way Heimlich valve or a water-seal device and used as a chest tube [16].

Primary spontaneous and iatrogenic pneumothorax may also be managed with a chest tube that is left in place for one or more days. This is much more frequently necessary in patients with severe emphysema, obstructive lung disease, or hyperinflation. Severe hypoxemia or hypotension can occur in patients with chronic obstructing pulmonary condition and be life-threatening [17, 18]; often hypercapnia also occurs, with the partial pressure of arterial carbon dioxide exceeding 50 mmHg. These features should advise implanting physicians to carefully evaluate and rule out a significant underlying pulmonary disease before scheduling a central venous implant procedure, possibly choosing an alternative approach (e.g. venous cutdown, ultrasound-guided procedure or peripherally-inserted central venous catheters). A radiology series, investigating the risk of pneumothorax and chest tube placement in 307 patients undergoing CT-guided transthoracic lung biopsy for pulmonary lesions, found about 20% of pneumothoraxes (61/307), but only 10% of them (6/61) requiring chest tube placement [19]. In a similar setting also dealing with the transthoracic needle aspiration biopsy of the lung Cox et al. [20] reported 40% of pneumothorax and 17% of chest tube placement. Once again, the presence of emphysema was significantly correlated with an increased rate of pneumothorax (p=0.01) and an increased demand of tube thoracostomy. Because air leakage is usually minimal, a small-bore (7 to 14 French) chest catheter usually suffices [21]. The catheter can be attached to a one-way Heimlich valve, which allows ambulation or to a water-seal device. Routine application of suction

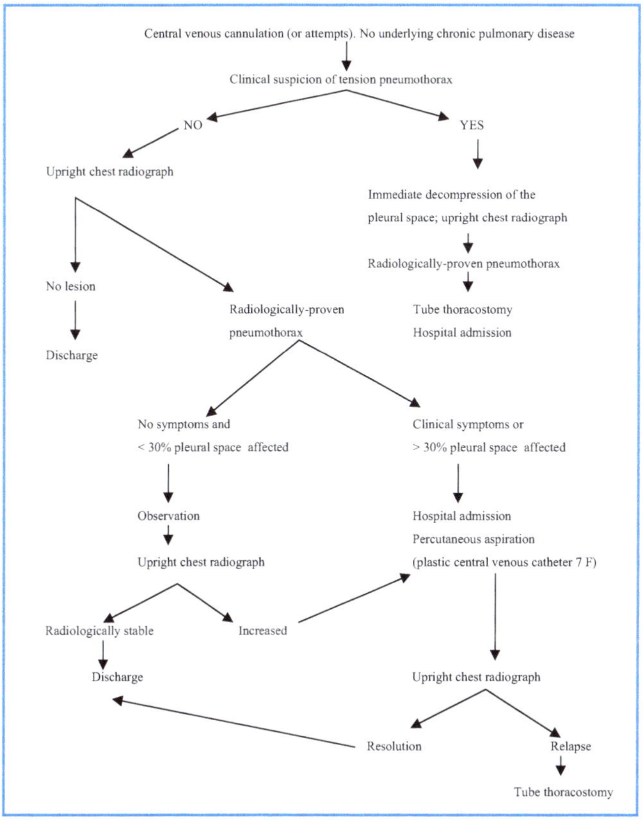

Fig. 11.1 Iatrogenic pneumothorax complicating central venous ports placement. Treatment flow-chart

(with a pressure of 20 cmH_2O) has not been shown to improve the outcome [22]. Complications of chest-tube drainage include pain [23], pleural infection, incorrect placement of the tube, hemorrhage, and hypotension and pulmonary edema due to lung re-expansion.

No persistent air leaks were observed in our clinical series; these are more common with secondary pneumothorax than with primary spontaneous or iatrogenic pneumothoraxes [24]. Seventy-five percent of air leaks in primary spontaneous pneumothorax and 61 percent of air leaks in secondary spontaneous pneumothorax resolve after 7 days of chest drainage, but 100 percent and 79 percent, respectively, resolve after 15 days [5].

In conclusion, patients suffering from pneumothorax following central venous cannulation and without a severe underlying pulmonary disease can be reassured, at the time of diagnosis, that surgery is usually unnecessary and tube thoracostomy is infrequently needed. The simple aspiration of the pleural air by means of a fine plastic catheter inserted percutaneously into the pleural space under local anesthesia should be considered, even if the amount of affected pleural space is more than 50%, before deciding on a formal tube-thoracostomy using small-bore tubes. A flow-chart summarizing the proposed approach is presented in Figure 11.1.

With respect to the prevention of this complication, routine use of real-time US guidance for central venous cannulation is able to minimize or nullify this problem [see Chapter 7].

References

1. Biffi R, De Braud F, Orsi F et al (1998) Totally implantable central venous access ports for long-term chemotherapy. A prospective study analyzing complications and costs of 333 devices with a minimum follow-up of 180 days. Ann Oncol 9:767–773
2. Aldrighetti L, Paganelli M, Arru M et al (2000) Complications of blind placement technique in 980 subcutaneous infusion ports. J Vasc Access 1:28–32
3. Lyon RD, Griggs KA, Johnson AM, Olsen JR (1999) Long-term follow-up of upper extremity implanted venous access devices in oncology patients. J Vasc Interv Radiol 110:463–471
4. Sarajego J, Bootorabi B, Matsumoto T, Kernstein M (1993) Major long-term complications in 1422 permanent venous access devices. Am J Surg 165:249–251
5. Sahn SA, Heffner JE (2000) Primary care: spontaneous pneumothorax. N Engl J Med 342:868–874
6. Biffi R, Pozzi S, Cenciarelli S et al (2001) Treatment of pneumothorax as a complication of long-term central venous port placement in oncology patients. An observational study. J Vasc Access 2:129-136
7. Dines DE, Clagett OT, Payne WS (1970) Spontaneous pneumothorax in emphysema. Mayo Clin Proc 45:481–487
8. Barton ED (1999) Tension pneumothorax. Curr Opin Pulm Med 5:269–274
9. Thomas CJ, Butler CS (1999) Delayed pneumothorax and hydrothorax with central venous catheter migration. Anaesthesia 54:987–990
10. Whitman DE (1996) Complications associated with the use of central venous access devices. Curr Probl Surg 4:309–378
11. Bradley M, Williams C, Walshaw MJ (1991) The value of routine expiratory chest films in the diagnosis of pneumothorax. Arch Emerg Med 8:115–116
12. Bourguin P, Couisineau G, Lemire P, Hebert G (1985) Computed tomography used to exclude pneumothorax in bullous lung disease. J Can Assoc Radiol 36:341–342
13. Northfield TC (1971) Oxygen therapy for spontaneous pneumothorax. BMJ 4:86–88
14. Soulsby T (1998) British Thoracic Society guidelines for the management of spontaneous pneumothorax: do we comply with them and do they work– J Accid Emerg Med 15:317–321
15. Martin T, Fontana G, Olak J, Ferguson M (1996) Use of pleural catheter for the management of simple pneumothorax. Chest 110:1169–1172
16. Minami H, Saka H, Senda K et al (1992) Small caliber catheter drainage for spontaneous pneumothorax. Am J Med Sci 304:345–347
17. Shields TW, Oilschlager GA (1966) Spontaneous pneumothorax in patients 40 years of age and older. Ann Thorac Surg 2:377–383
18. George RB, Herbet SJ, Shames JM et al (1975) Pneumothorax complicating pulmonary emphysema. JAMA 234:389-393
19. Laurent F, Michel P, Latrabe V et al (1999) Pneumothoraxes and chest tube placement after CT-guided transthoracic lung biopsy using a coaxial technique: incidence and risk factors. AJR 172:1049-1053
20. Cox JE, Chiles C, McManus CM (1999) Transthoracic needle aspiration biopsy: variables that affect risk of pneumothorax. Radiology 212:165–168
21. Ponn RB, Silverman HJ, Federico JA (1997) Outpatient chest tube management. Ann Thorac Surg 64:1437-1440
22. So SY, Yu DY (1982) Catheter drainage of spontaneous pneumothorax: suction or no suction, early or late removal. Thorax 37:46–48

23. Owen S, Gould D (1997) Underwater seal chest drains: the patient's experience. J Clin Nurs 6:215–225
24. Chee CB, Abisheganaden J, Yeo JK et al (1998) Persistent air-leak in spontaneous pneumothorax – clinical course and outcome. Respir Med 92:757–761

Hemothorax 12

Hasan Karanlik and Sidika Kurul

Abstract

The use of a totally implantable central venous access port provides long-term central venous access and thus simplifies the administration of chemotherapy, parenteral nutrition, and the repeated collection of blood samples. In contrast to the percutaneous central venous catheterization, dilators and peel-away sheaths are used to insert the catheter. In most cases, catheterization is done in the subclavian vein, but it can be done in the internal jugular vein, the external jugular vein, and the common femoral vein. Before the advent of real-time ultrasound guidance, cannulation used to be performed using anatomic landmarks alone. The aim of this section is to review hemothorax complication with regard to etiology, clinical presentation, and prevention during implantation of totally implantable venous access devices.

Keywords

Totally implantable venous access port • Complication • Hemothorax • Subclavian vein • Vascular injury • Thrombocytopenia • Catheter tip • Ultrasound guidance

12.1 Introduction

The use of a totally implantable central venous access port provides long-term central venous access and thus simplifies the administration of chemotherapy,

H. Karanlik (✉)
Department of Surgery, Institute of Oncology, Istanbul University,
Istanbul,Turkey
e-mail: hasankaranlik@yahoo.com

I. Di Carlo, R. Biffi (eds.), *Totally Implantable Venous Access Devices*,

parenteral nutrition, and the repeated collection of blood samples. In contrast to percutaneous central venous catheterization, dilators and peel-away sheaths are used to insert the catheter. In most cases, catheterization is done in the subclavian vein, but it can be done in the internal jugular vein, the external jugular vein, and the common femoral vein. Before the advent of real-time ultrasound guidance, cannulation used to be performed using anatomic landmarks alone. The aim of this section is to review hemothorax complication with regard to etiology, clinical presentation, and prevention during implantation of totally implantable venous access devices.

12.2 Etiology and Clinical Presentation

Vascular injury during an insertion of a subclavian catheter can be the result of three mechanisms that differ in both pathophysiology and clinical presentation. The most common vascular injury is inadvertent puncture or cannulation of the subclavian artery by a small- or large-bore needle. The incidence of such injuries ranges from 1 to 11% with a quoted average of 5% for small needle injuries, and 0.1 to 0.8% for large-bore needles or cannulas. Small needle injuries are usually self-sealing and require no further treatment [1, 2]. Large-bore needles or catheters have been associated with more serious complications. An expanding mediastinal hematoma can cause airway or venous obstruction; hemothorax can be massive, and arteriovenous fistulae or pseudoaneurysm may carry grave consequences [3–5]. The management of such injuries ranges from observation only to endovascular or surgical repair. Delayed diagnosis of vascular injury is very much different with an estimated incidence of only 0.17% but a mortality rate as high as 74% [6]. The proposed mechanism of injury is erosion of a vessel by the catheter tip, resulting in extravasation of blood or chemotherapeutic agents into the pleural cavity or the mediastinum. This is completely different from a needle injury and is not an immediate acute complication but becomes apparent 2.5–3.6 days after placement of the catheter [7]. This adverse event is preferably managed nowadays by endovascular stenting. Injury to the internal thoracic artery or its branches during catheter insertion is extremely rare [8]. Because the diagnosis can only be made by angiography, it is not clear whether such injuries are underreported, underdiagnosed, or simply extremely rare. The mechanism of such an injury is not entirely clear.

We believe that any patient presenting with hypotension during or immediately following insertion of a central catheter for totally implantable venous access devices should be suspected of having a massive hemothorax due to vascular injury. The diagnosis can be confirmed by a tube thoracostomy, which, if draining a considerable amount of blood, should lead to immediate angiographic visualization and embolization.

12.3 Frequency and Intervention

In the review of Di Carlo et al., 5 patients were found with hemothorax from a total of 6535 percutaneously inserted totally implantable venous access devices [9]. Published data on the nature and extent of complications are often rather vague. For example, *a number of hemothoraces occurred in subsequent cases performed by residents* [10, 11]. It is often unclear whether patients were at increased risk for complications, because of their medical history or local anatomy, and whether or not such factors were taken into account. In addition, definitions of specific complications may differ substantially. For example, some authors include all pneumothoraces and hemothoraces following catheter insertion as complications, including those that are very small, while others include only complications requiring intervention and treatment. Thus the incidence of hemothorax after port catheter insertion reported in the literature varies from 0-2%. It is therefore difficult to estimate the degree of risk for certain complications.

Venous bleeding, or arterial bleeding due to accidental cannulation of the carotid or subclavian arteries, occurs more frequently in patients with thrombocytopenia [10, 12]. Other coagulation disorders and a prolonged clotting time (i.e. due to the use of anticoagulants or liver disease) appear to be less important in this regard [10, 13 14]. Catheter insertion procedures in patients with platelet counts of 50.000/mm^3 or less should be performed by experienced physicians. The risk of the procedure should be weighed against the reason for catheter insertion. In our own experience, and as reported in studies dealing mainly with cancer patients, the risk of severe bleeding after catheter insertion is low, even in thrombocytopenic patients, provided these precautions are taken [9, 15]. When profuse and/or prolonged bleeding occurs, appropriate procoagulant therapy (administration of platelets, fresh frozen plasma, desmopressin and/or tranexamic acid) should be considered. The same procedures should be applied to patients receiving potent anticoagulant therapy such as streptokinase, urokinase, ticlopidine or clopidogrel [10].

12.4 Prevention

Prior to insertion of the introducing needle (usually 18 gauge), the presence of the vein and the optimal route for insertion can be established with a smaller needle (seeking needle) to assess the location of the vein and surrounding bony structures. This can be done, for example, during infiltration of local anesthetic prior to CVC insertion. In most patients it should be possible to aspirate venous blood with a standard 21 gauge, 0.8 mm (green) injection needle, especially if the insertion site is the subclavian or jugular vein. The sharper longer bevel of this needle causes much less collapse of easily compressible veins. Thus, when the larger introducer needle is subsequently inserted, the location of the vein and the distance over which the needle needs to be advanced are known; this can reduce the trauma caused by the insertion of the introducer needle. In addition, accidental puncture of an artery will have less serious consequences if this occurs with a smaller needle [9, 10].

The complication risk increases with each insertion attempt made. In general, it appears reasonable to limit the number of attempts made by inexperienced doctors to no more than two [16]. The catheter should not be advanced too far because of the increased risk of mechanical complications (including damage to the heart valves) and because of the severe consequences of catheter colonization and infection if the catheter tip is positioned inside the heart (endocarditis, intra-cardiac abscess). No force should be applied either during cannulation of the vein or during insertion and advancement of the guidewire and catheter.

The optimal position of the catheter tip for catheters inserted in the jugular or subclavian vein remains a matter of debate [17]. Various case reports describe the occurrence of cardiac tamponade due to atrial or ventricular perforation by a catheter tip located inside the pericardial sac. Based on such observations, most catheter packages contain strict warnings stating that the catheter tip must lie outside the pericardial sac. However, there are some problems with this advice. Firstly, the pericardium may ascend along the medial wall of the superior vena cava by up to 5 cm (mean 3 cm), so that placement of the catheter tip just proximal to the atrium does not obviate the risk of tamponade [18]. Moreover, the overall risk for this complication appears to be quite low and placing the tip in positions above the right atrium may be associated with a higher risk for other, more frequently occurring, complications such as perforation of a central vein and thrombosis [17–19].

The risk of perforation appears to be directly related to the angle of the catheter to the vessel wall: the more perpendicular the catheter, the higher the risk of perforation [17–19]. Thus, if the catheter tip is perpendicular to the vessel wall, the catheter should be moved to a different position, even if this means that it is sited in the upper right atrium. Prevailing evidence suggests that the catheter tip may be safely sited in the upper right atrium provided it does not pass through the tricuspid valve or into the coronary sinus, and provided its position is parallel to the atrial wall. The routine use of 30 cm length catheters that are fully inserted is likely to result in placement deep inside the heart. The average insertion depth for placement in the upper superior vena cava is approximately 16 cm. This distance is somewhat shorter on the right side than on the left side. Thus, when inserting a catheter via the subclavian or jugular veins, 20 cm (left side) or 16 cm (right side) length catheters should be used in the majority of adult patients [10, 19, 20].

Ideally, the tip should be located just outside the heart and parallel with the long axis of the vein in which it is located. The carina can be used as a radiologic landmark, located approximately halfway along the superior vena cava and marking the beginning of the pericardial sac [18]. Another tool which may be useful in catheter positioning in the superior vena cava is the use of ECG-guided central venous catheters; in this instance, the catheter tip is advanced until an intra-atrial P-wave is observed, after which the catheter is withdrawn 3 cm back into the superior vena cava [10, 20]. Although this may be of value, especially in correctly positioning the catheter tip, it remains unclear whether mechanical complications of catheter placement can be prevented through its use. It is important to realize that there are complications associated with all tip positions, and to suspect catheter-related problems in cases of clinical deterioration.

In patients with severe coagulopathy (especially thrombocytopenia), administration of platelets or clotting factors may be considered prior to catheter insertion. It is difficult to give firm recommendations regarding the threshold to correct coagulopathy, as the risk of bleeding may be influenced by many of the factors discussed above and by the choice of insertion site. As a general rule, administration of platelets should be considered in elective procedures if the platelet count is below 50, particularly if other risk factors are present. Platelet administration should also be considered in situations where platelet function is impaired (uremia, use of aspirin, surgery with extracorporeal circulation, etc.). Fresh frozen plasma or clotting factors may be given if clotting levels are below 20% of normal values. The catheter should be inserted immediately after the blood products are administered.

The use of ultrasound for guidance of catheter insertion has been associated with reductions in complications, mean insertion attempts, and placement failure rates [21–23]. This includes arterial injury, specifically in patients with poor anatomic landmarks or coagulopathies. The point of the ultrasound device may be attached to the tip of the insertion needle (smart needle); however, results and experiences with this *smart needle* vary, depending on personal preferences and skills. Conventional Doppler ultrasonography can also be used. Ultrasound guidance may be helpful during difficult insertion procedures in high-risk patients, although the results of a randomized trial show only modest benefits [24]. The risk of accidental arterial puncture appears to decrease slightly through use of the Doppler-assisted technique. Gualtieri et al. reported that the success rate of central catheter placement by less experienced operators was improved by ultrasound guidance, but that this is much less obvious with experienced physicians [23]. More studies are needed to establish the role of sonography for subclavian vein catheter insertion, and perhaps future technology improvement will allow its routine use.

In many hospitals it is routine to order a chest radiograph after central catheter insertion to verify the catheter position and to check for complications. It is questionable whether this is really necessary. The risk of malposition after a procedure with no technical problems and no clinical signs of complications appears to be very small, especially if a catheter with small diameter lumen was used [10]. Thus, the value of post-procedural radiographs after catheter insertion appears to be limited.

In summary, the likelihood of hemothorax complication is determined to a large extent by patient factors (morbidity, underlying disease and local anatomy) and by the experience of the physician carrying out the insertion procedure. The insertion site should be chosen with care, taking into account factors such as the expected indwelling time, complication risks associated with different sites, the patient's local anatomy, underlying disease and co-morbidity, and the physician's personal experience and preferences. Insertion at a site where a catheter was previously placed should be avoided if possible, and a different insertion site chosen.

References

1. Mazeh H, Alaiyan B, Vald O et al (2010) Internal mammary artery injury during central venous catheter insertion for TPN: rare but fatal. Nutrition 26:849–851
2. Golden LR (1995) Incidence and management of large-bore introducer sheath puncture of the carotid artery, J Cardiothorac Vasc Anesth 9:425–428
3. Shah PM, Babu SC, Goyal A et al (2004) Arterial misplacement of large-caliber cannulas during jugular vein catheterization: case for surgical management, J Am Coll Surg 198:939–944
4. Eckhardt WF, Iaconetti J, Kwon JS et al (1996) Inadvertent carotid artery cannulation during pulmonary artery catheter insertion. J Cardiothorac Vasc Anesth 10:283–290
5. Nicholson T, Ettles D, Robinson G (2004) Managing inadvertent arterial catheterization during central venous access procedures. Cardiovasc Intervent Radiol 27:21–25
6. Walshe C, Phelan D, Bourke J, Buggy D (2007) Vascular erosion by central venous catheters used for total parenteral nutrition. Intensive Care Med 33:534–537
7. Inaba K, Sakurai Y, Furuta S et al (2009) Delayed vascular injury and severe respiratory distress as a rare complication of a central venous catheter and total parenteral nutrition. Nutrition 25:479–481
8. Eulmesekian PG, Pérez A, Minces PG et al (2007) Internal mammary artery injury after central venous catheterization, Pediatr Crit Care Med 8:489–491
9. Di Carlo I, Pulvirenti E, Mannino M, Toro A (2010) Increased use of percutaneous technique for totally implantable venous access devices. Is it real progress– A 27-year comprehensive review on early complications. Ann Surg Oncol 17:1649–1656
10. Polderman KH, Girbes AJ (2002) Central venous catheter use. Part 1: mechanical complications. Intensive Care Med 28:1–17
11. Matthews NT, Worthley LI (1982) Immediate problems associated with infraclavicular subclavian catheterization; a comparison between left and right sides. Anaesth Intensive Care 10:113–115
12. Doerfler ME, Kaufman B, Goldenberg AS (1996) Central venous catheter placement in patients with disorders of hemostasis. Chest 110:185–188
13. Lokich JJ, Bothe A Jr, Benotti P, Moore C (1985) Complications and management of implanted venous access catheters. J Clin Oncol 3:710–717
14. Fischer NC, Mutimer DJ (1999) Central venous cannulation in patients with liver disease and coagulopathy - a prospective audit. Intensive Care Med 25:481–485
15. Barrera R, Mina B, Huang Y, Groeger JS (1996) Acute complications of central line placement in profoundly thrombocytopenic cancer patients. Cancer 78:2025–2030
16. Karanlik H, Kurul S (2009) Modification of approach for totally implantable venous access device decreases rate of complications. J Surg Oncol 100:279–283
17. Fletcher SJ, Bodenham AR (2000) Safe placement of central venous catheters: where should the tip of the catheter lie? Br J Anaesth 85:188–191
18. Schuster M, Nave H, Piepenbrok S et al (2000) The carina as a landmark in central venous catheter placement. Br J Anaesth 85:191–193
19. Dailey RH (1998) Late vascular perforations by CVP catheters. J Emerg Med 146:487–490
20. Kurul S, Saip P, Aydin T (2002) Totally implantable venous-access ports: local problems and extravasation injury. Lancet Oncol 3:684–692

21. Peris A, Zagli G, Bonizzoli M et al (2010) Implantation of 3951 long-term central venous catheters: performances, risk analysis, and patient comfort after ultrasound-guidance introduction. Anesth Analg 111:1194–1201
22. Orsi F, Grasso RF, Arnaldi P et al (2000) Ultrasound guided versus direct vein puncture in central venous port placement. J Vasc Access 1:73–77
23. Gualtieri E, Deppe SA, Sipperly ME, Thompson DR (1995) Subclavian venous catheterization: greater success rate for less experienced operators using ultrasound guidance. Crit Care Med 23:692–697
24. Bold RJ, Winchester DJ, Madary AR et al (1998) Prospective, randomised trial of Doppler-assisted subclavian vein catheterization. Arch Surg 133:1089–1093

Air Embolism

13

Hasan Karanlik and Sidika Kurul

Abstract

Air embolism is a rare but potentially fatal complication of procedures involving totally implantable venous access devices. Air can enter the central venous system during puncture or through an opening in the intravenous infusion tubing during disconnection. This section provides a review of the pathopysiology and clinical presentation of this acute phenomenon, as well as an in-depth analysis and algorithms for favorable methods of detection, prevention, and treatment.

Keywords

Totally implantable venous access port • Complication • Venous air embolism (VAE) • Trendelenburg position • Hypoxemia • Pulmonary symptoms, central nervous system • HBO therapy

13.1 Introduction

Air embolism is a rare but potentially fatal complication of procedures involving totally implantable venous access devices. Air can enter the central venous system during puncture or through an opening in the intravenous infusion tubing during disconnection. This section provides a review of the pathophysiology and clinical presentation of this acute phenomenon, as well as an in-depth analysis and algorithms for favorable methods of detection, prevention, and treatment.

H. Karanlik (✉)
Department of Surgery, Institute of Oncology, Istanbul University, Istanbul,Turkey
e-mail: hasankaranlik@yahoo.com

I. Di Carlo, R. Biffi (eds.), *Totally Implantable Venous Access Devices*,

13.2 Pathophysiology

Intraoperative venous air embolism (VAE) can be a lethal event. The factors that determine the morbidity and mortality of any episode of VAE include the rate of air entrainment, the volume of air entrained, and the position of the patient at the time VAE occurred [1–3]. Experimental studies have been conducted using several animal models to assess the volume of VAE necessary to provoke circulatory collapse. In dogs, the lethal volume of air (LD_{100}) when injected rapidly is 7.5 mL/kg. In a smaller animal such as the rabbit, the LD_{50} is as low as 0.55 mL/kg. When the rate of entrainment is slow, a dog can tolerate as much as 1,400 mL of air over several hours. In humans, the volume of gas tolerated is unknown, but accidental injections of air of between 100 mL and 300 mL have been reported to be fatal [3–6]. The volume becomes clinically relevant when one considers that Flanagan et al. [7] calculated that 100 mL of air per second could flow through a 14-gauge needle with only a 5 cm pressure gradient.

The major cause of death from massive air embolism is due to circulatory obstruction and ultimately arrest resulting from air trapped in the right ventricular outflow tract [2]. Large emboli may cause paradoxical (arterial) embolization by acutely increasing right atrial pressure, facilitating a right to left shunting through a patent foramen ovale or across the pulmonary capillary bed. Micro air emboli can lodge in pulmonary vessels and either produce gradual obstruction to blood flow or undergo spontaneous resorption depending on the rate and volume of air entrained. In addition, the air-blood interaction may induce the production of fibrin clots or thrombosis and further obstruct right ventricular outflow of pulmonary blood flow. The severity of hypoxemia associated with VAE is variable and depends on the significance of the episode. The mechanism of this hypoxemia is the result of ventilation-perfusion (V/Q) maldistribution [6–10].

In many clinical settings venous air entrainment is insidious and the clinical signs nonspecific. In the absence of a high level of suspicion, VAE may be difficult to diagnose in this subacute setting.

13.3 Clinical Presentation

Vascular air embolism may have cardiovascular, pulmonary, and neurologic sequelae. The spectrum of effects is dependent on the rate and entrained volume of VAE, as well as two other additional factors: whether the patient is spontaneously breathing, yielding negative thoracic pressure during respiratory cycle with facilitation of air entrainment, or under controlled positive-pressure ventilation [11].

Cardiovascularly, tachyarrhythmias are common, and the electrocardiogram demonstrates a right heart strain pattern as well as ST–T changes. Myocardial ischemia may be observed, and in animal studies, peaking of the P wave is seen in the earlier stages. Blood pressure decreases as cardiac output falters. Pulmonary artery pressures increase as a consequence of increased filling pressures and reduction of cardiac output. The central venous pressure measurements also increase as a secondary effect of right heart failure, and jugular venous distension may be noted. As hypotension increases, shock ensues [3, 12].

Pulmonary symptoms in awake patients include acute dyspnea, continuous coughing, urgent complaints of breathlessness, lightheadedness, chest pain, and a sense of *impending doom* [12]. The common response of gasping for air as a consequence of dyspnea forces a further reduction in intrathoracic pressure, frequently resulting in more air entrainment. Pulmonary signs of VAE include rales, wheezing, and tachypnea. During anesthesia with respiratory monitoring, decreases in end-tidal carbon dioxide ($ETco_2$), and both arterial oxygen saturation (Sao_2) and tension (Po_2), along with hypercapnia, may be detected. Invasive cardiac monitoring commonly increases pulmonary airway pressure.

The central nervous system may be affected by VAE by one of two mechanisms. Firstly, cardiovascular collapse secondary to reduced cardiac output (from output obstruction, right ventricular failure, or myocardial ischemia) rapidly results in cerebral hypoperfusion. In mild form, acute altered mental status presents, but focal deficits related to cerebral hyperemia and cerebral edema leading to frank coma quickly follow. Secondly, direct cerebral air embolism may occur via a patent foramen ovale, a residual defect that is present in approximately 20% of the adult population. Mental status changes postoperatively should raise the suspicion of cerebral ischemia secondary to air embolism in at-risk individuals [1, 3, 13].

13.4 Prevention

It is common to use the Trendelenburg position during the insertion of central venous catheters in the jugular or subclavian veins. Nevertheless, even when using optimal positioning and techniques, air embolism has been reported in the interventional radiology literature at an incidence of 0.13% (15 episodes in 11,583 insertions). The criteria for confirmed VAE were such that only substantial volumes would have met the threshold: the hearing of audible suction or visualization of right ventricular air on fluoroscopy. One of the 15 patients died as a result of the embolism. In the authors' case series, the complication was commonly noted during insertion of a tunneled catheter through a peel-away sheath [1, 3]. This technique is frequently used in the operating room for insertion of hemodialysis access or the placement of portacaths. In such a scenario, it is common practice to stop ventilation during insertion of the finder needle to decrease the risk of a pneumothorax, especially with the subclavian site. Holding ventilation also reduces the negative intrathoracic pressure during the expiratory phase that may induce a suction effect, promoting VAE.

Similarly, increasing right atrial pressure during the tunneling phase of catheter insertion may also minimize the risk of air entrainment.

Regarding placement and removal of the popular temporary, nontunneled catheters, it is important for providers to understand that the conditions that can increase the risk of air embolism include fracture or detachment of catheter connections, failure to occlude the needle hub or catheter during insertion or removal, dysfunction of self-sealing valves in plastic introducer sheaths, presence of a persistent catheter tract following removal, deep inspiration during insertion or removal (increases the magnitude of negative pressure within the thorax), hypovolemia (reduces central venous pressure), and upright positioning of the patient (reduces central venous pressure). Removal of the catheter should be synchronized with active exhalation if the patient is cooperative. If the patient is on mechanical ventilation, one can apply positive end-expiratory pressure. The Valsalva maneuver has proven to be superior to breath holding for increasing central venous pressure and may be beneficial to reduce the incidence of air entrainment in awake and cooperative patients [14, 15].

Based on case report data, hospital safety-driven approaches toward development of protocols of central line care have been developed. The protocols emphasize incorporation of the Trendelenburg position during placement and removal of a central venous catheter. There are clinical situations where it may not be possible to have the patient in a Trendelenburg position for the duration of the procedure, as in the presence of increased intracranial pressure. In such circumstances, one may recommend transient Trendelenburg position during insertion of the guide wire or the catheter after the vein has been identified by the finder needle, and/or raising the legs by keeping pillows under the knees to increase the venous return and pressure in the right atrium. Debate exists as to whether the Trendelenburg position is necessary during catheter removal [3, 16, 17]. Careful attention toward occlusion of the entry site may be most important.

13.5 Management

The optimal management of VAE is prevention. Even after significant VAE, the greatest risk to the patient is continued entrainment of air. Attempts at aspiration of air from the right atrium seem prudent if a catheter is in place, and it is probably the only management strategy with demonstrated clinical efficacy. For catastrophic VAE with cardiovascular collapse, use of ionotropic support and, if necessary, cardiopulmonary resuscitation are standard measures that also may have a beneficial action in clearing residual air embolism. There is little evidence to support special patient positioning as a means of enhancing air dispersion. If paradoxical cerebral air embolism occurs in a patient with stable hemodynamic and respiratory status, the consideration of HBO therapy is appropriate [1, 3, 13].

13.6 Conclusions

Clinicians must be aware of this silent but dangerous entity that can occur during implantation of totally implantable venous access devices. Unfortunately, there remains a paucity of prospective, controlled trials to assess various preventative and treatment options.

Vascular air embolism may be detected by $ETco_2$ monitoring, and precordial Doppler ultrasound should be used in moderate- to high-risk patients undergoing high-risk procedures. Emphasis is given to the prevention (hydration, positioning) and prompt recognition of this event and to the use of all available tools (fluids, positive ionotropic agents) in the management of cardiovascular complications.

The use of invasive monitoring devices such as transesophageal echo and central venous catheters should be dictated by the presence of comorbidities, rather than as a primary tool to manage VAE. The use of hyperbaric oxygen is indicated depending on the severity and duration of the embolic sequelae, the presence of arterial embolism, and the availability of such a technique. Use of perfluorocarbons is an exciting new concept but has yet to be validated in humans.

References

1. Palmon SC, Moore LE, Lundberg J, Toung T (1997) Venous air embolism: a review. J Clin Anesth 9:251–257
2. Aldridge J (2005) Potential air embolus from a Level 1 Rapid Infuser. Anaesthesia 6012:1250–1251
3. Mirski MA, Lele AV, Fitzsimmons L, Toung TJ (2007) Diagnosis and treatment of vascular air embolism. Anesthesiology 106:164–177
4. Oppenheimer MJ, Durant TM, Lynch P (1953) Body position related to venous air embolism and associated cardiovascular-respiratory changes. Am J Med Sci 225:362
5. Heckmann JG, Lang CJ, Kindler K et al (2000) Neurologic manifestations of cerebral air embolism as a complication of central venous catheterization. Crit Care Med 28:1621–1625
6. Alper F, Kantarci M, Onbas O et al (2004) Three-dimensional spiral CT reconstruction in a patient with massive cerebral air embolism. Emerg Radiol 11:87–88
7. Flanagan JP, Gradisar IA, Gross RJ, Kelly TR (1969) Air embolus–a lethal complication of subclavian venipuncture. N Engl J Med 281:488–489
8. Vesely TM (2001) Air embolism during insertion of central venous catheters. J Vasc Interv Radiol 12:1291–1295
9. Peter DA, Saxman C (2003) Preventing air embolism when removing CVCs: An evidence-based approach to changing practice. Medsurg Nursing 12:223–228
10. Brouns R, De Surgeloose D, Neetens I, De Deyn PP (2006) Fatal venous cerebral air embolism secondary to a disconnected central venous catheter. Cerebrovasc Dis 21:212–214
11. Kolbeck KJ, Itkin M, Stravropoulos SW, Trerotola SO (2005) Measurement of air emboli during central venous access: Do "protective" sheaths or insertion techniques matter? J Vasc Interv Radiol 16:89–99
12. Souders JE (2000) Pulmonary air embolism. J Clin Monit Comput 16:375–383
13. Droghetti L, Giganti M, Memmo A, Zatelli R (2002) Air embolism: Diagnosis with single-photon emission tomography and successful hyperbaric oxygen therapy. Br J Anaesth 89:775–778

14. Andrews CM (2002) Preventing air embolism. Am J Nurs 102:34–36
15. Sing RF, Thomason MH, Heniford BT et al (2000) Venous air embolism from central venous catheterization: Under-recognized or over-diagnosed? Crit Care Med 28:3377–3378
16. Brederlau J, Greim C, Schwemmer U et al (2004) Ultrasound-guided cannulation of the internal jugular vein in critically ill patients positioned in 30 degrees dorsal elevation. Eur J Anaesthesiol 21:684–687
17. Wysoki MG, Covey A, Pollak J et al (2001) Evaluation of various maneuvers for prevention of air embolism during central venous catheter placement. J Vasc Interv Radiol 12:764–766

Accidental Arterial Puncture

14

Zhang Qinming

Abstract

Accidental arterial puncture is a rare complication that may occur during central venous catheter insertion. Arterial injury may be a potentially lethal problem of serious bleeding or large hematoma. The author described the incidence, predilection site, clinical presentation, prevention and management guideline based on the patient's clinical data. Central venous cannulation under the guidance may be an effective preventive technique for accidental arterial injury.

Keywords

Accidental arterial puncture • Carotid artery • Subclavian artery • Hematoma • Pseudo-aneurysm • Arterio-venous fistula • Ultrasound • Angiogram • Central venous cannulation

14.1 Introduction

Accidental arterial puncture during central venous catheter insertion is a potentially lethal problem. It is the most frequently described complication of internal jugular cannulation and the second most common complication of subclavian cannulation [1, 2]. Numerous studies have reported that the incidence of accidental arterial puncture or cannulation ranges from 0% to 15% [1–5].

The most commonly injured arteries during central venous access procedures are the carotid and subclavian arteries. Although carotid artery puncture

Z. Qinming (✉)
Pediatric Surgery, Beijing Children's Hospital affiliated to Capital University of Medicine, Beijing, China
e-mail: qzhang9611@yahoo.com

I. Di Carlo, R. Biffi (eds.), *Totally Implantable Venous Access Devices*,

is usually not dangerous, it can still result in life-threatening complications that may lead to death. Hematoma is reported as the most common complication of accidental arterial puncture. Hematoma may enlarge rapidly if the patient suffers from a coagulation disorder, or if a large puncture wound is produced by the introduction of the sheath itself into a major artery. A large hematoma around the artery and airway may cause compressing syndrome that may threaten life. Airway obstruction, pseudoaneurysm, arteriovenous fistula formation and retrograde aortic dissection have all been reported as a consequence of carotid puncture [6–9].

14.2 Management of Accidental Arterial Puncture

The management of accidental arterial puncture varies according to the arteries punctured. Accidental puncture of the carotid artery is usually managed easily by removing the needle and compressing the puncture site for a few minutes until bleeding has stopped. If accidental arterial cannulation has occurred, achieving hemostasis will be more difficult and a local hematoma may form because cannulation produces more severe bleeding than puncture.

In cases of accidental puncture of the subclavian artery, hematoma may form and spread quickly as the bleeding is hard to compress from the skin puncture site. Ultrasound (US) and computed tomography angiography are usually used to detect the size and location of the hematoma. Large persistent bleeding may need surgical intervention to suture the injured artery. Thrombotic obstruction of the subclavian artery following accidental arterial puncture has also been reported [10].

Central venous cannulation under US guidance has been recommended in recent years in order to avoid accidental arterial puncture. Many studies have concluded that US-guided venous catheterization is more effective than the landmark technique. However, the use of US for central venous catheterization in children has not obtained the same results [11]. The small caliber of veins in children is believed to be responsible for the failure of the US-guided procedure, although it may reduce accidental arterial injury. Due to the above results and the need for at least 3-6 months training in vascular ultrasound, the landmark technique is currently still a predominant procedure for central venous catheterization in children.

References

1. Mitchell SE, Clark RA (1979) Complications of central venous catheterization. Am J Roentgenol 133:467-476
2. Jobes DR, Schwartz AJ, Greenhow DE et al (1983) Safer jugular vein cannulation: Recognition of arterial puncture and preferential use of the external jugular route. Anesthesiology 59:353-355

3. Rosen M, Latto IP (1981) Handbook of percutaneous central venous catheterization. WB Saunders, Philadelphia, pp 76-113
4. Borja AR (1972) Current status of infraclavicular subclavian vein catheterization. Ann Thorac Surg 13:615-624
5. Anagnou J (1982) Cerebrovascular accident during percutaneous cannulation of internal jugular vein. Lancet ii:377-378
6. Knoblanche GE (1979) Respiratory obstruction due to haematoma following internal jugular vein cannulation. Anaesth Intensive Care 7:286
7. Shield CF, Richardson JD, Buckley CJ et al (1975) Pseudoaneurysm of the brachiocephalic arteries: A complication of percutaneous internal jugular vein catheterization. Surgery 78:190-193
8. Gobeil F, Couture P, Girard D, Plante R (1994) Carotid artery-internal jugular fistula: another complication following pulmonary artery catheterization via the internal jugular venous route. Anaesthesiology 80:230-232
9. Applebaum RM, Adelman MA, Kanschuger MS et al (1997) Transesophageal echocardiographic identification of a retrograde dissection of the ascending aorta caused by inadvertent cannulation of the common carotid artery. J Am Soc Echocardiogr 10:749-751
10. Min Gue Jung, Soon Im Kim, Sang-won Seo et al (2008) Thrombotic obstruction of the subclavian artery associated with inadvertent arterial puncture on attempted right internal jugular vein cannulation. Korean J Anesthesiol 55:95-98
11. Grebenik CR, Boyce A, Sinclair ME et al (2004) NICE guidelines for central venous catheterization in children. Is the evidence base sufficient? Br J Anaesth 92:827-830

15 Cardiac Arrhythmia

Adriana Toro and Isidoro Di Carlo

Abstract

Mechanical stimulation from the catheter can result in many types of atrial and ventricular arrhythmias. Possible reasons for delayed arrhythmias include catheter malposition at the time of placement and postplacement migration. If the cause of arrhythmia is the embolized fragment of the catheter, a fatal cardiac complication such as ventricular fibrillation and sudden cardiac death may occur. The correct catheter tip position is mandatory to avoid this complication. Optimal tip position is usually at the junction of the superior vena cava and right atrium.

Keywords

Cardiac arrhythmias • Supraventricular tachycardia • Ventricular arrhythmias • Atrial arrhythmias • Atrial fibrillation • Ventricular tachycardia • Cardiac perforation • Dysrhythmia • Synchronized cardioversion

15.1 Introduction

Mechanical stimulation from the catheter can result in many types of atrial and ventricular arrhythmias. Cardiac arrhythmias can occur during central venous catheter (CVC) insertion but are usually transient and rarely cause hemodynamic problems [1], although life-threatening supraventricular tachy-

I. Di Carlo (✉)
Department of Surgical Sciences, Organ Transplantation and Advanced Technologies,
University of Catania, Cannizzaro Hospital,
Catania, Italy
e-mail: idicarlo@unict.it

I. Di Carlo, R. Biffi (eds.), *Totally Implantable Venous Access Devices*,

cardia has been reported in the pediatric population [2]. In adults, the reported incidence of arrhythmias occurring during CVC insertion ranges from 23% to 25% for ventricular arrhythmias and 6% to 40% for atrial arrhythmias [3, 4]. Brothers et al. [5] reported a 0.9% incidence of serious arrhythmias requiring intervention of cardioversion in a series of 300 patients who underwent surgical insertion of 329 totally implantable venous access devices.

Possible reasons for delayed arrhythmias include catheter malposition at the time of placement and postplacement migration. Atrial fibrillation has also been reported in patients with central venous catheter embolisation [6].

The frequency of dislocation for CVC in the superior cava is around 2.5% [7]. This event may occur because of a variation in intrathoracic pressure, which may take place during cough or vomiting, or a variation in central venous pressure, cardiac congestive failure, and the formation of fibrin sleeve with initial dislocation of the tip [7].

Peripherally inserted central catheters (PICCs) are more likely to be malpositioned compared with other long-term vascular access devices [8]. In a series of 963 PICC insertion procedures, Ng et al. [9] described 4 patients (0.4%) who had delayed onset of palpitations, premature ventricular contractions, or ventricular tachycardia. There has been a case report of a PICC inserted deep within the right atrium becoming wedged in an artificial heart tricuspid valve, resulting in acute cardiac arrest and death [10]. Higher incidences of venous thrombosis with the tip of the PICC positioned in the upper superior vena cava have been documented [11]. The lower position of the tip deep in the right atrium increases the incidence of arrhythmias and cardiac perforation.

15.2 Clinical Manifestations

Symptomatic dysrhythmia induced by overinsertion of the guidewire or malposition of a catheter represents an acute complication of central venous access devices [12]. It is noteworthy that brief dysrhythmia induced by insertion of a catheter or guidewire is usually an indicator of direct irritation to the right endocardium. In the setting of symptomatic arrhythmia, immediate retraction of the guidewire or the catheter should be the first interaction [13]. Lightheadedness, shortness of breath, dizziness, chest discomfort and forceful or painful extra beats are commonly reported with various arrhythmias.

In contrast, if the cause of arrhythmias is the embolized fragment of the catheter, a fatal cardiac complications such as ventricular fibrillation and sudden cardiac death may occur [14, 15].

15.3 Treatment and Prevention

The correct catheter tip position is mandatory to avoid this complication. Optimal tip position is usually at the junction of the superior vena cava and right atrium [16].

Central venous catheter placement from the jugular approach has been reported to move in patient and cadaver studies with flexion and extension of the neck [17]. Also for CVC inserted peripherically it has been demonstrated that the tip of an antecubital central venous catheter can migrate with changes in body position.

There is a positive correlation with the height of the patient and the right subclavian position. Ventricular ectopy is significantly more common in shorter patients and when the catheter is inserted from the right subclavian position. This complication can be prevented by careful confirmation of the catheter tip position, and can be simply managed by re-insertion of the catheter.

Adenosine is a short-term acting drug that blocks AV node contraction; it terminates 90% of tachyarrhythmias [13]. Synchronized cardioversion can also be used immediately in patients who develop hypotension, pulmonary edema, or ischemic chest pain [13]. Other investigators have also suggested that arrhythmias can be prevented by using intravascular ECG monitoring during the advancement of the catheter even for catheters that are too short to reach the atrium [18, 19].

References

1. Polderman KH, Girbes AJ (2002) Central venous catheter use. Part 1: mechanical complications. Intensive Care Med 28:1-17
2. da Silva PS, Waisberg J (2010) Induction of life-threatening supraventricular tachycardia during central venous catheter placement: an unusual complication. J Pediatr Surg 45:E13-16
3. Stuart RK, Shikora SA, Akerman P et al (1990) Incidence of arrhythmia with central venous catheter insertion and exchange. JPEN J Parenter Enteral Nutr 14:152-155
4. Lee TY, Sung CS, Chu YC et al (1996) Incidence and risk factors of guidewire-induced arrhythmia during internal jugular venous catheterization: comparison of marked and plain J-wires. J Clin Anesth 8:348-351
5. Brothers TE, Von Moll LK, Niederhuber JE et al (1988) Experience with subcutaneous infusion ports in three hundred patients. Surg Gynecol Obstet 166:295-301
6. Faraj W, Zaghal A, El-Beyrouthy O, Kutoubi A (2010) Complete catheter disconnection and migration of an implantable venous access device: the disconnected cap sign. Ann Vasc Surg 24:692
7. Paoletti F, Ripani U, Antonelli M, Nicoletta G (2005) Central venous catheters. Observations on the implantation technique and its complications. Minerva Anestesiol 71:555-560
8. Vesely TM (2003) Central venous catheter tip position: a continuing controversy. J Vasc Interv Radiol 14:527-234
9. Ng PK, Ault MJ, Ellrodt AG, Maldonado L (1997) Peripherally inserted central catheters in general medicine. Mayo Clin Proc 72:225-233
10. Smyth SH, Zaetta JM (2000) Fatal complication of percutaneously inserted central catheter: extent of tip movement. J Vasc Interv Radiol 11:295-296
11. Steiger E (2006) Dysfunction and thrombotic complications of vascular access devices. JPEN J Parenter Enteral Nutr 30:S70-72
12. Cobb DK, High KP, Sawyer RG et al (1992) A controlled trial of scheduled replacement of central venous and pulmonary-artery catheters. N Engl J Med 327:1062-1068
13. Yavascan O, Mir S, Tekguc H (2009) Supraventricular tachycardia following insertion of a central venous catheter. Saudi J Kidney Dis Transpl 20:1061-1064

14. Gowda MR, Gowda RM, Khan IA et L (2004) Positional ventricular tachycardia from a fractured mediport catheter with right ventricular migration—a case report. Angiology 55:557-560
15. Suárez-Peñaranda JM, Guitian-Barreiro, Concheiro-Carro L (1995) Longstanding intracardiac catheter embolism. An unusual autopsy finding. Am J Forensic Med Pathol 16:124-126
16. Gupta S, Steiger E, Sands M (2006) Vascular access for the patient receiving parenteral nutrition. In: Buchman AL (ed) Clinical nutrition in gastrointestinal disease, SLACK, Thorofare, NJ, pp 409-419
17. Curelaru I, Linder LE, Gustavsson B (1980) Displacement of catheters inserted through internal jugular veins with neck flexion and extension. A preliminary study. Intensive Care Med 6:179-183
18. Pawlik MT, Kutz N, Keyl C ET AL (2004) Central venous catheter placement: comparison of the intravascular guidewire and the fluid column electrocardiograms. Eur J Anaesthesiol 21:594-599
19. Dionisio P, Valenti M, Cornella C /ET AL (1995) Monitoring of central venous dual-lumen catheter placement in haemodialysis: improvement of a technique for the practising nephrologist. Nephrol Dial Transplant 10:2118-2121

Heart Tamponade

16

Adriana Toro and Isidoro Di Carlo

Abstract

Pericardial tamponade caused by central venous catheter perforation of the heart or great vessels is an uncommon complication, but it remains potentially deadly with catastrophic consequences. The signs and symptoms of pericardial tamponade include confusion, pain or discomfort in the chest or epigastrium, nausea, dyspnea, tachycardia or bradycardia, engorgement of neck veins, pulsus paradoxus, hypotension, low-voltage electrocardiography and increase in the area of cardiac dullness. This complication can be prevented by the correct positioning of the catheter tip. When a clinical diagnosis of tamponade is made, treatment should be instituted without waiting for confirmation from radiographs, which may in any case be equivocal. Pericardiocentesis should be performed, and the catheter should be removed.

Keywords

Pericardial tamponade • Heart tamponade • Dyspnea • Tachycardia • Bradychardia • Hypotension • 'Greenall Criterion' • 'Right Main Bronchus Criterion'

16.1 Introduction

Myocardial perforation and tamponade by central venous pressure cannulae [1, 2] cardiac catheters [3] or pacemakers [3–6] are well known. In contrast

I. Di Carlo (✉)
Department of Surgical Sciences, Organ Transplantation and Advanced Technologies,
University of Catania, Cannizzaro Hospital,
Catania, Italy
e-mail: idicarlo@unict.it

I. Di Carlo, R. Biffi (eds.), *Totally Implantable Venous Access Devices*,

pericardial tamponade caused by central venous catheter perforation of the heart or great vessels is an uncommon complication, but one which remains potentially deadly with catastrophic consequences. The incidence of tamponade associated with central venous catheter (CVC) perforation [7, 8] depends on the reported series with a maximum rate of 10%. The frequency of cannulation, catheter material, dimensions and design also affect the likelihood of perforation [9–13]. There are no specific data present in the literature regarding totally implantable venous access devices and heart tamponade.

16.2 Clinical Manifestations

The signs and symptoms of pericardial tamponade include confusion, pain or discomfort in the chest or epigastrium, nausea, dyspnea, tachycardia or bradycardia engorgement of neck veins, pulsus paradoxus, hypotension, low-voltage electrocardiography and enlargement of the area of cardiac dullness.

Pulmonary symptoms such as chest tightness, shortness of breath, air hunger (up to 6 hours prior to significant changes in vital signs) are very common.

Patients affected by heart tamponade may develop EKG changes referable to wall ischemia or injury. In order to resuscitate these patients, intubation may be performed, but incorrect diagnosis may produce a sudden drop in their blood pressure after intubation.

16.3 Prevention

Cardiac tamponade is a devastating complication of a central venous catheter that should be preventable if proper procedure is used. This complication can be avoided by adherence to proper technique, ensuring that the catheter tip lies proximal to the cardiac silhouette, optimally in the superior vena cava, 2 cm proximal to the pericardial reflection [14].

The 'Greenall Criterion' [10] states that the tip should lie no more than 2 cm below a line joining the lower surfaces of the clavicular heads on a posteroanterior chest radiograph.

The 'Right Main Bronchus Criterion' by Rutherford et al. [15] states that that the tip should lie proximal to the angle formed between the right main bronchus and the trachea. This anatomical landmark represents the upper limit of the pericardial reflection over the lower superior vena cava.

Physicians who place these catheters and train others to do so must be aware of this issue and they must educate their trainees as well.

Radiologists must be educated so they know that a central venous catheter tip should not be within the pericardial silhouette on chest radiographs. They should call the inserting physician, or someone responsible for the patient, to let them know that the catheter is in too far and needs to be withdrawn a certain distance, which can be measured on a chest radiograph. A repeat radiographic examination must be performed after the catheter has been withdrawn to ensure proper location.

Any patient with a central venous catheter in place who develops unexplained hypotension, air hunger, shortness of breath, or chest tightness should have cardiac tamponade included in their differential diagnosis. If the radiograph shows the catheter tip within the pericardial silhouette, an emergency echocardiogram should be obtained. If the patient is very unstable, pericardiocentesis should be performed emergently. Only by thinking of the diagnosis can the patient be saved.

16.4 Treatment

When a clinical diagnosis of tamponade is made, treatment should be instituted without waiting for confirmation from radiographs, which may in any case be equivocal. Initially an attempt should be made to aspirate fluid through the catheter. The aspiration of fluid other than blood supports the diagnosis, and when no more fluid can be withdrawn the catheter should be removed. No more action need be taken if the patient's condition is satisfactory. Continuing clinical deterioration or failure to obtain aspirate from the catheter are indications for urgent pericardial needle aspiration. Pericardiocentesis should be performed, and the catheter should be removed, if feasible a pericardial window may be performed, cardiothoracic surgery consultation should be obtained early for possible thoracotomy.

Nitrates and intubation may be erroneously used if a wrong diagnosis is made. Nitrates reduce venous return and worsen the physiology of the cardiac tamponade. Cardiac tamponade must be considered in any patient with an indwelling central venous catheter who becomes more hypotensive with the use of nitrates.

Lastly, intubation may worsen a patient's hypotension shortly after being intubated. Prior to intubation, the patient with tamponade tends to be breathing deeply. This negative intrathoracic pressure pulls blood back to the heart as a compensatory mechanism for the tamponade. Intubation converts this negative pressure to positive pressure. This dramatically reduces the venous return to the heart and the cardiac output, and usually leads to a sudden drop in the patient's blood pressure [16].

References

1. Thomas CS Jr, Carter JW, Lowder SC (1969) Pericardial tamponade from central venous catheters. Arch Surg 98:217-218
2. Friedman BA, Jurgeleit HC (1968) Perforation of atrium by polyethylene CV catheter. JAMA 203:1141-1142

3. Gorlin R (1968) Cooperative study on cardiac catherization. Perforations and other cardiac complications. Circulation 37:III36-38
4. McHenry MM, Hopkins DM (1968) Cardiac tamponade as a result of infusion. A complication of transvenous pacing. JAMA 203:1071-1072
5. Mullen DC, Porter JM, Thompson HK, Silver D (1968) Cardiac tamponade from ventricular perforation by a transvenous pacemaker. JAMA 203:142-144
6. Goyanes AD, Lomanto C, Boyan CP (1969) Complications of catheterization for central venous pressure: a report of three cases. Anesth Analg 48:563-565
7. Karnauchow PN (1986) Cardiac tamponade central venous catheterisation. Can Med Assoc J 135:1145-1147
8. Burri C (1982) Invited commentary (on ref. 10). World J Surg 6:142-143
9. Sitzmann JV (1986) The technique of managing central venous lines. J Critical Illness 50-55
10. Greenall MJ, Blewitt RW, McMahon MJ (1975) Cardiac tamponade and central venous catheters. Br Med J 2:595-597
11. Krog M, Berggren L, Brodin M, Wickbom G. Pericardial tamponade caused by central venous catheters. World J Surg 6:138-143
12. Belani KG, Wilder RT, Campbell LM et al (1989) The new "Pig-tail" tipped central venous catheter – a design to eliminate vascular perforation. Anesth Analg 68:S20
13. Bersten A (1987) Role of catheter design in complications of central venous catheterisation. Anaesth Intens Care 15:241
14. Collier PE, Goodman GB (1995) Cardiac tamponade caused by central venous catheter perforation of the heart: a preventable complication. J Am Coll Surg 181:459-463
15 Rutherford JS, Merry AF, Occleshaw CJ (1994) Depth of central venous catheterization: an audit of practice in a cardiac surgical unit. Anaesth Intensive Care 22:267-271
16. Collier PE, Blocker SH, Graff DM, Doyle P (1998) Cardiac tamponade from central venous catheters. Am J Surg. 176:212-214

Brachial Plexus Injury

17

Walid Faraj and Ahmad Zaghal

Abstract

Brachial plexus injury during central venous catheter insertion is uncommon. Understanding the anatomy and the relationship between the brachial plexus and the neck veins and arteries is highly important. The brachial plexus, stellate ganglion, vagus, accessory, hypoglossal and phrenic nerves are all closely associated with the internal jugular vein. Any of these structures may be injured during cannulation attempts, with the most common complication occurring when local anesthetic injected at the time of cannulation transiently blocks these nerves.

Keywords

Brachial plexus • Central venous catheter

17.1 Introduction

Brachial plexus injury during central venous catheter insertion, though uncommon, has been described in the literature. Understanding the anatomy and the relationship between the brachial plexus and the neck veins and arteries is very important [1].

W. Faraj (✉)
American University of Beirut, Medical Center, Department of Surgery
Beirut, Lebanon
e-mail: wf07@aub.edu.lb

I. Di Carlo, R. Biffi (eds.), *Totally Implantable Venous Access Devices*,

17.2 Anatomy of the Brachial Plexus and Central Neck Veins

The brachial plexus is divided into roots, trunks, divisions, cords and branches. There are five terminal branches and many other collateral branches that leave the plexus at different points along its length.

The subclavian vein is a continuation of the axillary vein and it runs from the outer border of the first rib to the medial border of the anterior scalene muscle. From that point, it joins the internal jugular vein to form the brachiocephalic vein, also known as *innominate vein*. The subclavian vein follows the subclavian artery and is divided posteriorly by the insertion of the anterior scalene. The subclavian vein is separated from the subclavian artery and brachial plexus by the anterior scalene muscle.

The subclavian artery runs laterally, between the anterior and middle scalene muscles, with the anterior scalene on its anterior side and the middle scalene on its posterior. The subclavian artery has a higher and more posterior course than the vein and appears behind the anterior scalene muscle above the first rib along with the roots of the brachial plexus formed by the 5th, 6th, 7th, and 8th cervical nerves and the first thoracic nerve. This is in contrast to the subclavian vein, which travels anterior to the scalene anterior. If subclavian vein puncture is performed too far laterally or too deeply, the artery may be punctured or the brachial plexus roots may be injured. Neurological complications may result from subclavian artery puncture if local hematoma develops and compresses the brachial plexus.

The internal jugular vein (IJV) is another safe route for central venous access. At the root of the neck, the right IJV is close to the common carotid artery, and crosses the first part of the subclavian artery, while the left IJV usually overlaps the common carotid artery. The left vein is generally smaller than the right, and each contains a pair of valves situated about 2.5 cm above the termination of the vessel. Injury to the brachial plexus can happen from cannulation of the IJV. The advantage of the internal jugular vein over the subclavian vein for venous access has been proven and reported.

17.3 Brachial Plexus Injury

The brachial plexus, stellate ganglion, vagus, accessory, hypoglossal and phrenic nerves are all closely associated with the internal jugular vein [2-7]. Any of these structures may be injured during cannulation attempts, with the most common complication occurring when local anesthetic injected at the time of cannulation transiently blocks these nerves [2].

Subclavian vein cannulation may also be complicated by injury to the recurrent laryngeal nerve, phrenic nerve, and brachial plexus [8-9]; this complication can be avoided by following proper techniques in insertion of the central venous catheters.

17.4 Management

When a patient experiences intense paresthesia during central venous cannulation, careful examination of the site of the insertion should be performed. A magnetic resonance imaging or computed tomography scan can be used to confirm the presence or absence of a hematoma. Electromyography provides ideal confirmation of involvement of nerve and muscle in patients with pain. It can aid in localizing the level of injury and assess its severity. Nevertheless, in nerve injury during the first 5 to 8 days, it is difficult to identify the type of nerve injury with electromyography; it is best done at least three to four weeks after the onset of paresthesia.

References

1. Mossman DA (1975) The anatomy of infraclavicular subclavian vein catheterization and its complications. Surg Gynecol Obstet 141:769-772
2. Burns S, Herbison GJ (1996) Spinal accessory nerve injury as a complication of internal jugular vein cannulation. Ann Intern Med 125:700
3. Depierraz B, Essinger A, Morin D et al (1989) Isolated phrenic nerve injury after apparently atraumatic puncture of the internal jugular vein. Intensive Care Med 15:132-134
4. Vest JV, Pereira MB, Senior RM (1980) Phrenic nerve injury associated with venipuncture of the internal jugular vein. Chest 78:777-779
5. Paschall RM, Mandel S (1983) Brachial plexus injury from percutaneous cannulation of the internal jugular vein. Ann Emerg Med 12:58-60
6. Sylvestre DL, Sandson TA, Nachmanoff DB (1991) Transient brachial plexopathy as a complication of internal jugular vein cannulation. Neurology 41:760
7. Whittet HB, Boscoe MJ (1984) Isolated palsy of the hypoglossal nerve after central venous catheterization. Br Med J (Clin Res Ed) 288:1042-1043
8. Trentman TL, Rome JD, Messick JM Jr (1996) Brachial plexus neuropathy following attempt at subclavian vein catheterization. Case report. Reg Anesth 21:163-165
9. Porzionato A, Montisci M, Manani G (2003) Brachial plexus injury following subclavian vein catheterization: a case report. J Clin Anesth 15:582-586

Part IV

Early Complications: Diagnosis and Treatment

Hemoptysis 18

Alexandra Ozimek, Pierre A. Clavien and Antonio Nocito

Abstract

Hemoptysis following port catheter implantation is a rather rare complication. It may occur as a consequence of mechanical injury to the trachea or the upper pulmonary lobe during implantation. Hemoptysis manifesting any time after surgery ensues from cardiovascular or pulmonary pathologies (e.g. pulmonary embolism). Thus therapy of hemoptysis is directed at the underlying cause and may involve removal of the catheter, anticoagulation, interventional or surgical embolectomy and thrombolysis.

Keywords

Hemoptysis • Venous thrombosis • Right heart thrombosis • Pulmonary embolism • Pulmonary artery pseudoaneurysm • Pinch-off syndrome

18.1 Definition and Epidemiology

Hemoptysis is defined as an expectoration of blood or blood-stained sputum deriving from the larynx, trachea, bronchi or lungs. Hemoptysis following port catheter implantation is a rare complication with an estimated incidence of 0.03% [1]. Therefore it is not surprising that data on hemoptysis following implantation of indwelling catheters is sparse and almost exclusively limited to case reports.

A. Ozimek (✉)
Department of Surgery, University Hospital Zürich,
Zürich, Switzerland
e-mail: alexandra.ozimek@med.uni-muenchen.de

I. Di Carlo, R. Biffi (eds.), *Totally Implantable Venous Access Devices*,

18.2 Pathogenesis

Hemoptysis following implantation of indwelling catheters generally develops as a consequence of mechanical injury and cardiovascular or pulmonary diseases. It can occur early or late after port implantation.

To date, only two cases of early hemoptysis after port implantation have been reported [1]. Both were caused by an accidential injury of the upper pulmonary lobe.

Hemoptysis appearing late after port implantation is usually a result of deep venous thrombosis, right heart thromboembolus formation or pulmonary embolism [2, 3]. Indeed, catheter-related deep venous thrombosis is a frequent complication and occurs in up to 66% of adults. In patients with upper-extremity deep-venous thrombosis, subsequent pulmonary embolism remains asymptomatic in 15–36 % of the cases. However, 5–14% of the patients become symptomatic [4]. Similarly, right heart thromboembolism ensues in up to 12.5% and subsequent pulmonary embolism occurs in up to to 6% [2].

Various mechanisms leading to hemoptysis after thrombosis or embolism exist. Deep venous thrombosis of the superior vena cava results in a superior vena cava syndrome, which can induce hemoptysis due to venous congestion of collateral pathways. In contrast, right heart thrombi have a dangerous potential to embolize to the lungs, thus leading to hemoptysis due to hypertensive changes in the arterial and venous pulmonary microvasculature. Futhermore, pulmonary embolism can lead to the development of a pseudoaneurysm of the pulmonary artery with subsequent inflammation or rupture of the aneurysmatic sac, thus enhancing hemoptysis [2, 5].

While catheter-related thromboembolic complications are one of the most frequent complications after TIVAD implantation, pulmonary embolization of catheter fragments as a consequence of catheter fracture is less common. Its incidence ranges from 0.4% to 1% [5]. Lastly, endotracheal migration of the catheter or catheter fragments has also been described as a further rare cause of hemoptysis [6]. Figure 18.1 shows a summary of the possible pathomechanisms of hemoptysis following port catheter implantation.

18.3 Risk Factors

The incidence of catheter-related thrombosis is influenced by various factors. These include patient comorbidities, port system characteristics, cannulation site and rheologic properties of the infusates [2]. Of note, catheter size has a significant impact on the development of venous thrombosis. Thick catheters more often induce a disruption of the vascular endothelium, thus entailing a higher risk of thrombosis. The most frequent sites of catheter-related thromboses are the central veins of neck, chest (especially the left subclavian vein) and upper extremity, since these veins are mostly used to obtain a central venous access [4]. Further risk factors for deep venous thrombosis are catheter

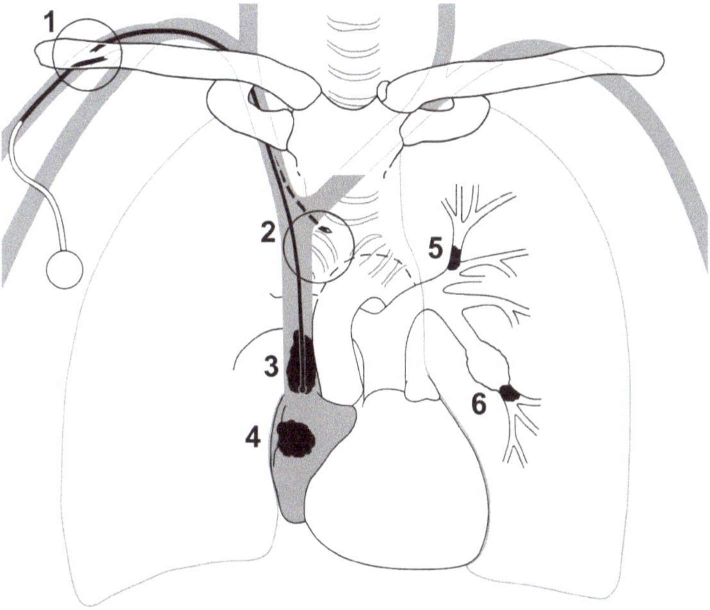

Fig. 18.1 Possible pathomechanism of hemoptysis following port catheter implantation. 1 Pinch-off syndrome; 2 Tracheal catheter migration; 3 Deep venous embolism; 4 Right heart embolism; 5 Pulmonary embolism; 6 Pulmonary artery pseudoaneurysm

malposition and previous catheter infections [4]. Similarly, catheter related right atrial thrombi are associated with catheter tip position in the right atrium, malignancy, concurrent infection, procoagulant states and cardiac structural abnormalities [2].

Catheter fractures mainly occur as a consequence of catheter compression between the first rib and the clavicle, the so-called *pinch-off* syndrome. The mechanical load first causes an intermittent occlusion and subsequently catheter fracture and fragment embolisation. Predisposing factors are a too medial catheter insertion, a shoulder trauma or an iatrogenic injury between the first rib and the medial part of the clavicle [5].

18.4 Diagnosis

As hemoptysis in patients with an implanted porth-catheter can be a sequel of a serious underlying disorder, a thorough clinical examination has to be performed immediately. Superior vena cava obstruction usually entails a swelling of the face, neck and upper extremity as well as a venous dilatation in the neck and on the chest wall. Furthermore dyspnea and cough and less commonly hoarseness, epistaxis, lingual swelling and upper gastrointestinal bleeding may be present [3].

The most common clinical features of pulmonary embolism are sudden-onset dyspnea, tachypnea, chest pain, cough and hemoptysis. More severe cases lead to cyanosis and hemodynamic instability [7].

Clinical symptoms of pulmonary artery pseudoaneurysm vary according to the localization and size of the pseudoaneurysm and include fever, chest pain and dyspnea. Importantly, hemoptysis is the most frequent presenting symptom [5, 7].

Apart from the clinical examination, diagnostic workup of hemoptysis always requires a laboratory test (e.g. complete blood count, coagulation profile, D-dimer, arterial blood gas study) a screening chest x-ray and if applicable a catheter-dye study to check for a correct catheter position. If the cause of hemoptysis remains unclear, further investigations including a spiral computertomography with angiography scan and a bronchoscopy should be evaluated. Especially in patients with endotracheal catheter migration bronchoscopy might reveal a catheter tip protruding into the catheter lumen [7].

When a catheter-related thrombosis or pulmonary embolism is suspected a complementary Doppler ultrasonography of the lower and upper extremities to detect deep venous thrombosis should be performed. In cases where a right atrial dilatation, dysfunction or right heart thromembolism is suspected, an echocardiogram should be obtained. In these cases a transesophageal echocardiography (TEE) is preferred over a transthoracic echocardiography (TTE) as TEE is more sensitive and allows a better characterization of clot morphology [2].

18.5 Therapy

Therapy of hemoptysis is directed at its underlying causes. In cases of catheter migration or even embolisation, the catheter has to be immediately removed via a percutaneous endovascular approach either in a radiologic suite or an operating room [6].

When a venous or right atrial thrombosis and / or pulmonary embolism is the underlying cause, anticoagulation should be initiated at once. Often further supportive treatment and surveillance in the ICU is necessary. In patients with catheter-related thrombosis in which the catheter is dysfunctional or not longer needed, the catheter should be removed 3–5 days after the initiation of anticoagulation, as recommended by the guidelines of the American College of Chest Physicians (ACCP) [4]. If a hemodynamic instability due to embolism ensues, the following therapeutic options should be evaluated: interventional radiology-guided clot retrieval, thrombolysis or surgical embolectomy [2].

Finally, the options for the treatment of pulmonary artery pseudoaneurysms are: bronchoscopic coagulation, angiographic embolization or surgical resection and repair [5].

References

1. Di Carlo I, Pulvirenti E, Mannino M et al (2010) Increased use of percutaneous technique for totally implantable venous access devices. Is it real progress? A 27-year comprehensive review on early complications. Ann Surg Oncol 17:1649–1656
2. Burns K, McLaren A (2009) Catheter-related right atrial thrombus and pulmonary embolism: A case report and systematic review of the literature. Can Respir J 16:163–165
3. Gopaluni S, Warwicker O (2009) Superior vena cava obstruction presenting with epistaxis, haemoptysis and gastro-intestinal haemorrhage in two men receiving haemodialysis with central venous catheters: two case reports. J Med Case Rep 3:6180
4. Baskin JL, Pui CH, Reiss U et al (2009) Management of occlusion and thrombosis associated with long-term indwelling central venous catheters. Lancet 374:159–169
5. Oz K, Demirhan R, Onan B (2008) Pulmonary artery pseudoaneurysm after a vascular access port catheter implantation. Ann Thorac Surg 87:295–297
6. Cattelani L, Bobbio A, Carbognani P et al (2006) Endotracheal migration of central venous catheter. J Cardiovasc Surg (Torino) 47:95–97
7. Goldhaber SZ (2005) Pulmonary thromboembolism. In: Kasper DL, Braunwald E, Fauci AS et al (eds) Harrison's Principles of Internal Medicine, 16th edn. McGraw-Hill, New York, pp 1561–1566i

Pocket Hematoma

19

Adriana Toro and Isidoro Di Carlo

Abstract

Pocket hematoma is an acute, relatively common complication that may occur after totally implantable venous access device (TIVAD) with an incidence ranging between 0% and 4.5%. A hematoma is assumed to be present if there is any palpable swelling of the TIVAD pocket exceeding the size of the device. The causes of the port hematoma may be intraoperative or postoperative. Intraoperative causes may be the consequence of a defective technique. Postoperative causes may also be the pharmacological therapy. In the event of hematoma the use of the port should be delayed until resorption in order to avoid the risk of infection. In case of doubt, this complication should be sonographically confirmed.

Keywords

Hematoma • Pocket hematoma • Subcutaneous pocket • Warfarin • Heparin • Aspirin therapy • Blood clots

19.1 Definition

Pocket hematoma is an acute, relatively common, complication [1] that may occur after totally implantable venous access device (TIVAD) implantation, with an incidence ranging between 0% [2] and 4.5% [3]. This complication occurs more frequently with the percutaneous technique than with the surgi-

I. Di Carlo (✉)
Department of Surgical Sciences, Organ Transplantation and Advanced Technologies,
University of Catania, Cannizzaro Hospital,
Catania, Italy
e-mail: idicarlo@unict.it

I. Di Carlo, R. Biffi (eds.), *Totally Implantable Venous Access Devices*,

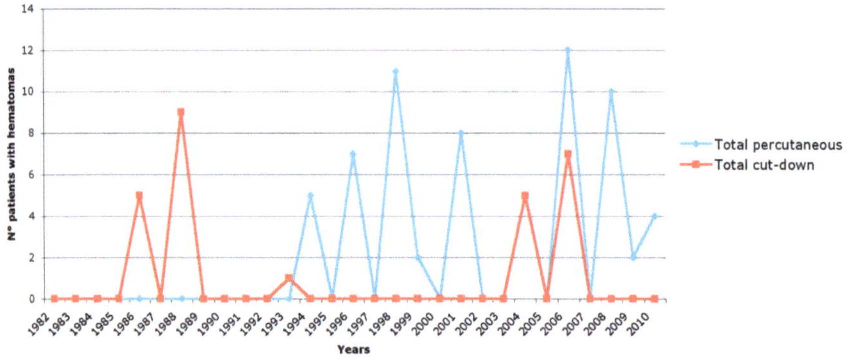

Fig. 19.1 Hematomas recorded in the literature from 1982 to 2010 with surgical cutdown (*red line*) and percutaneous approach (*blue line*)

cal technique (Fig. 19.1) [2, 4, 5]. The incidence of pocket hematoma also depends on the location of the port, which can be placed beneath the fascia of the pectoralis major muscle or above in the subcutaneous space. The incidence of pocket hematoma is more frequent in patients with the port in the subpectoral fascia than in the subcutaneous pocket.

19.2 Etiology

The causes of the port hematoma may be intraoperative or postoperative. A hematoma may develop at the pectoral region during local anesthetic infiltration which may result in failure of the procedure.

Intraoperative causes may be the consequence of a defective technique. TIVAD implantation should be a procedure without bleeding: if bleeding occurs, the technique is not adequate and hematomas can develop in the port pocket. During the procedure thorough hemostasis should be undertaken [6] to avoid this postoperative complication. The site of bleeding may be the pocket or back-bleeding around the lead venous entry site. The use of electrocautery is useful for minimizing pocket-related bleeding. Bleeding from the venous entry site usually subsides during the procedure but ongoing bleeding is controlled by a firm suture placed through and around the lead entry/pectoral muscle interface [1], or by directly suturing the vein more firmly if the surgical technique is adopted. In cases of percutaneous implant of TIVAD hematoma can usually be avoided by using ultrasound guidance [7]. Percutaneous venous intervention may be safely performed in patients without discontinuing anticoagulation therapy [8].

The only identifiable risk factor for pocket hematoma formation is the use of intravenous heparin. Patients who received heparin after TIVAD implant had a 5-fold and 10-fold greater risk of pocket hematoma formation than patients treated with warfarin alone or no anticoagulation, respectively. The risk is the same whether heparin therapy is initiated 6 h or 24 h after surgery. Aspirin therapy did not affect the risk of hematoma formation in patients undergoing TIVAD implantation [9]. The formation of hematoma may result in longer hospitalization. The partial thromboplastin time did not correlate with pocket hematoma formation, as might be expected, since the partial thromboplastin time value is an indicator of the degree of anticoagulation afforded by intravenous heparin. The use of warfarin alone conferred a much lower risk of pocket hematoma formation, perhaps because warfarin therapy usually requires at least three days to achieve a therapeutic level of anticoagulation [9].

Intraoperative bleeding is defined by protracted, diffuse bleeding of vascular, muscular, or subcutaneous origin, which cannot be stopped by surgical intervention including the use of local hemostyptic agents or required a non-prophylactic vacuum drainage. Risk is increased in anticoagulated patients. The use of heparin appears to be associated with a higher risk of bleeding than warfarin. It has been shown that continuation of warfarin with an international normalized ratio (INR) of about 2.0 is safe and without devastating complication over a 15 year experience [10] although in most cases, anticoagulation is discontinued for at least the duration of the procedure [1]. Usually there is no correlation between platelet count and hematoma or bleeding [11].

19.3 Treatment

In the event of hematoma the use of the port should be delayed until resorption in order to avoid the risk of infection. A hematoma is assumed to be present if there is any palpable swelling of the TIVAD pocket exceeding the size of the device. In case of doubt, this complication should be sonographically confirmed.

Usually, hematomas have clinical diagnosis, no re-operation is necessary [12] and they are managed conservatively unless expanding in size, tense or painful. In 3% of patients a hematoma became apparent, but these resolved spontaneously and caused no delay in treatment [13]. Severe pocket hematomas are classified by pain, prolonged hospitalization, or the need for reoperation [14]. In these cases, reoperation to evacuate the blood clots and identify and arrest the site of bleeding is required. Treatment is different in relation to the presence of wound infection. In cases of a simple hematoma which continues to discharge blood, removal of blood clots and irrigation of the pocket should be useful, and the port can be left in situ. In contrast, in cases of persistence of the hematoma and the absence of resorption the risk of infection becomes high and in the presence of clinical signs the port should be removed.

References

1. Pavia S, Wilkoff B (2001) The management of surgical complications of pacemaker and implantable cardioverter-defibrillators. Curr Opin Cardiol 16:66-71
2. Ku YH, Kuo PH, Tsai YF et al (2009) Port-a-cath implantation using percutaneous puncture without guidance. Ann Surg Oncol 16:729-734
3. Vardy J, Engelhardt K, Cox K et al (2004) Long-term outcome of radiological-guided insertion of implanted central venous access port devices (CVAPD) for the delivery of chemotherapy in cancer patients: institutional experience and review of the literature. Br J Cancer 91:1045-1049
4. Di Carlo I, Pulvirenti E, Mannino M, Toro A (2010) Increased use of percutaneous technique for totally implantable venous access devices. Is it real progress? A 27-year comprehensive review on early complications. Ann Surg Oncol 17:1649-1656
5. Sakamoto N, Arai Y, Takeuchi Y et al (2010) Ultrasound-guided radiological placement of central venous port via the subclavian vein: a retrospective analysis of 500 cases at a single institute. Cardiovasc Intervent Radiol 33:989-994
6. Kurul S, Saip P, Aydin T (2002) Totally implantable venous-access ports: local problems and extravasation injury. Lancet Oncol 3:684-691
7. Asch MR (2001) Venous access: options, approaches and issues. Can Assoc Radiol J 52:153-164
8. Gray RR, Sadler DJ, Shulman L et al (1999) Should anticoagulant therapy be stopped or reversed before venous intervention? Can Assoc Radiol J 50:306-309
9. Michaud GF, Pelosi FJ, Noble MD et al (2000) A randomized trial comparing heparin initiation 6h or 24 h after pacemaker or defibrillator implantation. J Am Coll Cardiol 35:1915-1918
10. Belott P, Reynolds D (2000) Permanent pacemaker and implantable cardioverter defibrillator implantation. In: Ellenboggen K, Kay G, Wilkoff B (eds) Clinical cardiac pacing and defibrillation. WB Saunders, Philadelphia, pp 573-644
11. Rouzrokh M, Shamsian BS, Tabari AKN et al (2009) Totally implantable subpectoral vs. subcutaneous port systems in children with malignant diseases. Arch Iranian Med 12:389-394
12. Knebel P, Fischer L, Cremonese E et al (2008) Protocol of an expertise based randomized trial comparing surgical venae section versus radiological puncture of vena subclavia for insertion of totally implantable access port in oncological patients. Trials 9:60
13. Poorter RL, Lauw FN, Bemelman WA et al (1996) Complications of an implantable venous access device (port a cath) during intermittent continuous infusion of chemotherapy. Eur J Cancer 32:2262-2266
14. Wiegand UKH, LeJeune D, Boguschewski F et al (2004) Pocket haematoma after pacemaker or implantable cardioverter defibrillator surgery: influence of patient morbidity, operation strategy, and perioperative antiplatelet/anticoagulation therapy. Chest 126:1177-1186

Wound Dehiscence

20

Alexandra Ozimek, Pierre A. Clavien and Antonio Nocito

Abstract

Wound dehiscence after implantation of a port catheter system occurs with an estimated incidence of 3%. It results either from poor surgical technique or from impaired wound healing. Any kind of wound complication demands an immediate cessation of the application of therapeutic agents via the port system and initiation of local wound care. In cases of early wound bursting a readaptation of the wound is possible. Delayed wound dehiscence neccessitates port removal and consequent antibiotic treatment in most cases.

Keywords

Wound dehiscence • Port erosion

20.1 Definition and Epidemiology

Wound dehiscence after port implantation is a postoperative complication with a reported incidence of 3% [1, 2]. It is defined as premature unintentional reopening of a wound along the surgical suture line after successful implantation of a subcutaneous port catheter system. This entity has to be clearly distinguished from port erosion – a spontaneous penetration of the port reservoir through the skin – which is often encountered in cachectic patients. A wound dehiscence after port placement represents a major cause of patient distress,

A. Ozimek (✉)
Department of Surgery, University Hospital Zürich,
Zürich, Switzerland
e-mail: alexandra.ozimek@med.uni-muenchen.de

I. Di Carlo, R. Biffi (eds.), *Totally Implantable Venous Access Devices*,

since it is associated with an interruption of chemotherapy, an additional surgical intervention and an increased risk of catheter related infections.

20.2 Pathogenesis and Risk Factors

A dehiscence of the skin after the implantation of a port reservoir is either the result of a poor surgical technique or impaired wound healing. While early postoperative wound-bursting points to a technical failure, such as incorrect port-placement, e.g. directly underneath the incision, incorrect knotting or broken suture material, a delayed dehiscence is rather related to wound healing problems. Apart from these factors, premature suture removal is one of the main causes of wound dehiscence [1, 2].

Impaired wound healing which leads to delayed wound dehiscence occurs as a consequence of poor blood supply or mechanical stress. Insufficient blood supply can result from local problems such as hematoma, inflammation, tight sutures as well as thin, fragile skin, or as a consequence of systemic factors such as nicotine abuse, diabetes mellitus or vascular diseases. Indeed local infection has been shown to be one of the most important risk factors for wound dehiscence. Pathogenic microorganisms are thought to inhibit fibroblast function, thus decreasing tensile strength and facilitating tissue destruction [3]. Similarly, collagen synthesis and consequently tensile strength is reduced in malnourished, hypoproteinemic patients.

Patients subjected to a TIVAD placement are often treated with different drugs, such as anti-inflammatory or chemotherapeutic compounds as well as steroids. These agents can dramatically impair wound healing. For instance, a higher incidence of wound healing complications after TIVAD placement was found in patients undergoing chemotherapy with bevacizumab, an antivascular endothelial growth factor antibody. In these patients, wound healing problems were almost exclusively detected when bevacizumab therapy was started within 10 days of port placement [2]. Additional risk factors for wound dehiscence are presented in Table 20.1.

Lastly, it is important to note that skin necrosis with consequent port erosion can occur at any time after port insertion. In many cases, gradual weight loss due to illness progression leads to cachexia thus reducing subcutaneous tissue and skin resistance. In addition, port erosion is further promoted by superficial port placement and inappropriate catheter selection.

20.3 Therapy

As a general rule, if a wound complication occurs, the application of therapeutic agents via the port system has to be immediately stopped and topical therapy has to be started. The therapeutic approach should be chosen according to the time delay and degree of wound dehiscence [1, 2].

Table 20.1 Risk factors for wound dehiscence after TIVAD implantation

Resulting from technical complications	Including failure to heal	
Surgery	Local factors	Systemic factors
Poor knotting/grabbing of stitches	Hemostasis	Malnutrition
Broken suture	Tight suture	Physical stress
Incision placed directly over the port system	Poor tissue vascularization	Anemia
Superficial port placement	Thin tissue	Malignancy
Hematoma/seroma	Local inflammation	Uremia
Wound closure under tension	Obesity	Hypertension
Too early suture removal		Medication
Inappropriate port catheter choice		Nicotine abuse
		Diabetes mellitus
		Vascular disease

In cases of early wound bursting, i.e. in the operation room or within 6 hours after TIVAD placement, a readaptation of the skin under maximum sterile conditions should be performed. Additionally, prophylactic antibiotic treatment should be installed. Delayed wound dehiscence due to a severe infectious complication mandates port removal at once and the initiation of antibiotic therapy. In cases of impending port erosion prophylactic removal is warranted. Salvage strategies for patients with a limited dehiscence include local wound care and the mobilization of a skin flap to cover the affected area [1, 2].

20.4 Prophylaxis

- To avoid postoperative local inflammatory complications the implantation of port catheter systems should always be performed in an operation room in aseptic environment under maximum sterile conditions (sterile gown, sterile gloves, a mask and a cap, disinfection of the operation area).
- Moderate hemostasis during port implantation avoids on the one hand postoperative hematoma and on the other wound ischemia.
- An appropriate choice of suture material and suture technique is essential. Tension free closure is recommended. Suture removal should be performed not earlier than 10–12 days after surgery.
- In cachetic patients a low profile vascular access port system should be chosen in order to prevent port erosion.

References

1. Kurul S, Salp P, DeVasher E (2002) Totally implantable venous-access ports: local problems and extravasation injury. Lancet Oncol 3:684-693

2. Zawacki WJ, Walker G, DeVasher E et al (2009) Wound dehiscence or failure to heal following venous access port placement in patients receiving bevacizumab therapy. J Vas Interv Radiol 20:624-627
3. Spiliotis J, Tsiveriotis K, Datsis A et al (2009) Wound dehiscence: is still a problem in the 21th century: a retrospective study. World J Emerg Surg 4:1-5

Reversal

21

Francesca Ratti, Marco Catena, Michele Paganelli and Luca Aldrighetti

Abstract

The technique of venous access port placement requires dissection of the pocket just above the level of the pectoralis fascia and then placement of nonabsorbable sutures through the holes in the reservoir base to secure it. A low rate of port inversion is reported when the port base is fixed to subcutaneous pocket.

However, series reporting both port fixation or no fixation show similar rates of reversal. Once identified, port reversal can be easily corrected by gentle rotation of the port. Rarely, reanchoring of the port is required.

Keywords

Reversal • Pocket size • Suture fixation

21.1 Introduction

The traditional technique of venous access port placement requires dissection of the pocket just above the level of the pectoralis fascia and then placement of nonabsorbable sutures through the holes in the reservoir base to secure it. The number of stitches recommended to avoid port dislocation varies depending on port type and number of holes in the reservoir (generally 3 or 4). At any rate at least two sutures should be placed even by surgeons with good expertise and only when a correct pocket size has been created.

F. Ratti (✉)
Department of Surgery, Hepatobiliary Surgery Unit, San Raffaele Hospital,
Vita-Salute San Raffaele University,
Milano, Italy
e-mail: ratti.francesca@hsr.it

I. Di Carlo, R. Biffi (eds.), *Totally Implantable Venous Access Devices*,

21.2 Diagnosis, Technical Considerations and Treatment

The pocket must be of sufficient size to accept the port without undue tension on the skin incision [1]. The purpose of this is to prevent inversion, flipping, twisting, or rotation within the pocket, since major risk factors for these complications include loose or redundant subcutaneous tissues and large pocket size, both of which would allow excessive mobility of the port [2]. Suture fixation of the port seems to decrease the incidence of port reversal (intending port rotation on its axis), particularly when the fibrous capsule has not yet formed, in the first one or two weeks after venous access placement [3]. Diagnosis of this complication is suspected when port puncture and subsequent blood withdrawal and fluid injection cannot be performed easily.

A low rate of port inversion is reported when the port base is fixed to the subcutaneous pocket [4, 5]. However, port inversion can occur despite suture fixation of the port to the pocket. In a series of 560 chest ports that were secured to the pectoralis muscle with two nonabsorbable sutures, three port rotations occurred (0.53%) and rotation is reported even when absorbable suture is used, because of a fixation that is not strong enough, especially when the device is not sutured to muscular fascia but to subcutaneous tissue [6].

Another reported cause of port reversal is direct trauma, even if an absorbable suture is present [7]. Many of the published series do not specify whether or not suture fixation of the port was performed. In many series, the port inversion rate ranged from 0 to 1% [8, 9]. In series where the port was not secured to the pocket routinely, the port inversion rate ranged from 0.2 to 1.6% [10, 11]. On the other hand, removal of a port that has been previously fixated results in a more difficult procedure, requiring more extensive dissection, because of the presence of a suture and of fibrous reaction. Although the resultant increase in morbidity, procedure time, and cost is probably minimal, it is not insignificant.

Cil et al. [10] made a report about 476 subcutaneous ports that were not routinely secured to the pocket (however, 3-0 sutures were placed to secure the port to the chest wall in patients with a large port pocket or with excessive and loose subcutaneous fat who were believed to be at high risk for port rotation, although the frequency of fixation is not reported in the study). One port inversion occurred (0.2%), which was thought to be caused by loose and excessive subcutaneous fat. It was not specified if this port had been sutured to the pocket at the time of initial placement.

McNulty et al. [12] reported a series of 534 chest port placements, none of which were secured to the pocket, with a port inversion rate of 0.2%: this rate is concordant with rates previously published in the literature of both sutured and nonsutured ports.

Once identified, port reversal can be easily corrected by gentle rotation of the port. Rarely, reanchoring of the port is required.

In conclusion, using anchoring sutures when required, securing port insertion and forming a small snug fitting pocket are procedures that may reduce the risk of catheter rotation.

References

1. Raaf JH, Heil D, Rollins DL (1994) Vascular access pumps and infusions. In: McKenna RJ, Murphy GP (eds) Cancer surgery. Lippincott Williams & Wilkins, Philadelphia, pp 51–53
2. Gebarski SS, Gebarski KS (1984) Chemotherapy port "Twiddler's syndrome". A need for preinjection radiography. Cancer 54:38–39
3. de Costa BR, Dickey K, Greenwood L (2000) A practical approach for repositioning flipped venous access ports. J Vasc Interv Radiol 11:213–214
4. Kock HJ, Pietsch M, Krause U et al (1998) Implantable vascular access systems: experience in 1500 patients with totally implanted central venous port systems. World J Surg 22:12–16
5. Shetty P, Mody M, Kastan D et al (1997) Outcome of 350 implanted chest ports placed by interventional radiologists. J Vasc Interv Radiol 8:991
6. Sánchez LY, Galbis Caravajal JM, Fuster Diana CA et al (2006) Protocol for the implantation of a venous access device (Port-A-Cath system). The complications and solutions found in 560 cases. Clin Translation Oncol 8:735–741
7. Forauer AR, Chen Y, Parks R (2005) A case of posttraumatic Twiddler's syndrome. J Vasc Interv Radiol 16:562–563
8. Charvát J, Linke Z, Horáèková M, Prausová J (2006) Implantation of central venous ports with catheter insertion via the right internal jugular vein in oncology patients–single center experience. Support Care Cancer 14:1162–1165
9. Harvey WH, Pick TE, Reed K et al (1989) A prospective evaluation of the Port-A-Cath implantable venous access system in chronically ill adults and children. Surg Gynecol Obstet 169:495–500
10. Cil BE, Canyiğit M, Peynircioğlu B et al (2006) Subcutaneous venous port implantation in adult patients: a single center experience. Diagn Interv Radiol 12:93–98
11. Lorch H, Zwaan M, Kagel C et al (2001) Central venous access ports placed by interventional radiologists: experience with 125 consecutive patients. Cardiovasc Intervent Radiol 24:180–184
12. McNulty NJ, Perrich KD, Silas AM et al (2010) Cardiovasc Intervent Radiol 33:751-755

Part V

Late Complications

Catheter-related Bloodstream Infection 22

Adriana Toro, Roberto Biffi and Isidoro Di Carlo

Abstract

The development of catheter-related septicemia is the most serious complication of venous access. Risk factors may be related to the patients, to the catheter or to the location in which the procedure is performed. The most common organism isolated from catheter tip cultures are skin flora such as *Staphylococcus epidermidis*, *Staphylococcus aureus* and *Streptococcus* species. Infection of the totally implantable venous access device (TIVAD) can occur without local signs, but with unexplained fever or systemic signs of sepsis. Most cases of catheter-related bacteremia can be successfully treated in situ with systemic antibiotics, more difficult to eradicate cases and early catheter removal should be considered seriously.

Keywords

Catheter-related bloodstream infection (CRBI) • Infection • Bacteremia • Sepsis • *Staphylococcus epidermidis* • *Staphylococcus aureus* • *Streptococcus species* • Antibiotic therapy • Peripheral blood culture

22.1 Introduction

The development of catheter-related septicemia is the most serious complication of venous access. Risk factors for totally implantable venous access device (TIVAD) infection may be related to the patient (immunocompetence,

I. Di Carlo (✉)
Department of Surgical Sciences, Organ Transplantation and Advanced Technologies,
University of Catania, Cannizzaro Hospital,
Catania, Italy
e-mail: idicarlo@unict.it

performance status, primary diagnosis of solid or hematologic tumor) or to the catheter (extraluminal obstruction from mural thrombus, fibrin sleeve or clot formation inside the catheter) or to the location in which the procedure is performed (operating room or interventional radiology unit) [1]. Early recognition, sensitive and rapid methods of diagnosis, and aggressive treatment are clearly necessary to avoid the potentially life threatening consequences of untreated bacteremia. Because most patients with cancer who have long-term indwelling venous catheters will experience periods of immune system compromise secondary to their disease or its treatment, it is not surprising that catheter-related bloodstream infections have been reported to range from 2.4% up to 16.0% [2, 3].

22.2 Etiology

The pathogenesis of catheter-related sepsis appears to be related primarily to the colonization of the intravascular portion of the catheter by bacteria, most commonly the patient's skin flora, which migrate along the external surface or the catheter from the exit site or are flushed through the lumen from the catheter hubs [4].

Several studies have shown that the most common organism isolated from cultures of catheter tips are skin flora such as *Staphylococcus epidermidis*, *Staphylococcus aureus*, and *Streptococcus* species [5].

Once bacteria gain access to the intravascular portion of the catheter, colonization may be facilitated by the presence of a biofilm which is typically present on long-term venous access catheters. By means of electron microscopy, bacterial colonization of Gram positive cocci has been observed in an adherent glycocalyx biofilm present on 13 of 15 (87%) long-term venous catheter lumens in cancer patients [6].

22.3 Diagnosis

A rapid and reliable method of diagnosing catheter-related bacteremia while the catheter remains *in situ* would be ideal and a number of studies have addressed this issue. Initially, other sources of infection based on clinical and laboratory findings should be excluded.

Infection of the TIVAD can occur without local signs, but with unexplained fever or systemic signs of sepsis. In this case, a quantitative blood culture should be obtained both through the TIVAD itself and from a peripheral vein. TIVAD site infection can be treated with local wound care and systemic antibiotics [7]. Antibiotic therapy is needed if the diagnosis of catheter-related bloodstream infection (CRBI) is performed. Based on available information the following criteria appear to be sufficient for diagnosing catheter-related infections: (1) the higher number of colony-forming units (CFU) of bacteria per milliliter of blood obtained through the device in comparison to the peripheral blood culture; (2) in the absence of peripheral blood culture, more than 1000 CFUs of bacteria obtained through the device; and (3) positive catheter tip culture after removal in the appropriate clinical setting [8–10].

In addition, if there is a relationship between the timing of catheter care (i.e. flushing) and the development of symptoms of bacteremia (i.e. fever and chills) there should be suspicion that manipulation of the catheter may have precipitated the episode.

Catheter sparing diagnostic methods, such as differential quantitative blood cultures and differential time to positivity (DTTP), have emerged as reliable diagnostic techniques. Paired blood cultures (aerobic and anaerobic) from a peripheral vein and the central catheter should be obtained. If the culture from the central catheter turns positive before the peripheral sample (diagnostic cut-off: 2 hours), this so-called DTTP can help to make the diagnosis of catheter-related infection [11].

22.4 Treatment

A number of studies have reported successful treatment of line sepsis while the catheter remains *in situ*.

In order of prevalence, the four most common pathogens are coagulase-negative staphylococci, *Staphylococcus aureus*, *Candida* species and enteric gram negative bacilli [12].

Cherifi et al. have shown that treatment was successful in 35 of 57 (56%) patients with antibiotics alone. Relapses were observed in 9 (16%) cases, while catheter-retaining treatment failed in 16 (28%) cases [13]. Successful treatment of line sepsis was defined as negative culture results after a course of antibiotics and failure was defined as persistently positive culture results after antibiotic therapy or the development of recurrent infections with the same organism.

It is reasonable to expect that in patients with line-related sepsis and without any local signs of infection, the likelihood of successful treatment with antibiotics alone even in the presence of neutropenia is high.

Catheter-related bacteremia was defined as a positive blood culture obtained from the central venous catheter in the presence of fever and no localizing signs.

A major question in the treatment of catheter-related bacteremia is: under what conditions should the infected catheter be removed? Clearly, a deteriorating clinical condition while the patient is on appropriate antibiotics should be treated with urgent catheter removal. Recurrent infections and persistently positive blood cultures after completion of treatment are other indications for catheter removal.

Therefore, although most cases of catheter-related bacteremia can be successfully treated *in situ* with systemic antibiotics, more difficult to eradicate

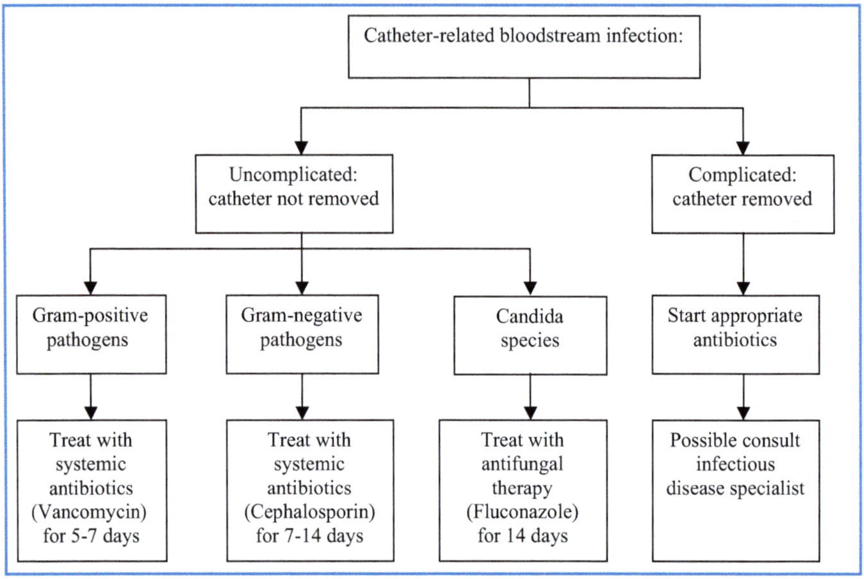

Fig. 22.1 Catheter-related bloodstream infection treatment pathway

cases and early catheter removal should be considered seriously. In all patients with catheter-related infection the decision to remove the catheter should be based on the close clinical assessment of the patient and response to initial antibiotic therapy. If there is persistent evidence of infection or any deterioration in the condition of the patient, the catheter should be removed (Fig. 22.1).

References

1. Di Carlo I, Toro A, Pulvirenti E et al (2011) Could antibiotic prophylaxis be not necessary to implant totally implantable venous access devices? Randomized prospective study. Surg Oncol 20:20–25
2. Silver DF, Hempling RE, Recio FO et al (1998) Complications related to indwelling caval catheters on a gynecologic oncology service. Gynecol Oncol 70:329–333
3. Biffi R, de Braud F, Orsi F et al (1998) Totally implantable central venous access ports for long-term chemotherapy. A prospective study analyzing complications and costs of 333 devices with a minimum follow-up of 180 days. Ann Oncol 9:767–773
4. Laurenzi L, Natoli S, Benedetti C et al (2004) Cutaneous bacterial colonization, modalities of chemotherapeutic infusion, and catheter-related bloodstream infection in totally implanted venous access devices. Support Care Cancer 12:805–809
5. Domingo P, Fontanet A (2001) Management of complications associated with totally implantable ports in patients with AIDS. AIDS Patient Care STDS 15:7–13
6. Tenney JH, Moody MR, Newman KA et al (1986) Adherent microorganisms on lumenal surfaces of long-term intravenous catheters. Importance of Staphylococcus epidermidis in patients with cancer. Arch Intern Med 146:1949–1954
7. Schwarz RE, Groeger JS, Coit DG (1997) Subcutaneously implanted central venous access devices in cancer patients: a prospective analysis. Cancer 79:1635–1640

8. Kurul S, Saip P, Aydin T (2002) Totally implantable venous-access ports: local problems and extravasation injury. Lancet Oncol 3:684–692
9. Greene JN (1996) Catheter-related complications of cancer therapy. Infect Dis Clin North Am 10:255–295
10. Wickham R, Purl S, Welker D (1992) Long-term central venous catheters: issues for care. Semin Oncol Nurs 8:133–147
11. Bouza E, Burillo A, Muñoz P (2002) Catheter-related infections: diagnosis and intravascular treatment. Clin Microbiol Infect 8:265–274
12. Safdar A, Mermel LA, Maki DG (2004) The epidemiology of catheter-related infection in the critically ill. In: O'Grady NP, Pittet D (eds) Catheter-related infections in the critically ill. Kluwer, Boston, pp 1–22
13. Cherifi S, Jacobs F, Strale H et al (2007) Outcome of totally implantable venous access device-related bacteraemia without device removal. Clin Microbiol Infect 13:592–598

Thrombosis

23

Zhang Qinming

Abstract

Catheter-related thrombosis is one of the late complications of totally implantable venous access port. Until now, few studies have introduced the practice of totally implantable venous access port in the clinical setting. On the basis of an extensive literature review, this chapter describes the definitions of various central venous catheter-related thrombosis, thrombogenic mechanism, clinical manifestations of thrombosis, diagnosis, prevention and treatment. The different incidence, catheter inserting technique, clinical presentations and treatment between adults and children are also demonstrated. The diagram, table and photographs from clinical cases are used to directly illustrate one of the most common complication of central venous access. The summary of both basic and clinical studies may help or serve as a guidance to provide clinical care for those in need of totally implantable venous access devices.

Keywords

Central venous catheter • Totally implantable venous access device • Thrombosis • Sleeve thrombus • Fibrin sheaths • Deep venous thrombosis • Thrombolytic agents • Anticoagulant • Heparin • Venography

23.1 Introduction

One of the most common complications of totally implantable venous access devices (TIVADs) is catheter-related thrombosis. This usually occurs later dur-

Z. Qinming (✉)
Pediatric Surgery, Beijing Children's Hospital affiliated to Capital University of Medicine
Beijing, China
e-mail: qzhang9611@yahoo.com

ing the port and catheter dwell time. The incidence of catheter-related thrombosis ranges from less than 1% to 56% in some reports [1], depending largely on the definitions used. Occlusion of the catheter and its connected port (unable to infuse or withdraw) due to thrombosis is the most common cause of failure in long-term TIVADs [2].

23.2 Types of Thrombosis

Thrombosis may occur both in the TIVAD and its dwelling vein. Sleeve thrombosis is the most common type and it tends to occur earlier [3–5]. The catheter sleeve becomes covered with an adherent coating of fibrin and collagen which envelopes the outer surface of the catheter and extends along the entire length of the catheter from the point of insertion in the vein to the tip. Sometimes it may extend beyond the tip and appear as a small freely floating tail suspended in the deep vein. Although the catheter sleeve presents a benign complication, it interferes with catheter function, is prone to developing local infection and sepsis, and may progress to a less common mural veno-occlusive thrombosis (Fig. 23.1).

Another rare type of thrombosis is clot formation inside the TIVAD – both the port chamber and catheter lumen – which leads to TIVAD dysfunction. The thrombosis may completely obstruct the lumen causing aspiration and flush failure. A compressed flush can cause catheter disconnection or migration as well as venous thromboembolism. Over 20 mL saline flush after infusion and blood drawing is the key-point for care providers to prevent thrombosis inside the TIVAD (Fig. 23.2).

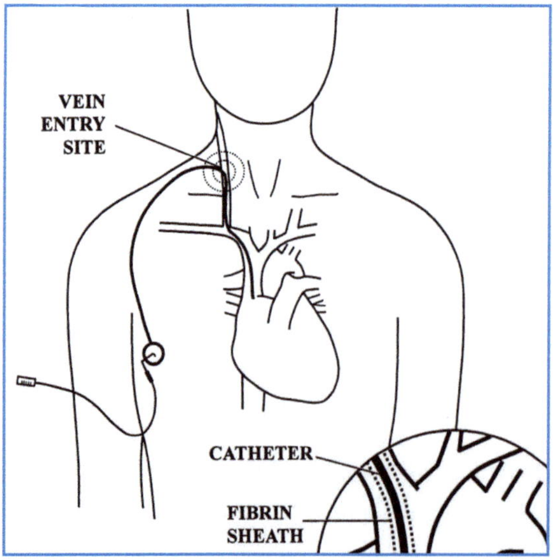

Fig. 23.1 Approach of central venous catheterization via external jugular vein cutdown. Detailed section shows the formation of sleeve thrombus

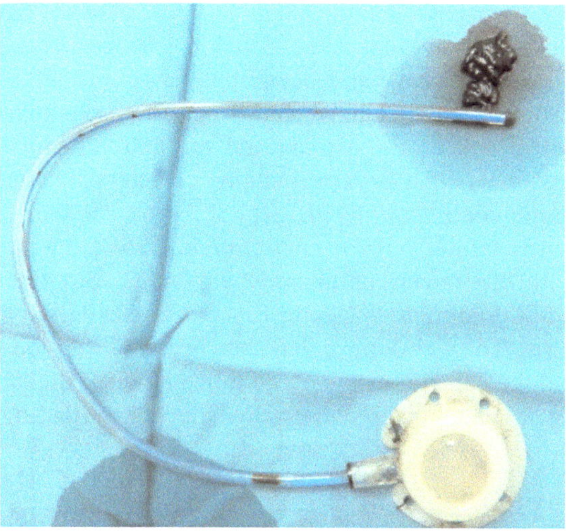

Fig. 23.2 Blood clots were washed from the TIVAD which was dysfunctional and was removed 305 days after insertion

A mural veno-occlusive thrombus occupying the lumen of the vein can result in partial or complete obstruction of the vessel. The thrombus becomes attached to the vessel wall where the catheter enters the greater part of its extent. For this reason, it is more adherent to the vein than a fibrin sheath and therefore less likely to be separated from it. The estimated incidence of mural thrombus has been found to be similar for both subclavian and jugular accesses [6]. However, catheterization through external jugular cutdown is less likely to cause thrombosis than through subclavian puncture [7].

23.3 Thrombogenic Mechanism

Many factors are believed to predispose a patient to thrombus formation. Vessel injury can be caused by catheterization, especially repeat blind venous puncture. Damage to the intimal layer of a vessel contributes to mural thrombosis. Intimal trauma may be caused by catheter insertion, the mechanical pressure of the stiff catheter from within (the narrower indwelling vessels are, the more crush injury may occur) and continuous infusion of chemotherapeutic agents. Slowing of indwelling venous blood flow also promotes thrombogenesis. It has been reported that cancer patients are usually in a hypercoagulable state: intrapulmonary or mediastinal tumor compression can lead to reduced blood flow in the venous system. Catheters with a long dwell time are more likely to generate thrombi than those with a short dwell time [8].

Catheter material has in recent years been recognized as a risk factor for developing thrombus. The biocompatibility of catheters (i.e. biochemical structure, diameter, rigidity, surface structure, and other additive agents) may play a certain role in thrombogenicity. Other impact factors like catheter tip position, side of insertion, insertion techniques and catheter-related complications (catheter dysfunction or infection) have also been hypothesized to affect thrombosis in some studies, but other studies have shown that there seems to be no relation between the incidence of thrombosis and the above factors. There has also been controversy on whether heparin-bonding catheters are able to significantly reduce thrombotic complications [9, 10].

The sleeve thrombus is usually termed a *fibrin sheath* to describe the well-formed translucent white sheath that covers chronically implanted catheters. The development of these sheaths coating the catheter first starts as a dark red sleeve thrombus containing fibrin. The sleeve thrombus then becomes a fibrous connective tissue sheath around the catheter as the dwell time elapses. Finally, the sheath completely encases the catheter, incorporating the freely floating clot at the catheter tip.

23.4 Clinical Manifestations of Thrombosis

Most patients with central venous catheter-related (CVC-related) thrombus are asymptomatic or have nonspecific clinical manifestations. Some studies have shown that only 6% of patients with CVC-related deep venous thrombosis (DVT) found by venography presented clinical manifestations [11].

Upper-limb DVT is more likely to have clinical presentations of arm swelling, erythema, pain, neck swelling, distal limb paresthesia, headache and congestion of subcutaneous collateral veins. Most cases with DVT are less symptomatic because thrombosis is not acute and less completely obstructive.

Catheter dysfunction may however be the common initial clinical manifestation of an otherwise asymptomatic CVC-related DVT. The presentation of acute respiratory failure indicates pulmonary embolism caused by the disconnection of thrombi from the catheter or DVT wall. Pulmonary embolism is the most serious complication of CVC-related DVT. The incidence of pulmonary embolism is estimated at approximately 12% in some reports [12]. Although pulmonary embolism rarely has clinical symptoms, patients with a CVC for total parenteral nutrition were reported to present a high incidence of this complication as the initial clinical presentation of venous thromboembolism.

A sleeve thrombus rarely produces any clinical symptoms. The fibrin sheaths covering the surface of the catheter or a free-floating clot at the catheter tip may produce a common problem found in long-dwelling catheters - *persistent withdrawal difficulty* - until aspiration fails completely. The preservation of the functions of infusing or flushing well is another characteristic which is symptomatic of sleeve thrombosis. When the fibrin sheath has completely encased the catheter, the catheter will be unable to function completely, i.e. neither be flushed nor aspirated. Fluid injected into the catheter can backtrack along the space between the catheter and the sheath and may cause pain to the neck or chest wall. In patients with a totally implanted venous access port, fluid may backtrack along the catheter resulting in extravasation into the tissue surrounding the port or catheter, even if the catheter and port have been disconnected.

23.5 Diagnosis of Thrombosis in TIVADs and Deep Veins

The most likely cause of TIVAD dysfunction is the obstruction of CVC or its dwelling vessels caused by thrombosis. Contrast venography is the definitive examination and considered the reference standard in detecting suspected thrombosis of both TIVADs and deep veins (Fig. 23.3). However, contrast venography is not recommended for diagnosis or investigation as a routine procedure due to its invasiveness, high cost and because the contrast material may aggravate existing thrombosis. Computed tomography of the chest may provide significant help for those with upper extremity deep venous thrombosis. Ultrasonography (US) with Doppler and color imaging has been recently used to confirm the diagnosis. The main findings of color-Doppler US are the visualization of mural thrombi (Fig. 23.4) or incompressible veins, the absence of normal blood flow or the presence of turbulent flow. The rhythmic pulsation produced by cardiac or respiratory motion may also disappear and show imaging signs of increased venous collateral circulation. Color-Doppler US is believed to be more sensitive in detecting the fibrin sheaths that cover the catheter surface by visualizing the thicker tip of the catheter or freely floating clot there. Despite its doubtless merit, the role of Doppler is still a matter of debate. Some studies have considered it unreliable because the superficial collateral vessels may be mistaken for normal deep venous blood flow. Recently,

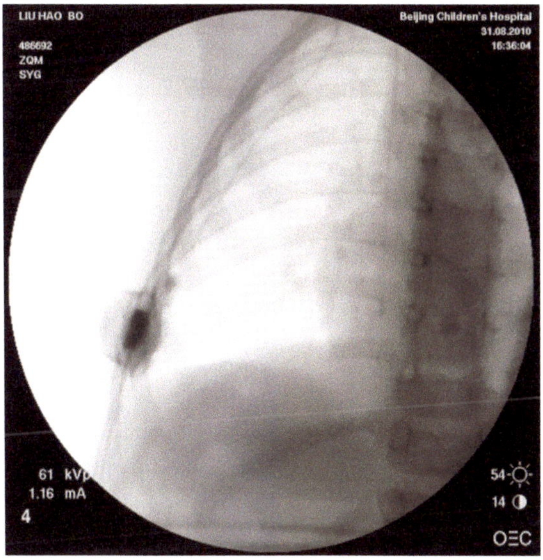

Fig. 23.3 Contrast venography shows thrombosis in the catheter blocking the passage of contrast agent into the atrium

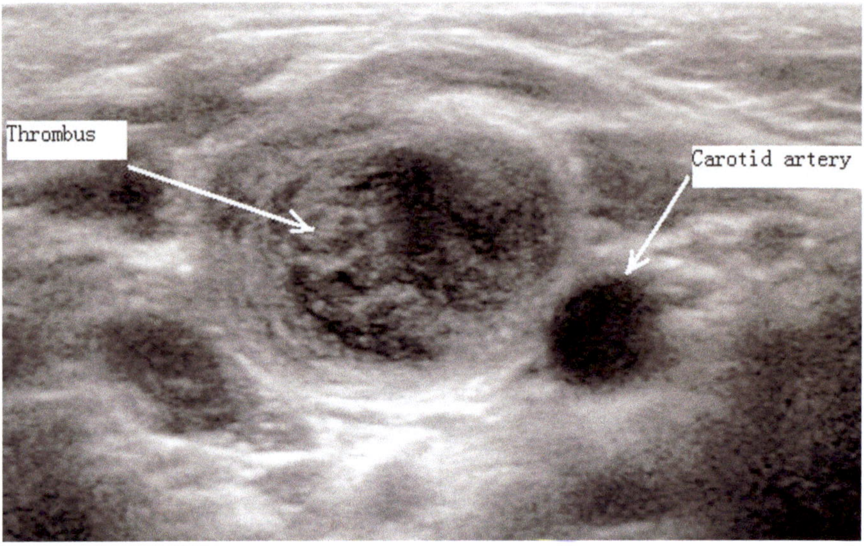

Fig. 23.4 Sonogram shows thrombus formed in right jugular vein. The patient presented mild swelling at the right neck two weeks after central venous catheterization

magnetic resonance venography and spiral computed tomography have been used both in the preinsertion evaluation of the central veins and in the diagnosis of suspected CVC-related deep venous thrombosis. However the role of these two imaging modalities in the diagnosis of CVC-related thrombosis needs to be confirmed by additional investigations using venography as a reference standard.

23.6 Prevention and Treatment

Various methods have been adopted to overcome the problem of catheter-related thrombosis. Minimizing frequent punctures and reducing injury to the central veins by using US guidance or choosing the cutdown procedure for catheterization are thought to be effective methods for preventing venous injury and reducing thrombosis. Central catheter insertion through peripheral veins such as the external jugular or basilic veins has been demonstrated to decrease the incidence of subclavian injury and reduce deep venous thrombosis [7]. The prophylactic use of oral anticoagulants, low-dose heparin and more than 20 mL normal saline flush for the entire TIVAD each time blood is drawn are believed to lower the rate of thrombus development.

Many studies [13–17] have been conducted on the prevention of CVC-related thrombosis during chemotherapy. Different types of anticoagulants, different dosage of anticoagulants and different subjects (adults and children) were included in these studies (Table 23.1). Both positive and negative results

Table 23.1 Clinical study of thrombosis prophylaxis in cancer patients with central venous catheter

Study	Study Design	No. of patients	Prophylactic regimens	Duration	Assessment	Thrombosis (%)	*p*
Bern (1990)	Prospective open-label, controlled	82	Warfarin 1 mg, No treatment	90 days	Venography	9.5 (37.5)	<.001
Monreal (1996)	Prospective open-label, controlled	29	Dalteparin 2500U, No treatment	90 days	Venography	6 (62)	0.002
Protekt (2001)	Randomized open-label, controlled	188 children	Reviparin 30-50U/kg Standard care	30+14 days	Venography	14.1 (12.5)	0.82
Reitchard (2002)	Randomized, double-blind, controlled	439	Dalteparin 5000U	16 weeks Placebo	Symptomatic events	3.7 (3.4)	0.9
Mismetti (2003)	Randomized, double-blind	57	Nodroparin 2850U Warfarin 1 mg	90 days	Venography	28.6 (16.7)	0.48

were obtained to demonstrate that the safety and effectiveness of daily prophylactic use of anticoagulants have not been confirmed and are still under debate. In our experience, avoiding damage to central veins and thoroughly carrying out post-insertion standard care are the key to preventing thrombosis rather than the prophylactic use of anticoagulants.

The management of CVC-related deep venous thrombosis should differ in the various clinical settings and it depends on clinical manifestations such as catheter dysfunction, local pain and swelling, and the risk of bleeding. Obstruction, causing failure to infuse through or withdraw blood from catheters, is common and occurs in up to 25% of catheters or ports in some studies [18, 19]. The purposes of treatment of CVC-related deep venous thrombosis are to reduce mortality and morbidity from the urgent situation and to minimize late complications. Once a thrombus has formed, it may occlude the catheter resulting in treatment delay, surgical replacement, patient discomfort, and increased cost of care. Management for a thrombus is more difficult. Urokinase was the only approved pharmacologic agent by the Food and Drug Administration for medical treatment of thrombosed venous catheters before 1999. However, given the concern of the potential to transmit infection, urokinase has been potentially replaced by streptokinase for clinical application. Urokinase or streptokinase are effective as a short course of intrathrombus infusion for an acute occlusion. However, as most clots develop gradually over time with or without mild clinical manifestation before being confirmed, the clinical effectiveness of these two agents is limited. Catheter function is often restored with 5000-unit intracatheter boluses of urokinase. Some studies have shown that repeated intracatheter boluses of urokinase have no significant impact on catheter function return and that the rate of catheter function return in the pediatric group was higher than in the adult group. William and Robert [20] reported a group of patients who were successfully treated for their catheter function return with 6-hour continuous urokinase infusion after failure of bolus urokinase. Urokinase and streptokinase have also been used for the treatment catheters occluded by fibrin sheaths. Thrombolytic agents would be more successful at the early stage of a thrombus attached to the tip of the catheter. However, once the free-floating thrombus is replaced by a fully encasing fibrous sheath, urokinase and streptokinase are unlikely to dissolve it. Many studies have demonstrated the efficacy and safety of low-molecular-weight heparin (LMWH) in treating upper or lower limb deep venous thrombosis and occluded catheters by 5 to 7 days intravenous administration plus continuous oral anticoagulation. There is no need for thrombolysis and catheter removal in patients with deep venous thrombosis without severe clinical manifestation or the risk of venous thromboembolism and catheter occlusion.

References

1. DeBona R (1999) Thrombotic complications of central venous catheters in cancer patients. Semin Thromb Hemost 25:147-155

2. Lokich JJ, Bothe A, Benotti P et al (1985) Complications and management of implanted venous access catheters. J Clin Oncol 3:710-717
3. Hoch JR (1997) Management of the complications of long-term venous access. Semin Vasc Surg 10:135-143
4. Martin C, Viviand X, Saux P et al (1999) Upper extremity deep vein thrombosis after central venous catheterization via the axillary vein. Crit Care Med 27:2626-2629
5. Xiang DZ, Verbeken EK, Van Lommel AT et al (1998) Composition and formation of the sleeve enveloping a central venous catheter. J Vasc Surg 28:260-271
6. Ruesch S, Walder B, Tramer MR (2002) Complications of central venous catheters: Internal jugular versus subclavian access—A systematic review. Crit Care Med 30:454-460
7. Zhang Qinming, Jiao Lii, Zhou Hong (2009) Comparison of implantable central venous ports with catheter insertion via external jugular cut down and subclavian puncture in children: single center experience. Pediatr Surg Int 25:499-501
8. Horattas MC, Wright DJ, Fenton AH et al (1998) Changing concepts of deep venous thrombosis of the upper extremity – Report of series and review of the literature. Surgery 104:561-567
9. Brismar BO, Hardstedt C, Jacobson S (1981) Diagnosis of thrombosis by catheter phlebography after prolonged central venous catheterisation. Ann Surg 194:779-783
10. Pierce CM, Wade A, Mok Q (2000) Heparin-bonded central venous lines reduce thrombotic and infective complications in critically ill children. Intensive Care Med 26:967-972
11. De Cicco M, Matovic M, Balestrieri L et al (1997) Central venous thrombosis: An early and frequent complication in cancer patients bearing long term silastic catheter—A prospective study. Thromb Res 86:101-113
12. Horattas MC, Wright DJ, Fenton AH et al (1988) Changing concepts of deep venous thrombosis of the upper extremity—report of a series and review of the literature. Surgery 104:561-567
13. Bern HM, Lokich JJ, Wallach SR et al (1990) Very low dose of warfarin can prevent thrombosis in central venous catheters: A randomized, prospective trial. Ann Inter Med 112:423-428
14. Monreal M, Alastrue A, Rull M et al (1996) Upper extremity deep venous thrombosis in cancer patients with venous access devices: Prophylaxis with a low molecular weight heparin (Fragmin). Thromb Haemost 75:251-253
15. Massicotte P, Julian JA, Gent M et al (2003) An open-label randomized controlled trial of low molecular weight heparin for the prevention of central venous line related thrombotic complications in children: The PROTEKT study. Thromb Res 109:101-108
16. Reichardt P, Kretzschmar A, Biakhov M et al (2002) A phase III, randomized, double-blind, placebo-controlled study evaluating the efficacy and safety of daily low-molecular-weight-heparin (dalteparin sodium) in preventing catheter-related complications (CRCs) in cancer patients with central venous catheters (CVCs). Proc Am Soc Clin Oncol 21:369a (abstr 1474)
17. Mismetti P, Mille D, Laporte S et al (2003) Low-molecular-weight heparin (nadroparin) and very low doses of warfarin in the prevention of upper extremity thrombosis in cancer patients with indwelling long-term central venous catheters: A pilot randomized trial. Haematologica 88:67-73
18. Raaf JH (1985) Results from the use of 826 vascular access devices in cancer patients. Cancer 55:1312-1321
19. Hurtubise MR, Bottino JC, Lawson M et al (1980) Restoring patency of occluded central venous catheters. Arch Surg 115:212-213
20. William DH, Robert PL (1992) Thrombosed central venous catheters: Restoring function with 6-hour urokinase infusion after failure of bolus urokinase. JPEN J Parenter Enteral Nutr 16:129-132

Superior Vena Cava Erosion and Perforation

24

Francesca Ratti, Michele Paganelli, Marco Catena and Luca Aldrighetti

Abstract

The most important predisposing factor to caval perforation is prolonged contact of the end of the catheter against the vein wall, as occurs more frequently in cases of catheter insertion through collateral vessels of the left innominate vein. The initial clinical manifestations of vascular perforation include cardiopulmonary symptoms (chest pain or dyspnea) or radiographic evidence of a new or rapidly progressive pleural effusion. The curved tip sign usually precedes other clinical and radiographic signs of perforation. Recognition of a gentle curve of the catheter tip should prompt readjustment or replacement of its position to avoid vessel perforation, which may result in hydrothorax and pneumothorax, hydromediastinum, and pericardial effusion, all potentially life-threatening complications. Once diagnosed, the catheter must be removed promptly.

Keywords

Erosion • Perforation • Superior vena cava • Curved-tip sign • Mediastinal effusion • Hydrothorax • Implantable venous port

24.1 Introduction

Erosion and perforation of the superior vena cava are uncommon complications that may occur after a variable length of time following totally

F. Ratti (✉)
Department of Surgery, Hepatobiliary Surgery Unit, San Raffaele Hospital,
Vita-Salute San Raffaele University,
Milano, Italy
e-mail: ratti.francesca@hsr.it

I. Di Carlo, R. Biffi (eds.), *Totally Implantable Venous Access Devices*,

implantable venous port positioning. Since the literature consists of isolated cases, the incidence of this rare complication cannot be defined with certainty, but it seems to approach 0.4-1.0% of catheter placements [1, 2]. At any rate, the true incidence may be considerably higher, considering the tendency of catheter erosion to remain unrecognized.

24.2 Pathogenesis

Pathogenesis is connected to a prolonged recumbency of the end of the catheter on the vein wall, leading to persistent trauma exacerbated by cardiac and respiratory movements [3]. The most important predisposing factor to caval perforation is prolonged contact of the end of the catheter against the vein wall, as occurs more frequently in cases of catheter insertion through collateral vessels of the left innominate vein. The left innominate vein joins the superior vena cava almost at right angles, so that by forcing the catheter especially in cases of access through the left jugular vein [4], the catheter takes a course which pushes the tip against the right margin of the caval wall [3]. The right innominate vein instead flows into the superior vena cava almost vertically, allowing the catheter a straight a course, with the tip almost parallel to the wall of the vena cava. For these reasons preferential port positioning in right veins is frequently suggested [3-6].

24.3 Diagnosis

The position of the catheter against the caval wall is radiologically detectable by the presence of an obtuse angle between the tip of the catheter and the right margin of the vena cava [6], also referred to as the curved-tip sign [2]. Several cases of perforation of the superior vena cava also by silicone and polyurethane catheters have been described [2], although it is considered that the risk is minimized by the use of these catheters [5, 7]. The intimal lesion that precedes perforation often leads to the development of thrombosis of the vessel wall: mural thrombosis is in fact described in the innominate-caval junction in 19% of autopsy reports of central venous catheter carriers [8]. Mural thrombosis, which may subsequently affect more or less extensively the lumen of the vena cava and its tributaries, is an element of protection from severe hemorrhage at the moment of perforation [6]. The *haemostatic effect* of the mural thrombus accounts for the typical presentation of [2] mediastinal effusion, hydrothorax with or without unilateral or bilateral effusion, secondary to the passage of infusions within the mediastinum, in contrast to bleeding complications due to injuries occurring during the positioning procedure, which may require surgical repair of the lesion [9]. The hemostatic parietal thrombus causes lesions which are often self-limiting, with the treatment of choice being the removal of the catheter and hydromediastinum/hydrothorax drainage [3].

Duntley et al. [1] reported outcomes from eight patients who developed superior vena cava perforation and erosion. The initial clinical manifestation of vascular perforation comprised cardiopulmonary symptoms (chest pain or dyspnea) or radiographic evidence of a new or rapidly progressive pleural effusion. Less common manifestations of patients include cough and Horner's syndrome. Symptoms may appear suddenly with rapid progression or as a nonspecific discomfort with an indolent evolution [10, 11]. Concomitant enlarging pleural effusions, mediastinal widening, increasing central venous pressure combined with progressive systemic hypotension, and curving or extravascular location of the distal catheter segment strengthen the suspicion of erosion. Inability to withdraw blood from the catheter support the hypothesis of perforation but the possibility of free blood return does not rule out the diagnosis.

Milky pleural fluid is a diagnostic profile in patients receiving intravenous fat emulsions without other causes of chylothorax, but biochemical features of pleural fluid in patients infused with nonlipid infusions are highly variable: a high pleural fluid to serum glucose ratio is suggestive of catheter erosion, whereas protein concentration is not useful in diagnosis since it may vary depending on the protein content of the infused fluids, the infusion rate, pleural inflammation or hemorrhage [1].

Diagnostic delay due to the nonspecific nature of symptoms, their delayed onset and the underlying medical and surgical conditions increase morbidity and mortality.

The curved-tip sign usually precedes other clinical and radiographic signs of perforation by hours or days [8]. Since it occurs after catheter insertion, catheter perforation of the caval wall is not usually considered to be a likely explanation for the patient's deterioration. The diagnosis may be further delayed by the observation of prompt return blood from the catheter. However, blood return does not rule out an extravascular position of the catheter tip, since most catheters haves side holes [3]. The central venous catheter should be placed in the superior vena cava distal to the last venous valve in the innominate vein and proximal to the pericardial reflection over the superior vena cava. In the chest radiograph this corresponds to the segment of the superior vena cava between the head of the clavicle and the arch of the azygos vein. The tip of the catheter should be parallel to the wall of the vessel. Catheter position should be checked periodically with chest radiographs in all patients with totally implantable venous access ports [12]. Since this sign may be most often visible on lateral chest radiographs, this view should be included in port follow-up. Recognition of a gentle curve of the catheter tip should prompt readjustment or replacement of its position to avoid vessel perforation, which may result in hydrothorax and pneumothorax, hydromediastinum, and pericardial effusion, all potentially life-threatening complications.

24.4 Treatment

Once diagnosed, the catheter must be removed promptly, allowing pleural fluid reabsorption, although thoracentesis may improve outcomes in some cases of patients with respiratory distress.

References

1. Duntley P, Siever J, Korwes ML et al (1992) Vascular erosion by central venous catheters. Clinical features and outcome. Chest 101:1633-1638
2. Ellis LM, Vogel SB III, Copeland EM (1989) Central venous catheter vascular erosions. Ann Surg 209:475-478
3. Tocino IM, Watanabe A (1986) Impending catheter perforation of superior vena cava. AJR 146:487
4. Iberti TJ, Katz B, Reiner MA et al (1983) Hydrothorax as a late complication of central venous indwelling catheters. Surgery 94:842
5. Sheep RE, Guiney WB (1982) Fatal cardiac tamponade. JAMA 248:1632
6. Russell SJ, Giles FJ, Edwards D (1987) Perforation of superior vena cava by indwelling central venous catheters. Lancet 94:842
7. Krog M, Berggren L, Brodin M et al (1982) Pericardial tamponade caused by central venous catheters. World J Surg 6:138
8. Ducatman BS, McMichan JC, Edwards WD (1985) Catheter-induced lesions of the right side of the heart: a one-year prospective study of 141 autopsies. JAMA 253:791
9. Sarajego J, Bootorabi B, Matsumoto T et al (1993) Major long term complications in 1422 permanent venous access devices. Am J Surg 165:249
10. Milam MG, Sahn SA (1988) Horner's syndrome secondary to hydromediastinum: a complication of extravascular migration of central venous catheter. Chest 94:1093-1095
11. Macksood MJ, Setter M (1983) Hydrothorax and hydromediastinum after use of an indwelling percutaneous catheter introducer. Crit Care Med 11:957-958
12. Aldrighetti L, Caterini R, Ronzoni M (1995) Ruolo dei sistemi totalmente impiantabili per accesso vascolare a lungo termine nel trattamento del paziente neoplastico. Minerva Chir 50:447

Catheter Obstruction

25

Francesca Ratti, Marco Catena, Michele Paganelli and Luca Aldrighetti

Abstract

Catheter obstruction is a venous access port related complication occurring when infusion and withdrawal of blood from the system are not possible and is caused by the formation of a blood clot or other substances precipitation.

Frequent infusion through the catheter of solutions containing heparin and positive-pressure locking techniques reduce occlusion incidence. A correct management of a suspected occlusion requires a chest radiograph to verify the correct positioning of the catheter and a Doppler Ultrasound or venography to evaluate the possibility of vascular thrombosis. Catheter obstruction is usually successfully treated by infusion of a fibrinolytic agent.

Keywords

Catheter obstruction • Infusion • Withdrawal • Withdrawal malfunction • Flushing • Positive-pressure locking techniques • Fibrinolytic agent

25.1 Introduction

Catheter obstruction is a venous access port related complication characterized by the impossibility to infuse substances and withdraw blood. This complication should be distinguished from simple withdrawal malfunction, which is the commonest type of catheter malfunction causing the loss of capacity to

F. Ratti (✉)
Department of Surgery, Hepatobiliary Surgery Unit, San Raffaele Hospital,
Vita-Salute San Raffaele University,
Milano, Italy
e-mail: ratti.francesca@hsr.it

I. Di Carlo, R. Biffi (eds.), *Totally Implantable Venous Access Devices*,

withdraw blood from the catheter without difficulty infusing through it [1, 2]. The reported frequency of totally implantable venous access port withdrawal malfunction varies from 0.8% to 5.0% [1, 2]. This problem is mainly connected to the development of a fibrin sheath around the tip of the catheter, acting as a one-way flap valve and hindering blood collection from the port. The impact of the catheter tip against the vein wall can also occur when aspiration pulls the wall against the catheter orifice. In over 90% of cases, withdrawal occlusion can be relieved by the acquirement of Trendelenburg position, saline infusion, or injection of fibrinolytic drugs [3].

25.2 Diagnosis and Prevention

Catheter occlusion, with an incidence reported in the literature ranging between 1.5% and 13% [4], can be quickly recognized when infusion and withdrawal of blood from the system are not possible: the most frequent cause is the reflux of blood in the catheter which results in the formation of a blood clot, although it also may be secondary to the infusion of substances with a high density (high-fat parenteral nutrition) or solutions containing substances that are incompatible, which may precipitate in the lumen of the catheter. In order to reduce the risk of catheter occlusion, some precautions should be taken. Firstly, infusion through the catheter of solutions containing heparin should be made after each injection, infusion or blood sampling and also in the intervals between one use and another. Flushing must be performed using the turbulent flush technique to prevent buildup or accumulation of fibrin and precipitated medication inside the catheter lumen [5]. The turbulent flush technique is achieved with a push-pause method. Secondly, in order to prevent blood reflux from the vein into the lumen of the catheter, positive-pressure locking techniques must be used. A previous study has shown that the positive-pressure technique is not widespread in all the centers where venous access ports are implanted [6], even though most series indicate that flushing must be performed every 4 weeks when the device is not in use [7]. However, a retrospective study suggests that less frequent flushing could be as safe and feasible [8]; indeed, the results from an Italian report show that flushing in some oncologic centers is performed at intervals greater than 30 days when the venous access port is not in use [6].

With regard to the failure of the device, incorrect positioning of a Huber needle (which is the most common cause of pseudo-obstruction of the system) and occlusion of the needle itself or the external connection need to be ruled out. The correct management of a suspected occlusion requires a chest radiograph to verify the correct positioning of the catheter and a Doppler ultrasound or venography to evaluate the possibility of vascular thrombosis.

25.3 Treatment

When a malposition or kinking that causes malfunction is observed on the chest radiograph, the system may have to be removed depending on the degree of dysfunction. Catheter obstruction is usually successfully treated by infusion of a fibrinolytic agent (streptokinase, 8,000-25,000 U, or urokinase, 5,000-250,000 U) [9] possibly followed by a second administration, after 5-6 hours, if the first attempt is ineffective [10]. The risk of breakage of the catheter secondary to the application of excessive pressure has to be taken into consideration when infusing solutions to remove the obstruction since pressures greater than 2000 mmHg can be exerted when using a syringe with less than 10 mL capacity.

Dal Molin et al. [11] carried out a multicenter prospective observational study in 26 Italian oncologic centers to analyze the outcome of 1082 patients. Of these 1076 oncologic patients with central venous access ports totally implanted entered the study. During follow-up, 515 patients were undergoing treatment while 561 patients required only flushing since chemotherapy treatment had been concluded. Occlusions were observed in both groups of patients. Eight patients in the first group and three in the second had occlusion, with an incidence of 0.24/1000 days and of 0.03/1000 days respectively. In their study, flushing was performed between 61 and 80 days in 22 devices and after more than 81 days in 81 cases with no recorded complications in these patients. These data, according to Kuo [8], suggest the possibility of flushing the totally implantable venous port at intervals greater than 4 weeks with no documented consequences on device functioning, even if more extensive trials should be carried out to validate this statement.

Obstruction, similar to other port related complications, can be avoided by the careful selection and preparation of the patient and by an attentive approach to implantation and subsequent handling.

References

1. Di Carlo I, Cordio S, La Gresa G et al (2001) Totally implantable venous access devices implanted surgically: a retrospective study on early and late complications. Arch Surg 136:1050–1053
2. Biffi R, De Braud F, Orsi F et al (2001) A randomized, prospective trial of central venous ports connected to standard open-ended or Groshong catheters in adult oncology patients. Cancer 92:1204–1212
3. Kurul S, Saip P, Aydin T (2002) Totally implantable venous-access ports: local problems and extravasation injury. Lancet Oncol 3:684-693
4. Aldrighetti L, Caterini R, Ronzoni M (1995) Ruolo dei sistemi totalmente impiantabili per accesso vascolare a lungo termine nel trattamento del paziente neoplastico. Minerva Chir 50:447
5. Gallieni M, Pittiruti M, Biffi R (2008) Vascular access in oncology patients. CA Cancer J Clin 58:323-346

6. Dal Molin A, Guerretta L, Mazzufero F et al (2009) The management of totally implanted venous ports in the ambulatory oncologic patient. J Vasc Access 10:22-26
7. Vescia S, Baumgartner AK, Jacobs VR et al (2008) Management of venous port systems in oncology: a review of current evidence. Ann Oncol 19:9-15
8. Kuo YS, Schwartz B, Santiago J et al (2005) How often should a port-A-cath be flushed? Cancer Inv 23:582-585
9. Brothers TE, Von Moll LK, Niederhuber JE et al (1988) Experience with subcutaneous infusion ports in three hundred patients. Surg Gynecol Obstet 166:295
10. Perrot D, Goullet D, Coiffier B (1987) Le systems d'access veineux implantables. Revue generale. Lyon-Pharmaceutique 38:237
11. Dal Molin A, Rasero L, Guerretta L et al (2010) The late complications of totally implantable central venous access ports: the results from an Italian multi center prospective observation study. Eur J Oncol Nurs 30:1-5

Catheter Rupture

26

Hong-Shiee Lai

Abstract

Catheter rupture after TIVAD insertion or during its removal is uncommon, but could become a severe late complication. Because catheter rupture is unexpected, the possibility of this complication should be always kept in mind during daily nursing care of TIVADs, especially when there is absence of blood return or resistance to flush is noted. The risk factors, ruptured sites, and possible symptoms and signs of catheter rupture should always be kept in mind during the setting, use, and removal of the TIVAD. Periodic routine chest radiography should be performed to check for rupture and proper positioning of the TIVAD catheter, especially before its removal. Once symptomatic or asymptomatic catheter rupture is identified, careful and total removal is always indicated to prevent further, more severe complications.

Keywords

TIVAD • Late complications • Catheter rupture • Risk factors • Subcutaneous tunnel • Removal • Infection • "Pinch-off" • Chest radiography • Portal-catheter junction • Extravasation • Adherence • Catheterization • Thrombosis • Venotomy

26.1 Introduction

Totally implantable venous access devices (TIVAD) currently play an essential role in chemotherapy agent injection and/or nutritional therapy. TIVADs are relatively safe and well accepted by both adult and pediatric patients,

H.-S. Lai (✉)
Department of Surgery, National Taiwan University Hospital,
Taipei, Taiwan
e-mail: hslai@ntu.edu.tw

although some early or late complications can occur. Among the late complications of TIVAD, catheter rupture is uncommon, but is relatively severe. The reported incidence of catheter rupture ranges from 0.1% to 2.1% [1, 2], but is most commonly reported to range from 1% to 1.9% [3, 4]. The true incidence may be higher, however, due to its underestimation in patients with no symptoms or signs, long-term TIVAD use to late-stage of malignant disease or even death. Catheter rupture can be asymptomatic; however, it also can result in severe local inflammation, thromboembolism, cardiac arrhythmia, or even sudden death. In this chapter, the risk factors, common sites, symptoms and signs, and management of catheter rupture are described.

26.2 Risk Factors for Catheter Rupture

Possible risk factors which cause catheter rupture include long-term use and repeated manipulations, manufacturing defects, material degradation, thromboembolism with deposition of fibrinous clots or calcium in the intravascular portion of the catheter, adhesion to the subcutaneous tunnel followed by difficult removal, acute angulation of the catheter, mechanical trauma especially during removal, infection with marked inflammation, frequent hemorrhagic episodes, and poor site for TIVAD insertion.

Long-term use and repeated manipulations can result in greater risk of catheter rupture, especially with rapid injection rates [5]. Difficult removing the TIVAD catheter could result in greater possibility of catheter rupture, which should be considered for catheters in situ for longer than 40 months [6]. A product guarantee of no manufacturing defects from a highly credible commercial company will prevent rupture due to poor materials and workmanship. Some practitioners report that TIVADs made of polyurethane appear to be unsuitable due to a high incidence of complications at the time of removal [6]. The thin plastic base of TIVADs results in a higher risk of TIVAD perforation, which is not seen with other devices [7]. Material fatigue followed with degradation may play a key role in catheter rupture [4, 8]. Deposition of fibrinous clots or calcium on the catheter increases the irregularity of the catheter surface, which then adheres to the vascular wall, making removal difficult. Catheter rupture is reported to occur either spontaneously or as a consequence of “pinch-off” syndrome caused by the compression of the catheter between the clavicle and the first rib due to poor site selection for insertion [9, 10]. Catheter rupture could also occur during forced removal from the vena cava or heart because of densely adherent calcification and obstruction of the catheter, causing the distal fragment to be retained in the vena cave or heart [6, 11, 12].

The TIVAD is usually inserted into the subclavian vein in adults or adolescents, with a smooth catheter curve into the vessel. In small children or infants, the external or internal jugular vein is commonly used for the site of catheter insertion. A subcutaneous tunnel from the neck to the subclavian area is then made for the extravascular part of the catheter. This procedure can result in fore-to-back 180° acute angulation of the catheter. Upon growth of the child, the angulation of the catheter could be changed and sometimes become more narrowed. Rupture of the catheter could occur due to high pressure resulting from the constant motion of the circulation within the acute angulation of the catheter, especially with frequent wide swinging of the arm and shoulder. Catheter rupture could also occur due to a local infection with inflammation or frequent pocket hematoma [6, 12]. A higher incidence of catheter rupture occurred with the subclavian route, often seen as the "pinch-off sign" on chest radiography [10]. Inadequate catheter length between the portal outlet tube and the vein entry site could cause shearing at the portal-catheter junction. Malfixation of the port to the local tissue may induce movement able to produce kinking at port-catheter junction, which might cause the catheter to rupture, especially in a small child. The subclavian portion of the catheter could be abraded and damaged by the clavicle with shoulder movement [3]. High pressure rapid pump infusion could cause either fluid extravasation (leakage) or catheter fracture and rupture [3, 13]. Very young patients under the age of one year old, small catheters, injection of caustic chemotherapeutic agents, and improper catheter care may also be risk factors for catheter rupture.

26.3 Sites for Catheter Rupture

Extravasation of fluid from a TIVAD catheter, which can be proven by contrast medium injection, could occur at the portal-catheter junction due to the catheter lock not being completely secured, at the port site due to use of too large a needle resulting in a large puncture hole, incorrect manipulation, or too frequent puncture, or at the catheter portion near the TIVAD-catheter junction directly due to rupture [7].

Catheter rupture sites are classified into four groups: (1) portal-catheter junction, (2) subcutaneous tunnel, (3) the site of catheter insertion into the venous system, and (4) the intravenous portion. The incidence of catheter rupture is higher at the portal-catheter junction (0.7%) than at the subcutaneous portion (0.3%) [3]. Biological inflammatory processes are one of the risk factors for catheter rupture, especially at the site of catheter insertion into the venous system [12]. Risk factors for catheter rupture occurring at the intravenous portion include adherence in situ to the local vein or migration into the vena cava, its tributaries, right heart, or the pulmonary arteries [9].

The catheter rupture site should be clearly demonstrated by chest radiography or by computed tomography (CT), as shown in Figure 26.1. The catheter rupture site at the portal-catheter junction (Fig. 26.2a), which occurs most frequently, can be clearly seen on chest radiography (Fig. 26.2b). Catheter rupture occurring in the intravenous portion or migrating into the vena cava, heart, or pulmonary artery is usually noted unexpectedly on routine chest radiography or CT, unless arrhythmia or sudden death occurred. The most common site for intravenous catheter rupture with a retained fragment was the subclavian

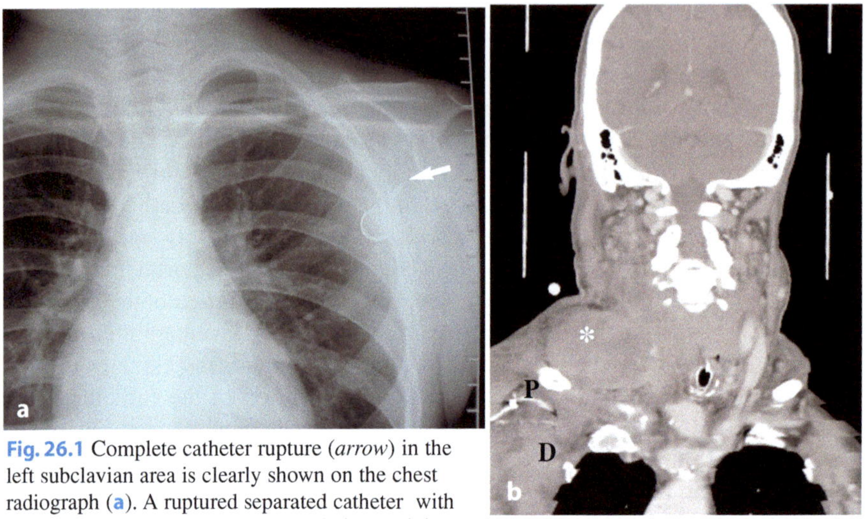

Fig. 26.1 Complete catheter rupture (*arrow*) in the left subclavian area is clearly shown on the chest radiograph (**a**). A ruptured separated catheter with fluid and hematoma accumulation (*) in the right lower neck area is shown on this computed tomogram (**b**). *P*, proximal; *D*, distal

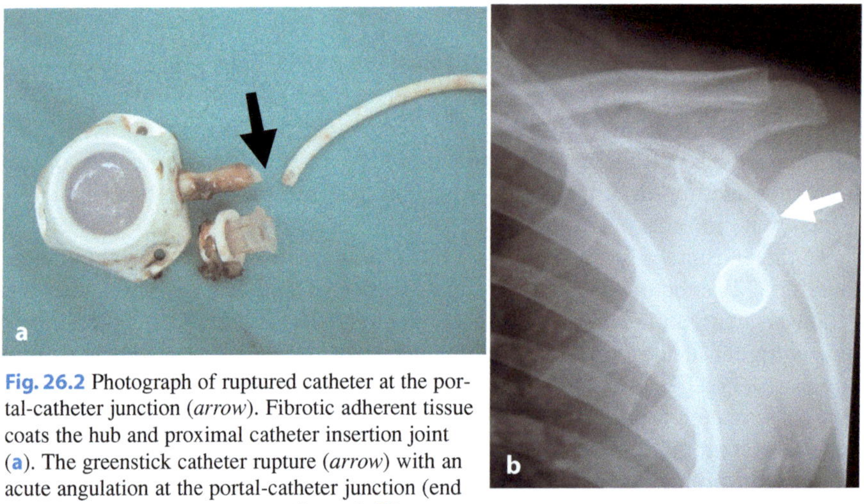

Fig. 26.2 Photograph of ruptured catheter at the portal-catheter junction (*arrow*). Fibrotic adherent tissue coats the hub and proximal catheter insertion joint (**a**). The greenstick catheter rupture (*arrow*) with an acute angulation at the portal-catheter junction (end of hub) is visible on the chest radiograph (**b**)

vein in situ, followed by migration into the superior vena cava, right atrium, right ventricle, and inferior vena cava. Only rare cases of ruptured catheter fragments migrating into the pulmonary artery are reported. Figure 26.3 shows an intravenous ruptured catheter that migrated into the superior vena cava, right atrium, and right ventricle. This ruptured catheter fragment was fortu-

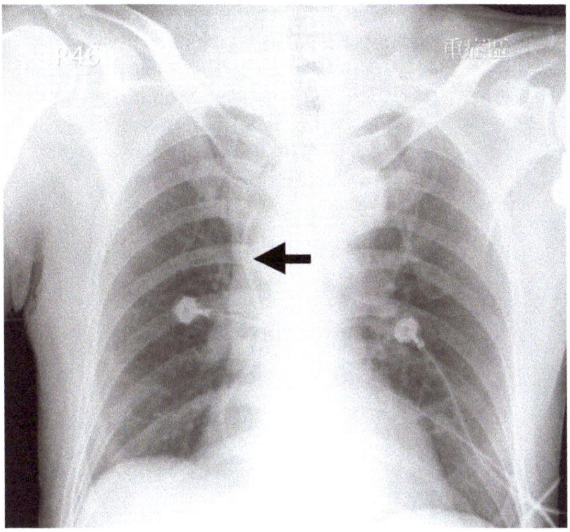

Fig. 26.3 Catheter rupture with distal fragment (*arrow*) migration into the superior vena cava and right heart is visible on the chest radiograph

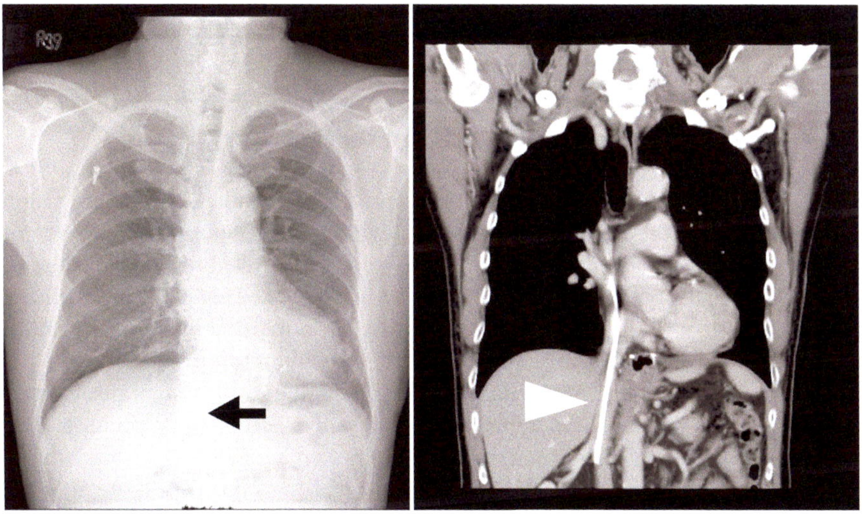

Fig. 26.4 Catheter rupture with distal fragment migration into the inferior vena cava is slightly visible (*arrow*) on the chest radiograph (**a**) and clearly visible on the computed tomogram (*arrowhead*) (**b**)

nately removed smoothly by transfemoral cardiac catheterization without any other complication. We treated one patient who experienced sudden arrhythmia, which occurred seven months after insertion of a TIVAD. Intravenous catheter rupture was suspected based on chest radiography, which vaguely showed a ruptured catheter fragment in the inferior vena cava (Fig. 26.4a). Further investigation by CT imaging clearly confirmed the catheter fragment was totally within inferior vena cava (Fig. 26.4b). The fragment was uneventfully removed by transfemoral catheterization.

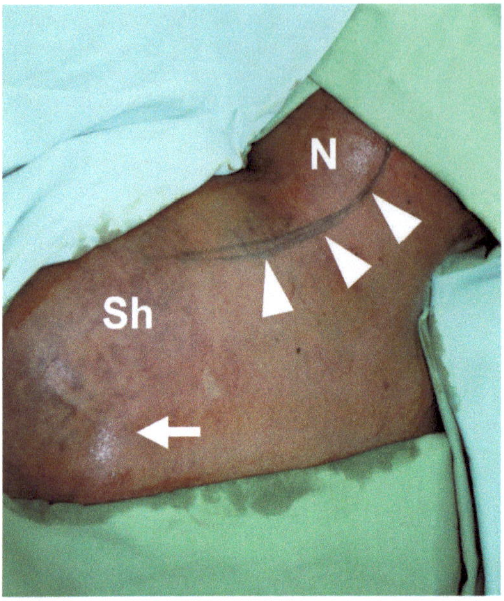

Fig. 26.5 Erythematous swelling and ecchymosis on the neck, shoulder, and port site (*arrow*). The distal fragment of the ruptured catheter is outlined (*arrowheads*) from the subclavian area to the venous insertion point in the neck. *N*, neck; *Sh*, shoulder

26.4 Symptoms and Signs of Catheter Rupture

For catheter ruptures occurring in the extravascular catheter portion, which includes the portal-catheter junction, subcutaneous tunnel, or the site of catheter insertion into the vein, extravasation of the infused fluid or leakage of a sanguineous discharge may occur, especially when the rupture site is near the superficial subcutaneous area, or particularly, in a malnourished patient with very thin skin, after insertion of the TIVAD. The symptoms and signs are the same for rupture sites occurring in the subcutaneous portion and portal-catheter junction. They include local swelling with fluctuating palpitation, erythematous skin, local pain, tenderness, and marked ecchymosis or hematoma. The local erythematous and hematomatous swelling could be more marked (Fig. 26.5) and more severely painful if the diagnosis of catheter rupture was delayed. Cellulitis and skin necrosis could also occur as a severe local complication if the catheter rupture is not managed well.

Infection, pulmonary abscess, arrhythmia, thrombosis with superior vena cava syndrome, erosion into contiguous structures, right atrium perforation, and sudden death have all been reported for catheter ruptures occurring in the intravenous portion [14]. Anemia due to bleeding from the rupture site could also be a systemic sign of catheter rupture. The catheter fragments retained within the central venous system could likely be related to thrombosis or catheter migration [14]. In a rare situation, pulmonary hypertension resulted from a retained TIVAD catheter fragment stuck within the pulmonary artery [9]. This patient died of pulmonary hypertension despite therapeutic anticoagulation and retrieval of the fragment via pulmonary artery catheterization.

Despite all the symptoms and signs of catheter rupture, most patients with intravenous catheter rupture are entirely asymptomatic because the ruptured catheter fragment adheres firmly to the vessel wall, prohibiting its migration [4, 6]. Some asymptomatic cases are found incidentally by routine chest radiography undertaken to determine progression of the underlying disease, even sometimes after removal of the TIVAD. For other asymptomatic but high risk patients, absence of blood return, or high resistance to flush fluid into the TIVAD should alert the clinician to the possibility of catheter rupture, and a chest radiograph should be obtained to verify its placement and patency.

26.5 Management of Catheter Rupture

Prevention of catheter rupture is always better than treatment for TIVAD catheter rupture. Careful selection of a good vessel for TIVAD insertion, suitable type, size, and quality of the TIVAD, and smooth angulation of the TIVAD catheter curve are important for preventing catheter rupture. Excessive arm swinging from the shoulder in small children should be avoided. Furthermore, proper nursing care is important for preventing catheter rupture: good skin disinfection, careful preparation for injection, avoiding high pressure infusion, and precise heparin concentration in normal saline irrigation to prevent thromboembolism help reduce the possibility of catheter rupture [15]. A chest radiograph should be obtained if there is absence of blood return, or high resistance to flush fluid into the TIVAD. All of these strategies are even more important in a patient with a TIVAD for chemotherapy to prevent inadvertent subcutaneous extravasation of potent chemotherapeutic agents.

Removal of a TIVAD is usually a simple procedure; nonetheless, chest radiography for showing the catheter position is always necessary before removal of a TIVAD. A careful check to verify whether the catheter has been completely removed is mandatory. A catheter that adheres firmly to a vessel wall can be left in situ, for it is not likely to migrate to the heart or lung [16], nonetheless, the potential consequences of a retained, fixed catheter fragment are uncertain. Venous thromboembolism [17], infection, induced endocarditis [18], and arrhythmia [6] are adverse events reported after the retention of catheters. For a stuck or retained, fixed catheter, venotomy or a cutdown technique is usually needed to retrieve the catheter. Endovascular intervention using a loop catheter has been successfully used to remove dislodged catheter segments, but difficulties can be encountered [19]. Under these circumstances, a second incision is sometimes required to remove the catheter segments successfully [6]. As severe complications can occur for the long-term consequences of leaving a catheter in situ for life or very long periods, and open heart surgery is a relatively invasive and risky procedure for removing a catheter, we insert a guide wire to straighten the catheter and then apply a "push-in" force to detach the adherent catheter from the vein and then remove the catheter uneventfully [11]. This technique can be a good option to remove a stuck TIVAD catheter.

For ruptured catheters that have migrated into the vena cava or right heart that venotomy or transfemoral cardiac catheterization has failed to retrieve, open heart surgery could be necessary to remove the retained catheter fragments. Percutaneous extraction of embolized catheter fragments has also been reported to be successful by radiologist and cardiologist [14]. However, removal of any retained catheter fragments by thoracotomy and open heart surgery is still strongly recommended for hard-to-remove catheter fragments, because severe pulmonary hypertension due to a ruptured TIVAD catheter fragment retained in the pulmonary artery can be fatal [9].

References

1. Kurul S, Saip P, Aydin T (2002) Totally implantable venous-access ports: local problems and extravasation injury. Lancet Oncol 3:684–692
2. Kock HJ, Pietsch M, Krause U et al (1998) Implantable vascular access systems: experience in 1500 patients with totally implanted central venous port systems. World J Surg 22:12–16
3. Ku YH, Kuo PH, Tsai YF et al (2009) Port-A-Cath implantation using percutaneous puncture without guidance. Ann Surg Oncol 16:729–734
4. Gebauer B, Teichgräber UM, Werk M et al (2008) Sonographically guided venous puncture and fluoroscopically guided placement of tunneled, large-bore central venous catheters for bone marrow transplantation-high success rates and low complication rates. Support Care Cancer 16:897–904
5. Sanelli PC, Deshmukh M, Ougorets I et al (2004) Safety and feasibility of using a central venous catheter for rapid contrast injection rates. Am J Roentgenol 183:1829–1834
6. Wilson GJ, van Noesel MM, Hop WC et al (2006) The catheter is stuck: complications experienced during removal of a totally implantable venous access device. A single-center study in 200 children. J Pediatr Surg 41:1694–1698
7. Dillon PA, Foglia RP (2006) Complications associated with an implantable vascular access device. J Pediatr Surg 41:1582–1587
8. Behrend M, Paboura E, Raab R (2002) Late embolization of an unfractured port catheter into the heart: report of a case. Surg Today 32:724–726
9. Espiritu JD, Stolar CG (2007) Pulmonary hypertension due to a retained totally implantable venous access device fragment. Chest 131:1574–1576
10. D'Silva K, Dwivedi AJ, Shetty A et al (2005) Pinch-off syndrome: a rare complication of totally implantable venous devices. Breast J 11:83–84
11. Huang SC, Tsai MS, Lai HS (2009) A new technique to remove a "stuck" totally implantable venous access catheter. J Pediatr Surg 44:1465–1467
12. Jones SA, Giacomantonio M (2003) A complication associated with central line removal in the pediatric population: retained fixed catheter fragments. J Pediatr Surg 38:594–596
13. O'Sullivan P, Brown M, Hartnett B et al (2006) Central line pump infusion and large volume mediastinal contrast extravasation in CT. Br J Radiol 79:e75–77
14. Surov A, Wienke A, Carter JM et al (2009) Intravascular embolization of venous catheter—causes, clinical signs, and management: a systematic review. J Parenter Enteral Nutr 33:677–685
15. Sanelli PC, Deshmukh M, Ougorets I et al (2004) Safety and feasibility of using a central venous catheter for rapid contrast injection rates. Am J Roentgenol 183:1829–1834
16. Jones SA, Giacomantonio M (2003) A complication associated with central line removal in the pediatric population: retained fixed catheter fragments. J Pediatr Surg 38:594–596

17. Anton N, Massicotte MP (2001) Venous thromboembolism in pediatrics. Semin Vasc Med 1:111–122
18. O'Grady NP, Alexander M, Dellinger EP et al (2002) Guidelines for the prevention of intravascular catheter-related infections. Healthcare Infection Control Practices Advisory Committee. Infect Control Hosp Epidemiol 23:759–769
19. Dillon PA, Foglia RP (2006) Complications associated with an implantable vascular access device. J Pediatr Surg 41:1582–1587

Catheter Migration

27

Walid Faraj and Ahmad Zaghal

Abstract

Catheter migration is a rare but important complication of the totally implantable venous access device (TIVAD), and is estimated to be in the range of 0.2% to 1.7%. While there are many causes of catheter disruption and migration, the commonest is chronic strain to the catheter due to compression between the clavicle and first rib – the so-called pinch-off syndrome. This compression can cause transitory obstruction of the catheter and may result in a split or even complete transection and migration of the catheter. Catheter migration is a rare but important complication of TIVAD. These disruptions may be asymptomatic but may cause significant consequences such as cardiac arrhythmias and even death. The recognition of the separation of the catheter and port on plain radiographs should lead to early intervention to prevent catheter migration.

Keywords

Catheter migration • Pinch-off syndrome

27.1 Introduction

Catheter migration is a rare but important complication of the totally implantable venous access device (TIVAD), with an incidence estimated to be in the range of 0.2% to 1.7% [1-4].

W. Faraj (✉)
American University of Beirut Medical Center, Department of Surgery, Beirut, Lebanon
e-mail: wf07@aub.edu.lb

Catheter tip migration, or sometimes called “secondary malposition” [5] is the change in the position of the tip of the catheter, whereas catheter embolisation occur after catheter rupture, or disconnection where the distal portion of the catheter travels freely in the vascular system.

27.2 Catheter Embolisation

While many reasons can cause catheter disruption and embolisation, the commonest is chronic strain to the catheter due to compression between the clavicle and first rib; the so-called pinch-off syndrome [6-9]. This compression can cause transitory obstruction of the catheter and may result in a split or even complete transection and embolisation of the catheter. A less common cause is the damage caused during its use by medical personnel, where inappropriate puncture of the catheter rather than the reservoir can lead to disruption. Another common cause for the detachment of the catheter from the reservoir is when medical personnel use a small gauge needle which can lead to high pressure within the system, a complication which can appear within 24 to 72 hours of insertion or first use of the system. Although these complications may be asymptomatic, they can be fatal in some cases. Disconnection of the port catheter from the port chamber is a further mechanism of catheter migration [10]. False locking of the port catheter connection has also been suggested [11]. Indeed the lock should be tested after it is applied, a procedure which is done with some traction. Many reports have shown that the cause of catheter fracture was attributed to trauma to the shoulder and excessive muscular exercises [12]. Catheters can embolize into the right atrium, right ventricle, pulmonary artery and coronary sinus [13, 14].

27.3 Catheter Tip Migration

The risk of catheter tip migration is increased when catheters are short and have their tips in the subclavian vein or upper third of the superior vena cava. Arm and shoulder movement, increased intrathoracic pressure caused by coughing or vomiting, congestive heart failure and forceful flushing can cause catheter movement; the catheter can loop, kink, coil, and curl. Catheters that loop at acute angles are at risk of fracture [15]. The catheter tip can migrate to locations such as the internal jugular vein in the neck or contralateral brachiocephalic vein [16-18]. Catheter tips that migrate to the internal jugular vein may cause pain or unusual sensation in the neck, ear, or shoulder areas and patients may report that they hear an odd sound when their catheters are flushed.

27.4 Clinical Presentation

The first sign of catheter dislocation is port dysfunction (46.3%); this can be followed by some cardiac symptoms due to catheter fragment migration into the pulmonary artery, right atrium and ventricle (7.3%). Fatal cardiac complications such as ventricular fibrillation and sudden cardiac death have also been reported [19], surprisingly, most patients are asymptomatic, and the most common symptom is pain or pressure during an attempt to use the damaged [20], other common symptoms are cough, palpitations, and swelling around the port site caused by fluid extravasation.

27.5 Management

The migrated catheter must be retrieved using guided interventional radiologic techniques in order to avoid thromboembolism [11, 21]. Thromboembolism can result from secondary migration into a vein adjacent to a catheter that was properly positioned initially. Medical personnel should be very careful in identifying any central venous catheter dysfunction that might lead to these complications.

27.6 Conclusion

Catheter migration is a rare but important complication of TIVAD. These disruptions may be asymptomatic but may cause significant consequences such as cardiac arrhythmias and even death. The recognition of the separation of the catheter and port on plain radiographs should lead to early intervention to prevent catheter migration. The radiologist should thoroughly examine chest radiographs in patients with functioning venous access devices and identify the locking system as well as the catheter and its anatomic position.

References

1. Ballarini C, Intra M, Pisani Ceretti A et al (1999) Complications of subcutaneous infusion port in the general oncology population. Oncology 56:97-102
2. Biffi R, de Braud F, Orsi F et al (1998) Totally implantable central venous access ports for longterm chemotherapy, a prospective study analyzing complications and costs of 333 devices with a minimum follow-up of 180 days. Ann Oncol 9:767-773
3. Lokich JJ, Bothe A Jr, Benotti P, Moore C (1985) Complications and management of implanted venous access catheters. J Clin Oncol 3:710-717
4. Sattari M, Kazory A, Phillips RA (2003) Fracture and cardiac migration of an implanted venous catheter. Interact Cardiovasc Thorac Surg 2:532-533
5. Gallieni M, Pittiruti M, Biffi R (2008) Vascular access in oncology patients. Cancer J Clin 58:323-346

6. Andris DA, Krzywda EA, Schulte W et al (1994) Pinch-off syndrome: a rare etiology for central venous catheter occlusion. JPEN J Parenter Enteral Nutr 18:531-533
7. Hinke DH, Zandt-Stastny DA, Goodman LR et al (1990) Pinch-off syndrome: a complication of implantable subclavian venous access devices. Radiology 177:353-356
8. Koller M, Papa MZ, Zweig A, Ben-Ari G (1998) Spontaneous leak and transection of permanent subclavian catheters. J Surg Oncol 68:166-168
9. Ouaknine-Orlando B, Desruennes E, Cosset MF et al (1999) The pinch-off syndrome: main cause of catheter embolism. Ann Fr Anesth Reanim 18:949-955
10. Behrend M, Paboura E, Raab R (2002) Late embolization of an unfractured port catheter into the heart: report of a case. Surg Today 32:724-726
11. Faraj W, Zaghal A, El-Beyrouthy O, Kutoubi A (2010) Complete catheter disconnection and migration of an implantable venous access device: the disconnected cap sign. Ann Vasc Surg 24:692
12. Iannelli A, Kianmanesh R, Msika S et al (2001) Post-traumatic fracture and migration in the pulmonary artery of the catheter of a totally implantable venous access device. Unusual complication. Minerva Chir 56:303-306
13. Burzotta F, Romagnoli E, Trani C (2008) Percutaneous removal of an embolized port catheter: description of a new coaxial recovery technique including a case-report. Catheter Cardiovasc Interv 72:289-293
14. Elkhoury MI, Boeckx WD, Chahine EG et al (2008) Retrieval of port-a catheter fragment from the main and right pulmonary arteries 3 years after dislodgment. J Vasc Access 9:296-298
15. Schulmeister L (2010) Management of non-infectious central venous access device complications. Seminars in Oncology Nursing, pp 132-141
16. Barnacle A, Arthurs OJ, Roebuck D et al (2008) Malfunctioning central venous catheters in children: a diagnostic approach. Pediatr Radiol 38:363-378
17. Binnebo¨ sel M, Grommes J, Junge K et al (2009) Internal jugular vein thrombosis presenting as a painful neck mass due to a spontaneous dislocated subclavian port catheter as long term complication: a case report. Cases J 9:7991
18. Jordan K, Behlendorf T, Surov A et al (2008) Venous access ports: frequency and management of complications in oncology patients. Onkologie 31:404-410
19. Gowda MR, Gowda RM, Khan IA et al (2004) Positional ventricular tachycardia from a fractured mediport catheter with right ventricular migration—a case report. Angiology 55:557-560
20. Lam AW, Chen YM, Yang KY et al (1999) Disconnection of a venous port-A-cath followed by embolisation, after saline flush, rare case report. Jpn J Clin Oncol 29:643-645
21. Surov A, Buerke M, John E et al (2008) Intravenous port catheter embolization: mechanisms, clinical features, and management. Angiology 59:90-97

Catheter Embolization

28

Franco Orsi

Abstract

Pulmonary embolization of fractured catheter is a really uncommon complication, mainly related to the port catheter system percutaneously implanted through the subclavian vein. The main reason seems to be related to a continuous mechanical stress between the catheter and the ligament connecting clavicle and the first rib, when the vein is too medially approached. Pinch-off sign is the typical radiological finding of this phenomenon and can be detected by a plain chest x-ray, immediately after an incorrect implantation. Embolized fragments of fractured catheter could be easily removed by means of a minimally invasive percutaneous procedure.

Keywords

Central venous catheters • Fractured catheter • Pinch-off syndrome • Foreign body removal

28.1 Introduction. Epidemiology and Diagnosis

Central venous catheters and totally implanted central venous access systems (port catheter system) play an important role in daily clinical practice and are widely used for parenteral nutrition and intravenous administration of chemotherapeutic agents, fluids, blood, blood products and for monitoring hemodynamic parameters [1-5]. The use of intravenous catheters is associat-

F. Orsi (✉)
Unit of Interventional Radiology, European Institute of Oncology,
Milan, Italy
e-mail: franco.orsi@ieo.it

I. Di Carlo, R. Biffi (eds.), *Totally Implantable Venous Access Devices*,

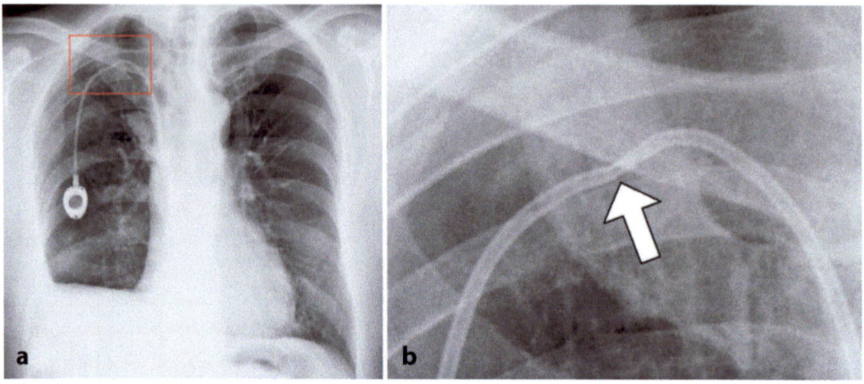

Fig. 28.1 a Chest radiograph clearly shows the bending catheter course (*within the red box*) in the infraclavicular region due to an overly medial percutaneous approach to the subclavian vein. **b** Image magnification shows the narrowing (*arrow*) of the catheter lumen due to compression from the ligament between the 1st rib and clavicle

ed with complications such as thrombosis or catheter-related sepsis. The incidence of dislodgement of the central venous catheter is rare, with an estimated rate of 0–3.1% [1]. When the fractured catheter migrates into the heart or other organs, distal embolization may happen and in rare cases lead to fatal complications. These rare events are sporadically reported in the literature as case reports.

Due to the improvement of catheter types and materials, the incidence of this complication nowadays seems lower than in the past, hence the available data are predominantly historical (the first report by Turner et al. goes back about half a century) [6]. A recent review of the literature reported a total of 215 patients with catheter embolization [1, 7]. In about three quarters of them, indication for catheter placement was intravenous chemotherapy and only one third of embolizations occurred in percutaneous venous catheters (CVCs), meanwhile the large majority of cases were associated with port catheter systems. The reason for this is probably related to the longer stay and usage of port catheters compared to CVCs. Moreover, the subclavian vein is more frequently associated with this complication than other access sites such as the jugular vein and other peripheral accesses and catheters are mainly fractured at the level of the infraclavicular region. This is due to the mechanical forces acting on the catheter between the clavicle and first rib, when a too medial approach to the subclavian vein is adopted, leading to lumen compression before and catheter fragmentation after [8]. Radiographic findings of this phenomenon are known as the pinch-off sign (Fig. 28.1) and it appears as the bending or deviation from a single curved catheter course or as a luminal narrowing while passing beneath the clavicle. The pinch-off syndrome has occurred significantly more frequently in the port catheter systems than in the CVC group. Catheter damage during explantation or catheter exchange is a

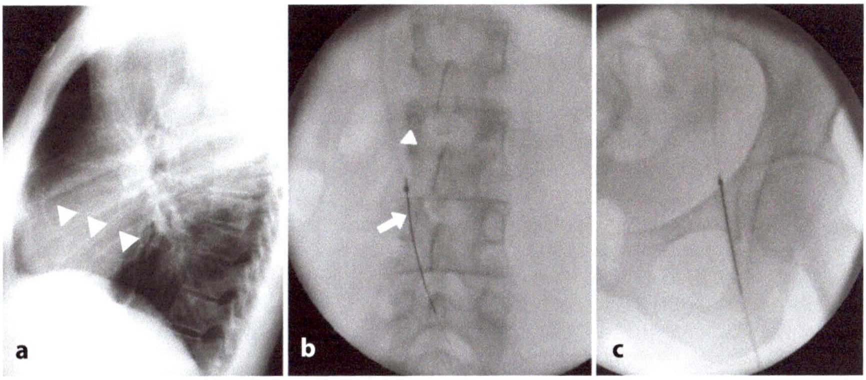

Fig. 28.2 a Chest radiograph clearly shows the embolized fragment (*arrowheads*) in the heart, between the right atrium and the ventricle. **b** The fragment (*arrowhead*) is firmly seized by the "snare loop" recovery system (*arrow*), then it is withdrawn through the left femoral vein (**c**) by the recovery system

less frequent cause of embolization. Whatever the reason of catheter fragmentation, the pulmonary artery and right atrium are the most common sites for fragment collection with no difference between CVCs and port catheter systems. Catheter malfunction is often the first sign of catheter embolization and local pain and/or subcutaneous swelling around the infraclavicular region is usually provoked when fluid is injected through the catheter in that situation [1, 9-11]. Catheter fragmentation and embolization is mainly diagnosed by routine chest radiograph (Fig. 28.2a), because patients are usually entirely asymptomatic. Palpitations, dyspnea, cough and thoracic pain are the most commonly reported manifestations in symptomatic patients.

28.2 Treatment

When embolized fragments are detected, their extraction should always be attempted using the percutaneous approach through the femoral vein (Fig. 28.2b) [12]; with dedicated catheters for foreign body removal (Fig. 28.2 b, c), interventional radiologists can usually achieve the goal in a short procedure time. Very few cases of surgical removal of embolized segments have been reported in the literature.

References

1. Surov A, Wienke A, Carter JM et al (2009) Intravascular embolization of venous catheter—causes, clinical signs, and management: a systematic review. JPEN J Parenter Enteral Nutr 33:677

2. Kurul S, Saip P, Aydin T (2002) Totally implantable venous-access ports: local problems and extravasation injury. Lancet Oncol 3:684-692
3. McGee DC, Gould MK (2003) Preventing complications of central venous catheterization. N Engl J Med 348:1123-1133
4. Ruesch S, Walder B, Tramer MR (2002) Complications of central venous catheters: internal jugular versus subclavian access—a systematic review. Crit Care Med 30:454-460
5. Polderman KH, Girbes AJ (2002) Central venous catheter use. Part 1: mechanical complications. Intensive Care Med 28:1-17
6. Turner DD, Sommers SC (1954) Accidental passage of a polyethylene catheter from cubital vein to right atrium. N Engl J Med 251:744-745
7. Richardson JD, Grover FL, Trinkle JK (1974) Intravenous catheter embolism. Experience with 20 cases and collective review. Am J Surg 128:722-727
8. Ballarini C, Intra M, Pisani Ceretti A et al (1999) Complications of subcutaneous infusion port in the general oncology population. Oncology 56:97-102
9. Bernhardt LC, Wegner G, Mendenhall J (1970) Intravenous catheter embolization to the pulmonary artery. Chest 57:329-332
10. Biffi R, De Braud F, Orsi F et al (1998) Totally implantable central venous access ports for long-term chemotherapy. A prospective study analysing complications and costs in 333 devices with a minimum 180 days of follow-up. Ann Oncol 9:767–773
11. Di Carlo I, Cordio S, La Greca G et al (2001) Totally implantable venous access devices implanted surgically: a retrospective study on early and late complications. Arch Surg 136:1050–1053
12. Fisher RG, Ferreyro R (1978) Evaluation of current techniques for nonsurgical removal of intravascular foreign bodies. AJR Am J Roentgenol 130:541-548

Withdrawal Obstruction

29

Alexandra Ozimek, Pierre A. Clavien and Antonio Nocito

Abstract

Withdrawal complications of port catheter systems include blood withdrawal malfunction as well as adverse events during port explantation. Blood withdrawal complications related to intermittent lumen occlusion can be relieved in more than 90% of the cases. Permanent lumen obstruction due to thrombosis requires infusion of thrombolytic agents. Technical problems can be detected by chest x-ray and usually require TIVAD removal. In cases where a TIVAD is stuck due to fibrous tissue, a venotomy should be perfomed.

Keywords

Withdrawal malfunction • Catheter occlusion • Fibrous tissue • Catheter fixation

29.1 Definition and Epidemiology

Withdrawal complications of TIVAD include blood withdrawal malfunction as well as adverse events during port explantation. While the reported frequency of withdrawal malfunction varies between 0.8 and 9%, literature on complications during port explantation is sparse [1, 2].

A. Ozimek (✉)
Department of Surgery, University Hospital Zürich,
Zürich, Switzerland
e-mail: alexandra.ozimek@med.uni-muenchen.de

I. Di Carlo, R. Biffi (eds.), *Totally Implantable Venous Access Devices*,

29.2 Pathogenesis

Withdrawal malfunction of TIVAD mainly refers to a sudden loss of the ability to withdraw blood from the catheter. To avoid resulting complications, technical problems such as malposition, kinking, disconnection, fracture and migration of the catheter should be immediately excluded by a chest radiograph [1].

In cases where the catheter line projection on the chest radiograph is correct, withdrawal failure is most likely related to intermittent or continuous catheter lumen obstruction. Intermittent obstruction is either caused by an abutment of the catheter tip against the venous wall during blood aspiration or by occlusion of the lumen by fibrous tissue around the tip acting as a one-way flap valve. In both cases the ability to withdraw blood is lost while liquid agents can be easily infused [1].

In contrast, permanent occlusion of the catheter lumen may be induced by blood clots, catheter thrombosis and precipitation of total parenteral nutrition, drugs, intravenous solutions or particles released from the port reservoir. Continuous occlusion can be easily recognized since it is characterized by the inability of both infuse liquid and withdraw blood [1].

Usually, a TIVAD can be easily explanted after the subcutaneous tissue has been dissected. However, removal becomes more complex or unsuccessful when the catheter is stuck in the central vein. In these cases harsh manipulation of the catheter can lead to catheter rupture and hence migration. Further complications occurring during port explantation include venous air embolism or bleeding. Venous air embolism during TIVAD removal is a potentially life-threatening and unfortunately poorly recognized complication. Typically, air embolism occurs when the port catheter is removed during the inspiration phase of the respiratory cycle, when intrathoracic pressure decreases below atmospheric pressure and thus air can be entrained into the venous circulation [2].

Bleeding after port catheter removal may result from excessive tissue damage with insufficient hemostasis or due to an underlying coagulopathy, platelet disorder or vascular disorder.

Unsuccessful removal of the port catheter is usually due to an adhesion of the catheter line to the vessel. In some cases parts of the catheter can even be integrated in the vascular wall. These catheters are stuck in strong fibrous tissue. These fibrous adhesions are thought to arise from pericatheter thrombus formations that are subsequently organized into a fibrous connective tissue matrix. Thus catheter-induced thrombosis with occlusion of the superior vena cava is often found in cases of unsuccessful catheter removal. In contrast, fibrin sheaths and pericatheter calcifications – occasionally developing around central venous catheters when the vascular wall or the smooth surface of the catheter is damaged [1, 2] – usually do not lead to catheter line adhesions. Therefore, these encapsulated catheter lines can easily be removed by gently sliding them out of the sheath.

Catheter adhesion may lead to catheter line rupture during removal. Usually, the catheter ruptures proximal to the point of entrance into the vein. Rupture should always be suspected when a resistance during removal is felt or the length of the retrieved catheter line is too short [3]. If undetected, catheter rupture can induce severe complications including embolization, vessel stenosis, dysrhythmia, sepsis and endocarditis.

29.3 Risk Factors

The mechanisms causing catheter adherence within the vessel are not well understood. Indwelling time and catheter material are thought to be the most important risk factors. However, no solid data on the maximum length of indwelling time for TIVAD can be found. The vast majority of TIVADs are removed within the first years after implantation. However, few patients need a permanent vascular access for several years. So far the only existing consensus is that catheters which are no longer used should be removed [4].

Besides indwelling time, the nature of the catheter-material is also an important risk factor for withdrawal complications. It appears that especially polyurethane is prone to adhere to vessels, thus complicating catheter removal. Indeed all case reports on stuck indwelling catheters involve TIVAD made of polyurethane. In contrast, no reports on stuck silicone catheters can be found.

29.4 Therapy

Intermittent catheter occlusion can be relieved in more than 90% of the cases by placing the patient in the Trendelenburg position or by infusing saline. In 40% of patients with long-term occluded catheters the patency may be re-established by infusion of thrombolytic agents (e.g. streptokinase, urokinase, alteplase) [1]. When withdrawal dysfunction is related to a technical problem as detected by chest radiograph, removal of the TIVAD is indicated.

In patients with a stuck TIVAD the catheter should be released by a venotomy. Catheter fragments resulting from catheter line rupture should be immediately removed by a percutaneous endovascular approach.

29.5 Prophylaxis

- Intermittent catheter occlusion can be relieved using the Trendelenburg position or saline infusion. The patency of permanently occluded catheters may be regained by infusion of thrombolytic agents.
- For removal of port catheters, patients should be placed in the Trendelenburg position to decrease the risk of air embolism. The catheter

line should be removed during expiration, when intrathoracic pressure is greater than atmospheric pressure.

- To avoid bleeding firm pressure should be applied for at least one minute following port removal.
- The length of the catheter line should be measured after removal in order to detect incomplete removal and consequently catheter fragments.
- Catheters that are no longer in use should be removed.

References

1. Kurul S, Saip P, Aydin T (2002) Totally implantable venous access ports: local problems and extravasation injury. The Lancet 3:684-692
2. Jones S, Giacomantonio M (2003) A complication associated with central venous line removal in pediatric population: retained fixed catheter fragments. J Ped Surg 38:594-596
3. Colon-Casanovas N, Lugo-Vincente H (2008) Distal fragmented port catheters: case report and review of literature. Bol Asoc Med P R 100:70-75
4. Mortensen A, Afshari A, Henneberg S (2010) Stuck long-term indwelling central venous catheters in adolescents: three cases and short topical review. Acta Anaesthesiol Scand 54:777-780

Skin Necrosis

30

Adriana Toro and Isidoro Di Carlo

Abstract

Risk factors for skin necrosis include local infection, metastatic carcinoma to the skin, body mass index or extravasation. Local infection may be the result of needle access site infections and port pocket infection. The site of metastatic carcinoma of the skin can influence the port site. The body mass index can cause an inadequate surgical procedure. In fact, in thin patients the port should be positioned under the muscle, whereas in obese patients an excess of subcutaneous adipose tissue should be reduced. Skin necrosis from the infiltration of soft tissue is a rare but potentially devastating complication of intravenous therapy. Irritant drugs cause only inflammation or pain at the site of extravasation, but vesicant drugs can produce severe soft-tissue necrosis and non-healing ulceration requiring surgical treatment. Treatment recommendation includes immediately interrupting the infusion. Local instillation of the appropriate antidote may be promptly used.

Keywords

Skin Erosion • Extravasation • Access site infections • Port pocket infections • Metastatic carcinoma • Surgical procedure • Obese patients • Anticancer drugs • Antracycline • Necrotic and ulcerated epidermidis • Dexrazone • Saline flush-out • Hyperbaric oxygen therapy

I. Di Carlo (✉)
Department of Surgical Sciences, Organ Transplantation and Advanced Technologies,
University of Catania, Cannizzaro Hospital,
Catania, Italy
e-mail: idicarlo@unict.it

I. Di Carlo, R. Biffi, *Totally Implantable Venous Access Devices*,

30.1 Introduction

In patients with a totally implanted venous access device (TIVAD) skin erosion generally results from either local infection, carcinoma metastatic to the skin, inappropriate surgical technique and extravasation. All these situations may cause port extrusion.

30.2 Local Infection

Local infection can be classified as needle access site infections and port pocket infections. In both cases the nursing of the site is a fundamental conditions to avoid these complications. Needle access site infections occur at the skin through the needle to the port. Local tenderness, pain, erythema and edema are the most frequent symptoms. Usually orally administered antibiotic therapy, with local wound care and associated with non-use of the port may have a beneficial effect. In cases of patients not responding to therapy who have persistent fever and positive cultures, the port should be removed. The port as the source of the pocket infection should be removed immediately and local wound care, along with oral antibiotic treatment, should be administered as soon as possible [1].

30.3 Metastatic Carcinoma

Metastatic carcinoma of the skin may affect the port site. In this case, if life expectancy is long the port can be removed and placed elsewhere. In cases of diffuse disease and/or reduced life expectancy the site may be abandoned.

30.4 Inadequate Surgical Procedure

The surgical procedure should be carefully performed, especially in thin and obese patients. In the first case the position of the port should be carefully evaluated and in cases of the absence of subcutaneous fat the port should be placed under the muscle.

Creation of a superficial port pocket and choice of a large profile port chamber in thin patients can cause skin erosion over the port chamber. Although creation of a superficial port pocket is most likely related to the experience of the operator, one may have to place the port under the pectoral fascia or muscle to avoid skin erosion [1]. When a subpectoral fascia pocket is created, skin with its underlying fascia has a better blood perfusion and less chance of skin erosion, necrosis and subsequent port exposure [2]. This solution may be adopted in very thin patients if a low profile port cannot be used.

In contrast, in obese patients an excess of subcutaneous adipose tissue should be reduced, with no more the 2 cm in depth being left in place. In this case hemostasis needs to be very thorough.

30.5 Extravasation

Extravasation is the most frequent cause of port extrusion and its estimated incidence of injuries ranges from 0.1% to 6% [3–5]. The implantation of a TIVAD is intended to create safe access to the venous system and thus avoid the likelihood of extravasation [6, 7]. However, the use of TIVAD may reduce but does not eliminate the risk of extravasation [8–11].

Skin necrosis from intravenous infiltration of soft tissue is a rare but potentially devastating complication of intravenous therapy. Several different chemicals, such as nutrients, electrolytes, chemotherapeutic agents and vasoconstrictors can produce intravenously induced skin injury [12].

The most frequent etiological agent of skin erosion and consequent port extrusion is extravasation of anticancer drugs. The causes of extravasation are: needle dislodgment, inadvertent puncture, leakage from a port membrane or port-catheter connection site, damaged or defective catheter, catheter embolisation, catheter occlusion, catheter fracture or disconnection, and malposition of the catheter tip. However, the most important and frequent cause of extravasation is when a puncture is made outside the port reservoir or when a needle dislodges from the port membrane. The puncture of the site should always be performed by an experienced nurse; after puncture catheter patency should be assessed before administration of chemotherapy. Only needles manufactured for the TIVAD should be used. A non-coring needle may reach the port but usually cannot be stabilized. When a correct needle is used for the TIVAD infusion, the major causes of extravasation could be the position of the port. In fact if the TIVAD is placed over a mobile muscle near the shoulder, the movement of the arm and the shoulder may cause decannulation. In addition, stabilization of the needle is difficult if the Huber needle is too long outside of the skin.

Another cause of extravasation can be the presence of excessive adipose tissue above the port which makes needle stabilization difficult. In this way during the surgical procedure the pocket in which the port will be located and fixed should be freed from the excessive fat. This maneuver should be carefully performed to leave in place the right amount of adipose tissue in order to prevent skin devascularization and erosion [13].

Lastly, extravasation from the port can result from a membrane which has worn out due to excessive use. In this case the cytostatic agents may ooze out under pressure through microscopic fragmentation sites of the port membrane.

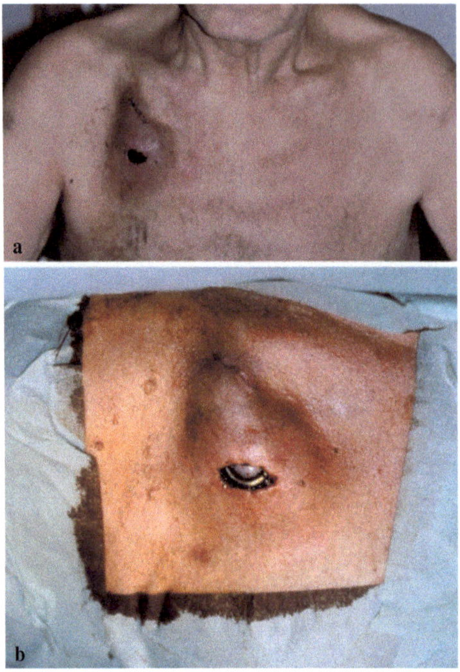

Fig. 30.1 a, b Skin necrosis due to anticancer drug extravasation, with port extrusion

30.6 Clinical Manifestations

Irritant drugs cause only inflammation or pain at the site of extravasation, but vesicant drugs can produce severe soft-tissue necrosis and non-healing ulceration requiring surgical treatment. Tissue damage can range from mild inflammation to widespread necrosis extending to the periosteum. Chronic ulcer and necrosis may progress because chemotherapeutic drugs cannot be locally metabolized or removed from an affected area by lymphatic circulation (Fig. 30.1).

Pain, burning, tingling or itching, discoloration of the overlying epidermis in the clavicular or port-pocket area during or after infusion make up the most common symptoms. Patients using a TIVAD for infusion who report vague discomfort should not be ignored, because symptoms of extravasation such as warmth, erythema, swelling or subcutaneous nodule formation may begin a few days later. In this case infusion should be promptly stopped and a chest X-ray should be done. If the result is negative other complications should be excluded before restarting the infusion. Therefore, a catheter dye study should be performed to search for a fibrin-sleeve formation, a catheter fracture or a disconnection. A dye study must be repeated if the symptoms persist even in the presence of a negative initial study.

Different grades of pain depend on the substance extravasated. An anthracycline extravasation is characterized by swelling and redness and is often very painful. Anthracyclines can persist in the tissue for weeks or even months after extravasation, so for this reason the local area of extravasation is at high risk of infection both for local necrosis and impaired immunological conditions of the patients.

Histologic examination of tissue shows a necrotic and ulcerated epidermis while the dermis shows ischemic necrosis with vascular obliteration and collagen necrobiosis [14].

The extent of affected tissue is clinically difficult and can be assessed by magnetic resonance imaging [15] and an intravenous fluorescein test should be performed in cases of anthracycline extravasation.

30.7 Treatment

Treatment recommendations include immediately interrupting the infusion and sudden aspiration of 3-5 ml of blood from the catheter. The latter maneuver is considered dangerous, by some authors because it may deepen the level of tissue damage by disseminating the agent throughout tissue planes and affect skin vascularity [16]. Local instillation of the appropriate antidote may be promptly used (Tables 30.1, 30.2). In case of extravasation of anthracyclines dexrazoxane is effective in diminishing tissue damage. The treatment should be performed within 5 hours of extravasation. The mechanism is unknown. The 3-day treatment schedule with dexrazoxane consists of a daily dose of 1000 mg/m^2 on day 1 and 2 and 500 mg/m^2 on day 3. Dexrazoxane should be

Table 30.1 Vesicant and irritant anticancer drugs

Vesicant drugs	
Alkylating agents	Mechlorethamine
Antitumor antibiotics	Mitomycin C
(Anthracyclines):	Daunorubicin
	Doxorubicin
	Epirubicin
	Idarubicin
	Actinomycin D
Vinca alkaloids:	Vincristine
	Vinblastine
	Vinorelbine
Taxanes:	Docetaxel
	Paclitaxel

(cont.) →

Table 30.1 (continued)

Irritant drugs (non vesicant)	
Alkylating agents:	Cyclophosphamide Ifosfamide Melphalan Carmustine Dacarbazine Thiotepa
Antimetabolites:	Methotrexate 5-Fluorouracil Cytarabine Fludarabine Gemcitabine
Antitumor antibiotics:	Bleomycin
Epipodophyllotoxin:	Etoposide
Platinum analogs:	Cisplatinum Carboplatin Oxaliplatin

Table 30.2 Antidotes and their indications in various cytotoxic drug extravasations

Drugs	*Antidote*	*Treatment*
Anthracycline and mitomycin C	Dimethyl sulfoxide (DMSO)	1–2 mL of 1 mM 50–99% DMSO, TID * 1–2 weeks. Apply topically in the affected area and leave to dry
Vinca alkaloids, anthracycline, paclitaxel and epipodophyllotoxin	Hyaluronidase	150–1500U intravenous or subcutaneous. Contraindicated in infective and cancerous site
Anthracycline	Dexrazoxane	1 g/m^2 within five hours of extravasation, repeated again on second day in same dose and 500 mg/m^2 on third day
Mechlorethamine (Mustine HCl) and cisplatine	Sodium thiosulfate	Mix 4 mL of 10% sodium thiosulfate with 6 mL of sterile water and inject 2 mL of this solution for 1 mg of mechlorethamine or 100 mg of cisplatine in the existing cannula. 1 mL of sodium thiosulphate is injected subcutaneously and repeated several times over 3–4 hours. 0.1 mL of drug should be injected subcutaneously around the leakage site

administered as an intravenous infusion over 1 to 2 hours in a large caliber vein in the contralateral arm. Cooling procedures should be removed from the area of extravasation at least 15 minutes before the infusion of dexrazoxane in order to allow sufficient blood flow in the area of extravasation. On the second and third day the treatment should start at the same time (+3 hours) as on the first day. Patients with impaired creatinine clearance should have a 50% dose reduction. If no antidote can be immediately used, saline flush-out with or without suction therapy can be a safe and effective procedure in preventing skin and soft tissue necrosis [17–20]. To keep the inflammatory response to a minimum, a general recommendation is the use of cold compression and steroid creams. Hyperbaric oxygen therapy has been proposed with the aim of preventing or reducing tissue necrosis.

The future of the TIVAD depends on the extent of the lesion. Small lesions usually allow the device to be kept in place, otherwise the TIVAD should be eliminated. If the port is to be eliminated a local flap can be used for reconstruction; in this case the anticancer drugs used should be carefully considered together with the local wound properties and blood count due to the fact that some chemotherapeutic agents can affect wound healing [16–20].

References

1. Cil BE, Canyiğit M, Peynircioğlu B et al (2006) Subcutaneous venous port implantation in adult patients: a single center experience. Diagn Interv Radiol 12:93-98
2. Rouzrokh M, Shamsian BS, KhaleghNejad Tabari A et al (2009) Totally implantable subpectoral vs. subcutaneous port systems in children with malignant diseases. Arch Iran Med 12:389-394
3. Lemmers NW, Gels ME, Sleijfer DT et al (1996) Complications of venous access ports in 132 patients with disseminated testicular cancer treated with polychemotherapy. J Clin Oncol 14:2916-2922
4. Strum S, McDermed J, Korn A, Joseph C (1986) Improved methods for venous access: the Port-A-Cath, a totally implanted catheter system. J Clin Oncol 4:596-603
5. Viale PH, Yamamoto DS, Geyton JE (1999) Extravasation of infusate via implanted ports: two case studies. Clin J Oncol Nurs 3:145-151
6. Jordan K, Behlendorf T, Surov A et al (2008) Venous access ports: frequency and management of complications in oncology patients. Onkologie 31:404-410
7. Held-Warmkessel J (2007) Accidental anthracycline extravasation. Nursing 37:72
8. Langstein HN, Duman H, Seelig D et al (2002) Retrospective study of the management of chemotherapeutic extravasation injury. Ann Plast Surg 49:369-374
9. Schulmeister L (2008) Managing vesicant extravasations. Oncologist 13:284-288
10. Uges JW, Vollaard AM, Wilms EB, Brouwer RE (2006) Intrapleural extravasation of epirubicin, 5-fluouracil, and cyclophosphamide, treated with dexrazoxane. Int J Clin Oncol 11:467-470
11. Langer SW (2008) Treatment of anthracycline extravasation from centrally inserted venous catheters. Oncol Rev 2:114-116
12. Dufresne RG Jr (1987) Skin necrosis from intravenously infused materials. Cutis 39:197-198
13. Di Carlo I, Cordio S, Privitera G et al (2001) Totally implantable venous access devices implanted surgically: a retrospective study on early and late complications. Arch Surg 136:1050-1053
14. Rudolph R, Larson DL (1987) Etiology and treatment of chemotherapeutic agent extravasation injuries: a review. J Clin Oncol 5:1116-1126

15. Yama N, Tsuchida Y, Nuka S et al (2001) Usefulness of magnetic resonance imaging for surgical management of extravasation of an antitumor agent: a case report. Jpn J Clin Oncol 31:122-124
16. Shenaq SM, Abbase EH, Friedman JD (1996) Soft-tissue reconstruction following extravasation of chemotherapeutic agents. Surg Oncol Clin N Am 5:825-845
17. Gault DT (1993) Extravasation injuries. Br J Plast Surg 46:91-96
18. Vanwijck R (1993) Liposuction to radiologist's rescue. Plast Reconstr Surg 92:175
19. Harris PA, Bradley S, Moss AL (2001) Limiting the damage of iatrogenic extravasation injury in neonates. Plast Reconstr Surg 107:893-894
20. Vandeweyer E, Heymans O, Deraemaecker R (2000) Extravasation injuries and emergency suction as treatment. Plast Reconstr Surg 105:109-110

Extravasation

31

Lisa Dougherty

Abstract

Extravasation of vesicant drugs from a port is a real risk caused by catheter damage, incomplete insertion or dislodgement of the needle from the port or fibrin sheath. The focus must be on safe techniques of administration, early detection by close monitoring of the patient and the port and immediate and appropriate management. Accurate and contemporaneous documentation is vital along with education of the patient following extravasation.

Keywords

Extravasation • Vesicants • Cytotoxic • Chemotherapy • Implanted ports • Central venous access devices

31.1 Definition

Extravasation literally means *leaking into the tissues*, but it has been linked with vesicants to describe a process that requires immediate action if local tissue damage is to be prevented [1, 2]. A vesicant is any solution or medication that causes the formation of blisters with subsequent tissue necrosis and may be DNA and non-DNA binding [1, 3, 4]. Extravasation is a well-recognized complication of intravenous (IV) chemotherapy administration, but in general it is a condition which is often underdiagnosed, undertreated and under-reported. The incidence of extravasation is estimated to be between 0.5 and

L. Dougherty (✉)
Nurse Consultant IV Therapy, The Royal Marsden NHS Foundation Trust, Surrey, UK
e-mail: lisa.dougherty@rmh.nhs.uk

I. Di Carlo, R. Biffi (eds.), *Totally Implantable Venous Access Devices*,

6.0% of cytotoxic drug administration [5-8]. Central venous access devices (CVADs) have decreased the incidence of extravasation, but it can still occur and the incidence is estimated at up to 6% with ports [7]. However, whilst the incidence is lower with CVADs, the severity of injuries is far greater as detection tends to occur later [1]. Early detection and treatment are crucial if the consequences of an untreated or poorly managed extravasation are to be avoided, since resulting injuries can lead to possible hospitalization and plastic surgery, delay in the treatment of disease and psychological distress for the patient [3, 9, 10].

31.2 Possible Causes of Extravasation

Causes of extravasation include:

- catheter leakage, rupture or fracture;
- separation of the catheter from the portal body of an implanted port;
- incomplete insertion of the needle into the implanted port;
- needle dislodgement from an implanted port [11] or fibrin sheath [12] – leading to backflow of drug along the outside of the catheter to the insertion site [3].

31.3 Prevention of Extravasation

The focus should be on safe intravenous technique and implementing strategies to minimize risk [13]. A number of strategies such as knowledge of patients at risk, types and location of device, sequencing and methods of administration relate to peripheral drug administration. However, monitoring the site and early recognition of extravasation is key. Once the port has been accessed, correct needle position must be confirmed by aspirating blood and then flushing with 0.9% sodium chloride solution with at least 5–10 mL prior to administration of vesicants and frequent monitoring thereafter [8, 13].

Extravasation should be suspected if:

1. The patient complains of burning, stinging pain or any other acute change at the injection site, although this is not always present [1, 4]. Any change of sensation warrants further investigation [8].
2. Swelling is a common symptom [1]. Induration or leakage may also occur at the injection site. Swelling may not always be immediately obvious if the port is sited in an area of deep subcutaneous fat [9].
3. Erythema can occur around the injection site but this is not usually present immediately [4].
4. In CVADs there should always be blood return and if this is absent steps should be followed to be able to verify correct tip and needle position or resolve a fibrin sheath.
5. Resistance is felt on the plunger of the syringe if drugs are given by bolus [3].

6. There is absence of free flow when administration is by infusion, once other reasons have been excluded [1].
7. Leaking around the implanted port needle [1].

Note: one or more of the above may be present. If extravasation is suspected or confirmed, the injection or infusion must be stopped immediately and action must be taken [1, 13].

31.4 Management of Extravasation

31.4.1 Stopping Infusion/Injection and Aspirating the Drug

It appears that most authors are agreed that aspirating as much of the drug as possible, as soon as extravasation is suspected, is beneficial [1, 13, 14] and may help lower the concentration of the drug in the area [8].

31.4.2 Application of Hot or Cold Packs

Cooling appears to be a better choice, with the exception of the vinca alkaloids and taxanes, than warming [15, 16].

31.4.3 The Use of Antidotes in the Management of Extravasation

A number of antidotes are available, but again there is a lack of scientific evidence to demonstrate their value and their role is still not clear [1]. There appear to be two main methods: (1) localize and neutralize (using hyaluronidase) [16]; and (2) spread and dilute (using an antidote).

Hyaluronidase (dose 1500 IU) [15, 17, 18] should be injected within 1 hour of extravasation, ideally through the intravenous device delivering the enzyme to the same tissue [13, 19] for extravasation of vinca alkaloids and taxanes.

Injectable corticosteroids appear to have little benefit and data now discourages use as there is little evidence to support their use [15, 19, 20], although as a cream they can help to reduce local trauma and irritation.

Topical dimethyl sulfoxide (DMSO) can be effective and well tolerated in managing anthracycline extravasation [15].

Dexrazoxane (Savene), is given IV daily for 3 days and it appears to reduce the wound size and duration with anthracyclines [21-23].

31.4.4 Surgical Techniques

It is now recognised that a plastic surgery consultation be performed as part of the management procedure in order to remove the tissue containing the drug.

The flush out technique is a less traumatic and cheaper procedure than surgery. A number of small stab incisions are made and large volumes of 0.9% sodium chloride are administered which flush out the extravasated drug [19] and it is more successful if performed within 24 hours of extravasation.

31.4.5 Documentation

An extravasation must be reported and fully documented as it is an accident and the patient may require follow-up care [24]. The ONS lists the key elements of vesicant extravasation documentation [1] (Table 31.1). Information may also be used for statistical purposes to monitor and analyse the incidence, degree, causes and corrective action [24] or may be required in case of litigation [7, 18, 25].

31.5 Ongoing Care

Patient follow up will be dependent upon the patient's needs and the degree of damage. Assessment should include inspection and management of the area of extravasation, skin integrity, the presence of pain and other symptoms, as well as the mobility and sensation of the limb [1].

Table 31.1 Key elements of vesicant extravasation documentation

Date and time the extravasation occurred
Type and size of vascular access device
Length and gauge of needle (ports only)
Location of device
Details of how patency was established before and during administration (description and quality of blood return)
Number and location of all cannulation attempts
Vesicant administration method e.g. bolus, infusion
Estimated amount of extravasated drug
Symptoms reported by the patient
Description of device site e.g. swelling, redness etc
Assessment of limb (where applicable) for range of movement
Immediate nursing interventions
Follow up interventions
Patient information
Photographs of extravasation site

31.6 Education of Patient and Relevant Others

Patients should always be informed when an extravasation has occurred and be given an explanation of what has happened and what management has been carried out [2]. An information sheet should be given to patients with instructions of what symptoms to look out for and when to contact the hospital during the follow-up period [2].

References

1. Polovich M, White JM, Kelleher L (2009) Chemotherapy and biotherapy guidelines and recommendations for practice, 3rd edn. Oncology Nursing Press, Pittsburgh, PA
2. Schulmeister L (2009) Antineoplastic therapy. In: Alexander M, Corrigan A, Gorski L et al (eds) Infusion therapy: an evidence based approach. Saunders Elsevier, Philadelphia, chapter 18, pp 366–367
3. Hyde, L, Dougherty, L, Schorstein R (2011) Safe handling of cytotoxic drugs. In: Dougherty L, Lister S (eds) The Royal Marsden NHS Foundation Trust manual of clinical nursing procedures, 8th edn. Wiley Blackwell Publishing, Oxford
4. Hayden BK, Goodman M (2005) Chemotherapy: principles of administration. In: Henke Yarbro C, Wujcik D, Holmes Gobel B (eds) Cancer nursing – principles and practice, 6th edn. Jones and Bartlett, Boston, MA, pp 351–411
5. Khan MS, Holmes JD (2002) Reducing morbidity from extravasation injuries. Ann Plast Surg 48:628–632
6. Lawson T (2003) A legal perspective on CVC-related extravasation. J Vasc Access Devices 8:25–27
7. Masoorli S (2003) Extravasation injuries associated with the use of central vascular access devices. JVAD 8:21–23
8. Goolsby TV, Lombardo FA (2006) Extravasation of chemo-therapeutic agents: prevention and treatment. Semin Oncol 33:139–143
9. Dougherty L (2008) Intravenous therapy: recognising the differences between infiltration and extravasation. J British Nurs 17:896–901
10. EONS (2007) Extravasation guidelines European Oncology Nursing Society
11. Schulmeister L (1989) Needle dislodgement from implanted venous access devices – inpatients and outpatient experiences. J Intraven Nurs 12:90–92
12. Mayo DJ (1998) Fibrin sheath formation and chemotherapy extravasation: a case report. Supp Care Cancer 6:51–56
13. Weinstein S (2007) Antineoplastic therapy. In: Plumer's principles and practices of intravenous therapy, 8th edn. Lippincott, Williams & Wilkins, Philadelphia, pp. 486–573
14. Rudolph R, Larson DL (1987) Etiology and treatment of chemotherapeutic agent extravasation injuries: a review. J Clin Oncol 5:1116–1126
15. Bertolli G (1995) Prevention and management of extravasation of cytotoxic drugs. Drug Saf 12:245–255
16. CP Pharmaceuticals (1999) How quickly could you act? CP Pharmaceuticals, Wrexham
17. Few BJ (1987) Hyaluronidase for treating intravenous extravasations. MCN Pharmacopoeia 12:23
18. Doellmann D, Hadaway L, Bowes-Geddes LA et al (2009) Infiltration and extravasation: update on prevention and management. J Infusion Nurs 32:203– 211
19. Gault D, Challands J (1997) Extravasation of drugs. Anaesth Rev 13:223–241
20. Wickham R, Engelking C, Sauerland C, Corbi D (2006) Vesicant extravasation part II: evidence based management and continuing controversies. ONF 33:1143–1150

21. Langer SW, Sehested M, Buhl Jensen P (2000) Treatment of antracycline extravasation with dexrazoxane. Clin Cancer Res 6:3680–3686
22. Mouridsen HT, Langer SW, Butter J et al (2007) Treatment of anthracycline extravasation with Savene (dexrazoxane): results from two prospective multicentre studies. Ann Oncol 18:546–550
23. Schulmeister L (2007) Totect. A new agent for treating anthracycline extravasation. Clin J Oncol Nurs 11:387–395
24. RCN (2010) Standards for infusion therapy. Royal College of Nursing, London
25. Dougherty L (2003) An expert witness working within the legal system in the United Kingdom. J Vas Ass Net 8:29–37

Pocket Infection

32

Alexandra Ozimek, Pierre A. Clavien and Antonio Nocito

Abstract

Pocket infections are local inflammatory complications after implantation of port catheter systems and occur with an estimated incidence of 2.5%. The main etiology for local catheter related infections is bacterial contamination either during implantation or clinical use of the device. Usually the diagnosis is made based on the typical clinical signs of inflammation. Therapeutic modalities include immediate wound care combined with intravenous antibiotic treatment or explantation of the TIVAD.

Keywords

Catheter related infection • Pocket infection • Bacterial contamination

32.1 Definition and Epidemiology

Catheter-related infections (CRIs) account for 0.2-27% of all complications after implantation of subcutaneous port catheter systems, thus causing considerable morbidity and substantial financial costs [1–4]. Importantly, up to 55% of CRIs result in TIVAD removal [4, 5]. CRIs are generally classified as either local or systemic [1]. Pocket infections belong to the group of local CRIs and occur in 0.8–2.5% of patients [4]. Clinical signs of pocket infection include induration, erythema and tenderness around the implantation site. In addition, an exsudation of pus at the needle entry site can be found or a culture-positive fluid is aspirated out of the port pocket [4].

A. Ozimek (✉)
Department of Surgery, University Hospital Zürich, Zürich, Switzerland
e-mail: alexandra.ozimek@med.uni-muenchen.de

32.2 Pathogenesis

Bacterial contamination and consequently overgrowth are at the root of the problem of pocket infection. Although rare, early postoperative infections are due to a contamination of the port catheter system during implantation [3]. Adopting a strict antiseptic surgical technique can easily prevent these cases [1].

Potential portals of entry for microorganism responsible for mid- and long-term pocket infections are the intact skin (needle passage), catheter lines and infusion solutions. Thus the colonization by physiological skin flora or pathogenic microorganisms represents the major risk factor, since penetration of the skin and subcutaneous tissue is always required to access the port reservoir. Apart from the usual needle passages, skin lesions related to impaired wound healing as well as port erosion due to suboptimal device selection or cachexia are additional factors which compromise the protective integrity of the skin and thus facilitate pocket infection [2]. In contrast to systemic central venous CRIs, for which coagulase-negative staphylococci are mainly responsible, *Staphylococcus aureus* and *epidermidis*, followed by coagulase-negative staphylococci and *Candida* species represent the causative agents for local port catheter infections [2, 6].

32.3 Risk Factors

Since port catheter systems are completely implanted under the skin, hence the term totally implantable venous access device (TIVAD), they are associated with lower infection rates than central venous catheters [4, 6]. While neither the utilized vein (catheter placement in the subclavian vein vs. internal jugular vein) [4, 6] nor the surgical technique [7] have been shown to influence complication rate, the number of skin punctures needed to obtain central venous access was identified as a risk factor of CRIs [5]. In addition, administration of high-caloric parenteral nutrition and a high frequency of port manipulation are further risk factors [2]. Moreover, younger patients with hematologic neoplasms as well as immunocompromised patients are more prone to CRIs [8].

32.4 Diagnosis

In clinical practice the diagnosis of CRIs is based on clinical signs and microbiologic analysis of blood or catheter tips. The prevailing symptoms in pocket infections are the classical features of local inflammation. These comprise pain, induration, tenderness, heat, and erythema around the implantation site. In addition, purulent fluid either exudates out of the needle access site or can be aspirated out the port reservoir. Signs of a concomitant systemic infection such as fever, chills, and/or hypotension may or may not be present.

When a local infection is suspected, microbiologic analyses of wound secretions as well as paired blood cultures (anaerobic and aerobic) obtained from both a peripheral vein and the port catheter should be immediately obtained [1]. Consequently, therapy should be instantaneously started, since if left untreated, a systemic CRI with deleterious effects can ensue [2].

32.5 Therapy

Port reservoir and catheter removal is always indicated in patients with a CRI due to *Staphylococcus aureus* (Level of Recommendation / Evidence A II), *Candida* species (B II) and in clinically unstable patients [2]. Patients presenting with early signs of pocket infection should be immediately subjected to wound care and intravenous antibiotic treatment in order to eradicate the infection [3]. Antibiotic treatment should cover a broad spectrum of Gram-positive and Gram negative bacteria, including *Staphylococcus* species and *Pseudomona aeruginosae* (aminoglycoside and vancomycin plus aztreonam or a third generation cephalosporin). Subsequently, this empiric therapy is adjusted according to culture and susceptibility results. However, in case of a persistence of clinical signs or a progression to a manifest port site infection, explantation of the port catheter system is warranted (B III) [2, 3].

32.6 Prophylaxis

Several sequential steps are recommended to reduce CRIs in central venous catheterization and port catheter implantation (Evidence Level 1b) [1–6; 9]:

1. Implantation of port catheter systems should always be performed in an operation room under aseptic conditions.
2. Maximum sterile precautions are essential. All surgeons should wear a sterile gown, sterile gloves, a mask and a cap. Before gloves are pulled over, an alcohol-based sanitizer or antimicrobial soap should be used.
3. Skin sterilization should be performed for at least 30 seconds. The solution should be allowed to dry for at least two minutes. 2% chlorhexidine based preparations reduce CRI most effectively. As alternatives, 70% alcohol solutions, iodophor or tincture of iodine can also be used.
4. Ultrasound guidance of port catheter placement has been shown to reduce the incidence of CRIs.
5. Single-dose preoperative antibiotic prophylaxis prior to the placement of totally implanted venous access ports decreases infection rates in several patients particularly at risk (e.g. patients with hematologic neoplasms or immunsuppression). There is no evidence for perioperative antibiotic prophylaxis during port catheter implantation in general.
6. In cachectic patients a low profile vascular access port should be used in order to prevent skin lesions due to port erosion.

7. Catheter site care with antiseptics and strict adherence to sterile precautions (skin-disinfection, use of sterile needle and gloves) when accessing the port catheter system is essential. The needle can be usually kept in place for 72 hours. However, in case of administration of blood products or lipid emulsions it should be replaced after 24 hours.
8. If the vascular access port is not used for a long time, the system should be flushed with 10 mL of 0.9% saline solution and 1 mL of heparin every 4 to 6 weeks and again before therapy is started.

References

1. Vesica S, Baumgärtner AK, Jacobs VR et al (2008) Management of venous port systems in oncology: a review of current evidence. Ann Oncol 19:9-15
2. Wolf HH, Leithäuser M, Maschmeyer G et al (2008) Central venous catheter-related infections in hematology and oncology. Guidelines of the Infectious Diseases Working Party (AGIHO) of the German Society of Hematology and Oncology (DGHO). Ann Hematol 87:863-786
3. Jan HC, Chou SJ, Chen TH et al (2010) Management and prevention of complications of subcutaneous intravenous infusion port. Surg Oncol [Epub ahead of print] doi:10.1016/j.suronc.2010.07.001
4. Biffi R, Orsi F, Pozzi S et al (2009) Best choice of central venous insertion site for the prevention of catheter-related complications in adult patients who need cancer therapy: a randomized trial. Ann Oncol 20:935-940
5. Scaife CL, Gross ME, Mone MC et al (2010) Antibiotic prophylaxis in the placement of totally implanted central venous access ports. Am J Surg 200:719-723
6. Beckers MMJ, Ruven HJT, Seldenrjik CA et al (2010) Risk of thrombosis and infections in central venous catheters and totally implanted access ports in patients for Cancer. Thrombosis Research 125:318-321
7. Nocito A, Wildi S, Rufibach K et al (2009) Randomized clinical trial comparing venous cutdown with the Seldinger technique for placement of implantable venous access ports. Br J Surg 96:1129-1134
8. Peris A, Zagli G, Bonizzoli MG et al (2010) Implantation of 3951 long-term central venous catheters: performances, risk analysis, and patient comfort after ultrasound-guidance introduction. Anesth Analg 111:1194-1201
9. Di Carlo I, Toro A, Pulvirenti E et al (2011) Could antibiotic prophylaxis be necessary to implant totally implantable venous access devices? Randomized prospective study. Surgical Oncology 20: 20-25

Nursing of Vascular Access: Highlights of Hot Issues

33

Paul L. Blackburn and Ton J. H. van Boxtel

Abstract

Totally implanted ports represent a novel technology that is capable of providing reliable vascular access for patients who are receiving a variety of infusates, for a variety of diagnoses, and over an extended length of time. Nursing care of these devices is aimed at providing longevity of the device, while allowing the patient to safely receive their therapy. The nurse clinician must be aware of multiple aspects of the port device, care, maintenance and potential complications in order to offer the highest level of care. The nurse must clearly understand the principles of port and access site assessment, preparation of the access site for access, port identification, available needle types and styles, flushing, and care and maintenance such as dressing changes. Additionally the clinician needs to be aware of potential complications and methodologies to prevent such complications.

Keywords

Access site • Skin flora • Flushing • Locking • Power injection • Patient education • Central venous catheter • CVC • Totally implantable venous access port • Nursing care • Port access • Huber needle

33.1 Assessment

Nursing assessment starts with information from the inserting expert, including technique of vein entry, tip position, depth of the septum, type of

P.L. Blackburn (✉)
Clinical Education Bard Access Systems,
Salt Lake City, Utah, USA
e-mail: paul.blackburn@crbard.com

I. Di Carlo, R. Biffi (eds.), *Totally Implantable Venous Access Devices*,

port and catheter (e.g. power injectable) and possible complications during insertion. Assessment of the patient also includes the elements listed below.

33.1.1 Depth of Septum

After hand disinfection, palpation of the shape of the port, depth of the septum and position of the port (not flipped) provide invaluable information for the clinician.

33.1.2 Site of the Port

Depending on available veins, skin integrity and patient circumstances, the totally implantable venous access device (TIVAD) can be placed in the thorax (most common), arm or in the flank. Positioning the TIVAD on the thorax can influence clothing (e.g. bra, open shirt) and activities (like wearing a safety belt). Young patients often prefer the flank for cosmetic reasons. Arm ports do not really have many benefits in functionality and care. Access of arm ports may be easy, but removing the needle without external help is difficult.

33.1.3 Port Identifiers

Each port insertion kit includes information about the port care and functionality. One way to inform the patient and healthcare providers about the brand and type of port is the identification card. This card contains information about the patient and port, including an identification number and the date of insertion. Some manufacturers provide additional information when a power injectable port is inserted. This information can include a purple arm band, palpable marks on the port septum or a radiopaque mark on the port that is visible on a radiograph.

33.2 Preparing the Access Site

The epidermis covering the access site is the body's last line of defense from bacteria and therefore should be meticulously prepared. Additionally, the epidermis is made up of multiple layers of cells that provide a home for bacteria, commonly called skin flora. There are approximately 1000 species of bacteria living on human skin. Most of these bacteria are found in the superficial layers of the epidermis and hair follicles. Skin flora are usually non-pathogenic, however, skin flora can cause life-threatening diseases if they are allowed to enter the bloodstream, especially in immunosuppressed people [1]. In the 2011 revision of the *Guidelines for the Prevention of Intravascular Catheter-related Infections* the CDC recommends the use of >0.05% chlorhexidine preparation with alcohol before central venous catheter access [2]. Apply the chlorhexidine preparation using a back-and-forth motion for at least 30 seconds [3]. Completely wet the treatment area with antiseptic. Allow the area to dry for approximately 30 seconds. Do not blot or wipe away. If the patient has an allergy to chlorhexidine, alcohol, or is younger than the minimum age suggested for chlorhexidine use, povidone-iodine can be used by applying the swabsticks in a concentric circle beginning at the center of the access site, moving outward. Povidone-iodine must remain on the skin for at least two minutes or longer to dry completely for adequate antisepsis. The following procedure can be used:

1. Perform hand hygiene
2. Verify patient's identity
3. Explain the procedure to the patient
4. Gather supplies
5. Assess skin over the implanted port, palpate to locate septum
6. Don mask and sterile gloves
7. Cleanse access site as described above
8. Proceed with access based on manufacturer's recommendations or according to institutional policy

Implanted vascular access ports should only be accessed with a Huber needle. If the device is to be used for power injection of contrast media, the Huber needle must be approved for power injection of contrast media, as should the port.

33.3 Port Access

One of the most important and sometimes difficult nursing aspects in TIVAD is access through the septum of the TIVAD into the central vasculature. If the septum can easily be palpated or even be seen through the skin, access can be fairly easy. In obese patients the septum can be very difficult to palpate and hard to access using a Huber needle with a length of 38 mm or even 50 mm.

Nurses should therefore be involved in the pre-insertion information to the patient and assessment of the patient situation. A TIVAD can be used right after insertion and confirmation of functionality and tip position. Most protocols state that a Huber needle is inserted at the end of the insertion procedure. This prevents painful access in a bruised area and enables therapy to be started immediately.

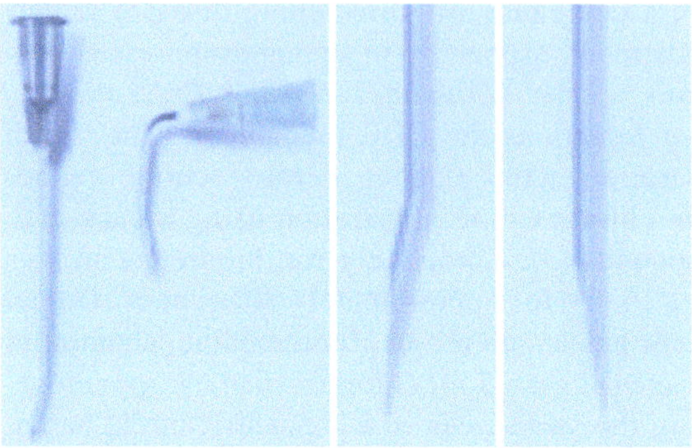

Fig. 33.1 Huber needle for port access with distal opening on the side

33.4 Needle Type

For port access the only type of needle that should be used is a needle with the distal opening on the side (Fig. 33.1). This is called a noncoring or Huber needle. Depending on the therapy and position of the port, the Huber needle varies in size, length and shape.

The size is always in Gauge (G) varying from 23 G for young children, 22 G for low flow infusion, 21G for blood sampling and hyperhydration and 19 G for high flow infusion and blood transfusion.

The length of the Huber needle is largely depending on the skin layer over the port septum. For a superficial septum a length of 19 mm will allow the needle tip to go through the septum to reach the bottom of the port. To reduce the risk of needle dislodgement during access, the Huber needle should be of a length that allows the needle to sit flush to the skin and securely within the port [4]. Huber needles are available in lengths of 16, 19, 25, 32, 38 and 50 mm. The Huber needle has a 90 degree angle but is also available as a straight needle for short access e.g. monthly flushing.

33.5 Flushing the Totally Implanted Venous Access Device

Flushing the TIVAD, when done correctly, can prolong the life of the device, while ensuring that the functional flow of the port and catheter is maintained. Additionally, regular flushing and locking of the TIVAD and catheter can potentially prevent catheter fracture due to partial or complete occlusion and over pressurization. A TIVAD can become occluded due to fibrin build-up intraluminally, precipitate formation due to inadequate flushing, and of course via a thrombus that forms in the end of the port catheter. All of these issues can be prevented in most patients, through the use of proper port flushing and locking.

Catheter design should be carefully considered when determining the frequency of the flush and lock procedure as well as the solution used to lock the port catheter. Additionally, the clinician performing the flush and lock procedure must be familiar with the patient's medical history, specifically looking for previous and current reactions to heparin. If present or suspected, heparin and all sources of heparin should be discontinued [5].

The clinician should review the patient's medical record or other available information to determine the type of port and catheter implanted in the individual patient. Flushing protocols vary and are dependent upon the catheter type, open-ended or distally valved, as well as single lumen versus dual lumen catheters. Flushing frequency, solutions, and technique should be described in institutional policy. Institutional policy is developed based on manufacturer's recommendations, universally accepted standards, and institutional experience. Flushing and locking a port and catheter is not necessary when the port and catheter are in continuous use. Flushing and locking a port and catheter should take place during intermittent use, or periodically during periods of non-use. A port and catheter should be flushed with a minimum of 10 mL of preservative-free 0.9% sodium chloride after each injection to help prevent interaction between incompatible drugs. If the port and catheter are not currently in use, the open ended port and catheter should be flushed and locked with heparin lock solution 100 units/mL [6] at least once every four weeks. For dual lumen catheters, each lumen should be flushed and locked with heparin as described above. A sterile normal saline lock may be used for port catheters with a distally located valve.

The technique a clinician chooses to use for the port and catheter flush and lock procedure is based on clinician experience, manufacturer's recommendations, and institutional protocol. No one technique has been thoroughly studied, therefore clinicians should select a technique that works for them. At minimum, a turbulent push-pause flushing method should be used. This method could potentially dislodge infusates and/or blood products that may cling to the catheter lumen and port body. Additionally, the clinician should use a positive pressure disconnect to ensure negative displacement of fluid does not occur upon removal of the Huber needle.

33.6 Dressing Change

Transparent semipermeable dressing (TSD) should be changed every 5-7 days or more frequently if the site is moist or the TSD is loosened. Dressing change should be performed every 2 days if gauze is used [7]. Skin integrity and the site of the port influence the type of dressing to choose. Skin integrity can be supported by removing the semi permeable folio through stretching and not pulling the folio. Daily evaluation of the insertion site for redness, exudate, swelling, pain or discomfort should be performed and reported.

33.7 Complications

Nurses should be aware of possible complications such as *pinch-off syndrome* which can influence functionality or even lead to leakage of the port catheter causing major extravasation. The position of the patient's arm can allow better infusion or blood sampling. Prior to infusion of irritant medication, the nurse should assess functionality. Pinch-off syndrome can be prevented by changing the site of insertion in such a way that the subclavian vein is avoided in favor of the jugular or axillary veins. Additionally, the use of ultrasound for vascular access has been shown to decrease insertion complications. Other complications the nurse should be aware of include:

- blood clot
- partial blockage
- infection
- thromboses.

These complications have been dealt with in previous chapters.

33.8 Power Injection

In recent years, several *power injectable* TIVADs have been introduced to the vascular access market. Each of these products come to the market with certain restrictions aimed at preventing patient injury and port/catheter damage during power injection of contrast media. One of the major concerns is the access device that is being used with a power injectable port. All manufacturers recommend that a Huber needle that has been designed specifically for power injection of contrast media be used with a power injectable TIVAD when power injecting contrast media. A maximum pressure of 300 psi has proven effective as has flow rates that vary from 2 mL to 5 mL per second. Maximum flow rates are usually dictated by the needle gauge size. Additionally, the prudent clinician will ensure that the port and catheter have been checked for patency prior to power injection of contrast media. This is easily done by attaching a 10 mL syringe filled with sterile normal saline. The clinician should first attempt to aspirate blood, followed by a vigorous push-pause flushing technique. If no resistance is felt, the catheter lumen is most likely free of occlusion and will therefore tolerate power injection of contrast media.

33.9 Patient Education

Patient education is one of the most important aspects of caring for an implantable port and catheter. This education should begin at the first sign that the patient may need a vascular access device. The education at minimum should include:

- device types
- efficacy of specific device types
- applicability of device types for their therapy based on infusate, length of therapy, and risk to patient and
- risks associated with the insertion procedure.

Once the choice of vascular access device has been made, the clinician should provide education that will help the patient understand the role they play in the care and maintenance of their port and catheter. This is particularly important if the patient and/or a caregiver will be providing care outside of the hospital. An educational plan should be developed that covers, at minimum, the following:

- proper care of the port and catheter
- precautions for preventing infection and other complications
- signs and symptoms to report and
- ensuring that healthcare providers are employing proper infection prevention methods [8].

Lastly, a discussion should occur regarding placement position for the TIVAD. This discussion should include such issues as convenience for accessing the device, cosmetic issues, personal appearance, body habitus and personal preference.

A fully informed patient is empowered with the ability to make healthcare decisions that may very well enhance the outcome of the treatment regimen prescribed by their physician.

References

1. Wikipedia (2011) Skin flora. http://en.wikipedia.org/wiki/Skin_flora. Accessed 27 May 2011
2. O'Grady NP, Alexander M, Patchen Dellinger E et al (2011) Guidelines for the prevention of intravascular catheter-related infections. CDC p.64 http://www.cdc.gov/hicpac/pdf/guidelines/-bsi-guidelines-2011.pdf. Accessed 27 May 2011
3. Infusion Nurses Society (2011) Policies and procedure for infusion nursing, 4th edn. Infusion Nurses Society, p. 90
4. Gorski L, Perrucca R, Hunt M (2010) Central venous access devices: care, maintenance and potential complications. In: Alexander M, Corrigan A, Gorsk L et al (eds) Infusion nursing: an evicence-based approach, 3rd edn. Saunders/Elsevier, St Louis, pp. 495-515
5. Infusion Nurses Society (2011) Infusion nursing standards of practice. J Infusion Nurs 34[Suppl 1]:S60
6. Infusion Nurses Society (2011) Infusion nursing standards of practice. J Infusion Nurs 34[Suppl 1]:S61
7. Infusion Nurses Society (2011) Infusion nursing standards of practice. J Infusion Nurs 34[Suppl 1]:S63
8. Infusion Nurses Society (2011) Infusion nursing standards of practice. J Infusion Nurs 34[Suppl 1]:S16

Paul L. Blackburn, RN, BSN, MNA, VA-BC is employed by Bard Access Systems as the Director of Clinical Education. Additionally, Paul serves on the Association for Vascular Access Board of Directors, the Wise Foundation Board of Directors and the Carolina Vascular Wellness Board of Directors.

Power Technology: How to Safely Use Ports and Central Catheters to Deliver Contrast Medium in Radiology Procedures

34

Roberto Biffi

Abstract

The use of totally implantable venous access devices in radiology may be associated with a number of complications, including occlusion of the system, infection, extravasation of contrast media into the soft tissues, sub-intimal venous or myocardial injection, or serious damage to the device itself due to the high-pressure administration of contrast medium by automatic injectors (so-called "power injectors"). In this chapter state-of-the-art knowledge on this topic is presented; results of experimental and clinical studies are fully discussed, focusing on preventive measures and educational needs.

Keywords

Central venous catheters • Power injection • CT scan • Contrast medium • RECIST criteria

34.1 Introduction

The use of totally implantable venous access devices in radiology may be associated with complications such as occlusion of the system (because of the high density of some contrast), infection (if the port is not handled in aseptic conditions, using proper barrier protections), and mechanical complications due to the high-pressure administration of contrast by automatic injectors (so-

R. Biffi (✉)
Division of Abdomino Pelvic Surgery, European Institute of Oncology, Milan, Italy
e-mail: roberto.biffi@ieo.it

I. Di Carlo, R. Biffi (eds.), *Totally Implantable Venous Access Devices*,

called "power injectors"): extravasation of contrast media into the soft tissues, subintimal venous or myocardial injection, or serious damage to the device itself (breakage of the external connections, dislocation of the non-coring needle, or breakage of the catheter). The latter problem – i.e. damage of the device from a *power injection* – is not an unjustified fear, but a reality. A warning by the U.S. Food and Drug Administration first issued in July 2004 [1] reported around 250 complications of this kind, referring to both Port and CVC and PICC catheter systems, which occurred over a period of several years; in all cases, the damage occurred during the injection of contrast by means of "power injectors" for computed tomography (CT) or magnetic resonance imaging (MRI) procedures. In addition to the obvious loss of a vascular access and the need for repositioning a new device, in some cases the breakage of the catheter may cause an extravasation of contrast into the patient's soft tissues, and/or an embolization of catheter fragments in the central venous or pulmonary arterial circulation (which may result in the need to retrieve them by interventional radiology). Typical mechanical damage includes: breakage of the extension of the non-coring needle or its detachment from the needle; sudden expulsion of the non-coring needle from the silicone septum and thus from the port chamber; breakage of the silicone portal septum. The more fragile the system is, even in one of its components, the lower the injection pressure at which mechanical damage may occur.

Secondary contamination of healthcare personnel due to contact with patient blood [2] has also been reported. Complications of this kind may be even more frequent than reported, since in the USA the obligation to report the event, exists only in the event of patient death or *serious injury*.

The FDA warning of 2004 thus concludes with the recommendation to use *power injection* only with vascular devices [3] specifically certified for such use [4]. It is also important to stress that some devices, even if apparently intact, might have been irreparably damaged by the excessive pressures to which they were subjected, and damage or malfunctioning may appear some time later.

Though the risk associated with the use of ports in radio-diagnostics is thus clear, it has been suggested that administration of the contrast via the port may have some advantage in terms of image quality. This contention is not supported by the evidence, as many CT exams (the only ones to require high flow rates of viscous contrast) are routinely performed using peripheral veins with excellent qualitative results. Nonetheless, the use of a power injectable device may be associated with increased comfort for the patient (i.e. by avoiding an additional cannula being inserted into a peripheral vein) and maybe more accurate reproducibility of the patient's own follow-up exams. In addition, since many cancer patients who need frequent CT studies already have totally implantable systems, it would seem reasonable to try to define how and when such systems may be safely used.

A recent Consensus of the GAVeCeLT (Italian Study Group on Long Term

Central Venous Accesses) has addressed this topic, and most of the conclusions here reported are a part of this Consensus [5].

34.2 Diagnostic Radiology Use of Central Venous Devices and Related Problems

With regard to totally implantable venous ports, the risk of pressure damage is closely related to the dynamics of the high-flow rate infusion which takes place through the whole system. The pressure preset on the injectors is usually 300-325 PSI, a value established as appropriate for the injection of contrast media in a peripheral vein via a 18-G short cannula connected to an extension tube of slightly more than 1 meter in length; the extension tube is normally supplied by the manufacturer of the power injector and both its strength and its flow capacity are compatible with the pressure required.

In the case of ports, the extension tube coming from the power injector is connected to a shorter tube, of smaller caliber, directly connected to the non-coring needle, which may be of variable caliber and length. When the internal caliber of one or more of these various components is smaller, in order to maintain an appropriate flow rate, the initial pressure generated by the power injector should be increased; nevertheless, in clinical practice, the power injector is programmed with a maximum pressure ceiling so that when the resistance of the system increases, the pressure applied is automatically reduced and the injection proceeds at a slower flow rate. Since the injection cannot be interrupted, an increase in the resistance within the system may cause excessive pressure leading to detachments, damage or bursting of some system components. Therefore, as a power injector is applied to a totally implanted venous port, the high resistance created by the presence of the non-coring needle needs to be taken into account, as this is the segment with the smallest caliber along the entire infusion line and it acts as a *bottleneck* in the system. In order to infuse an adequate volume of contrast media at high flow (5-6 mL/s) through the entire system, the power injector must inevitably generate a very high pressure upstream of the non-coring needle (even more than 300 PSI). This explains why most of the mechanical damage created by high-pressure/high-speed infusion occurs on the infusion line upstream of the connection between the non-coring needle and the reservoir.

Contrast media imaging parameters that may influence the quality of a CT image are flow rate, total volume of dye, and the distance of the injection site to the right atrium.

1) **flow**: flow rate influences the blood concentration of the contrast media (high rates = high concentrations, low rates = low concentrations).
2) **total volume**: this correlates with the duration of the injection of contrast media at a certain constant flow. In addition, after the passage into the pulmonary circulation, it represents the length of the contrasted blood *column* that will reach the organ to be studied. The longer the column is, the greater

the transit time, and thus the time available for studying the organ. The use of increasingly fast machines has reduced the total volume of the contrast media needed for these exams.

3) **injection site distance**: this element may influence the time between the start of the infusion of contrast media and the *arrival* of the contrasted blood column into the organ to be studied. The greater the distance from the right atrium is, the greater the dilution of the contrast media in the blood. Therefore, at equal flow rates, an injection performed at a shorter distance from the right atrium (i.e. via a central venous line) will produce a greater blood concentration.

Therefore, the execution of CT for parenchymatous abdominal organs preferably requires forced injection (flow rates between 2.5 and 5 mL/s) to obtain a high blood concentration and enhance the contrast media resolution of the parenchyma in the arterial phase. Better resolution will improve diagnostic accuracy; in particular, the contrast media imaging dynamics in the various phases (early arterial, late arterial, portal, and late phase images) will offer a better identification of the focal alterations of the liver, as well as an assessment of their nature.

The key point is whether the *power injection* method through the port is complication-free; once this point is settled in favor of the substantial safety of the procedure (i.e. adopting devices designed and constructed to tolerate the high pressures generated by power injection), the use of a venous port already present might be more cost effective and more comfortable than the search for a suitable peripheral vein, which may not always be easy to find. In this regard, the scientific literature offers only indirect information.

The cost-effectiveness of the use of ports in long-term therapies in cancer patients has been addressed in several papers, but its value is biased by the fact that randomized trials comparing ports vs. repeated venous accesses may be conducted exclusively in patients with an uncompromised peripheral venous system who are undergoing cycles of bolus chemotherapy [6]. In patients with peripheral veins that are already compromised at the initial assessment, or in patients who require infusion chemotherapy, there is a strong recommendation for the insertion of a venous port: therefore, these patients cannot be randomized in studies of adequate statistical power, thus limiting the possibility of achieving Level I scientific evidence [7]. At the present state of scientific knowledge, there is objective evidence that the implantation and use of a port is a safe and effective strategy for long-term venous access in cancer patients, and that this strategy is able to reduce several problems (anxiety, pain, costs) connected with repeated searches for peripheral venous access [8–10].

Among the potential advantages of the use of ports in radiodiagnostics, worthy of note is the possibility for a better standardization of infusion techniques, both among the various patients and within the framework of the follow-up during and/or after therapy in the same patient. Moreover, the infusion of contrast media through a central venous catheter (tip in proximity of the cavoatrial junction) would allow the use of lower flow rates and lower volumes vs. those needed during the infusion in a peripheral vein.

At the present state of knowledge, based on the reports in the scientific literature of the sector, it is not possible to define when the infusion of contrast media via a venous port is contraindicated. In contrast, there are some clinical situations in which infusion of contrast media via the port is strongly indicated, for the purpose of detecting device-related complications such as occlusion or damage of the reservoir and/or of the catheter (so called 'catheter-gram' or 'line-o-gram').

In addition, numerous clinical and experimental studies have described the use of a venous port for radiodiagnostic purposes, without appreciable complications. There is a growing number of studies reporting that the administration of contrast media by power injector into a central venous catheter can be performed safely, with the sole precaution of limiting the injection pressure [11–15]; this is particularly true in pediatric patients, where a smaller volume of contrast is required. It should also be pointed out that the FDA warning refers generically to any type of device (CVC, PICC, and ports), whereas obviously there are significant differences among the different types of access in terms of resistance to pressure damage. In a study which is extremely detailed from the technical standpoint, carried out by a pediatric radiology unit at the Children's Memorial Hospital in Chicago [15], no complication from power injection was observed in 63 children who underwent a CT body scan; care was taken to set the injector at a pressure limit of 25 PSI (172 kPa), i.e. the minimum for this type of injector (Medrad EnVision), in accordance with previous indications from other groups [16]. The authors chose 30 kg as the cut-off body weight to apply the above protocol, since the greatest impact of power injection on the quality of the exam was observed in children with weight below 30 kg. In this study, tunneled catheters performed better – in terms of contrast enhancement – than ports and PICCs.

However, considering the reports of serious damage derived from the use of *power injection* with central venous access devices not specifically equipped for that purpose and the fact that they have also been the subject of the already-mentioned warning of the U.S. Food and Drug Administration in July 2004 [1] – the panel of experts in the GAVeCeLT Consensus prudently recommended that before using a port for radiodiagnostic purposes, the physician and/or the nurse should assess the specific constructive features of the device (as documented for FDA approval or for CE mark) [4].

It was the panel's opinion that the use of a safe venous access device for radiodiagnostic purposes, designed to tolerate the high flows and pressures generated by *power injection*, may be advantageous for the patient (avoidance of a new peripheral or central vein puncture).

Lastly, there is another specific application for power injectable central venous access devices. There are clinical oncologic studies (phase I or II) on the use of innovative experimental drugs, in which the evaluation of the response is made on the basis of RECIST criteria (response evaluation criteria in solid tumor), which are universally recognized and documented [17].

In these cases, an optimal radiologic assessment is of paramount importance; for example, the RECIST Committee recommends that the lymph nodes used as parameters for the definition of the response should be measured in their short axis, rightfully considering this more significant. In such cases, for obvious ethical and cost/benefit reasons, an optimal quality of the radiologic documentation is mandatory. The impossibility of obtaining adequate peripheral venous access (patients with already-compromised peripheral veins, obese patients, etc.) and/or the presence of a central venous access system that cannot be used – because it is not certified for *power injection* - could pose a limit to the performance of this type of more refined assessment.

34.3 Final Recommendations

How to prevent mechanical damage/infectious complications from *power injection*.

- Mechanical damage can be effectively prevented using devices characterized by specific features of design and construction which make them safe for power injection. The manufacturer indication that a totally implantable central venous port is safe for power injection is to be considered an essential requirement when high-flow contrast media infusion is indicated. Since the *power injectability* of the device is normally tested in vitro, the manufacturer's data should be coupled with the actual clinical data (implantation technique, type of contrast media, temperature of injection, needle used to access the system, etc.).
- All the components of the system should be *power injectable* (including the non-coring needle and its extension tube). The *power injectable* port as well as the other *power injectable* components (connectors, non-coring needle, etc.) should be easily recognizable (with clinical and/or radiologic methods: color code of the external components, structural features of the reservoir, etc.), even in absence of the paper documentation.
- Before the actual pressure injection, checking the anatomic location of the catheter and its tip is also recommended (utilizing the so called frontal *scout* view), to rule out malpositions, kinking or other abnormalities which may affect the flow rate and hinder power injection.
- Positioning and stabilization of the non-coring needle should be performed exclusively by medical or nursing personnel specifically trained in this procedure.
- The device must be checked for patency (infusion and withdrawal function) prior to connection to the power injection.
- In order to minimize the risk of infection/needle dislocation/catheter occlusion, the average level of skills in the use of implanted venous ports in radiology departments should be as high as in oncology departments.
- When using a port for contrast medium injection, systematic protocols of interventions for early detection and early management of potential com-

plications should be adopted in the radiologic suite.

- All radiologic units using contrast infusion through venous ports should adopt specific protocols (or 'bundles') for prevention of infective and mechanical complications, and should implement an educational strategy including training courses for the healthcare personnel working with venous access devices [18].
- It is recommended that all future studies defining local strategies for optimal use of ports in radiodiagnostics, should focus on the following endpoints: patient safety (minimization/elimination of complications); cost-effectiveness (best clinical outcome with minimal risk and minimal costs); efficiency (maximal economic yield with minimal use of resources).

References

1. FDA - Center for Devices and Radiological Health (2009) Reminders from FDA regarding ruptured vascular access devices from power injection. http://www.fda.gov/MedicalDevices/-Safety/AlertsandNotices/TipsandArticlesonDeviceSafety/ucm070193.htm. Accessed 20 May 2011
2. Eakle M, Lange S (2010) Device safety. Power injectors put I.V. lines under pressure. http://www.fda.gov/MedicalDevices/Safety/AlertsandNotices/TipsandArticlesonDeviceSafety/ucm225493.htm Accessed 20 May 2011
3. Health Devices (2004) A high-pressure situation: conventional I.V. sets can burst when used with CT contrast injectors. Health Devices 33:100-102
4. ACR (2004) Manual on contrast, 5th edn. American College of Radiology, Reston VA
5. GAVeCeLT (2011) Consensus on the correct use of totally implantable venous access devices for diagnostic radiology procedures. J Vasc Access [Epub ahead of print] doi: 10.5301/JVA.2011.7736
6. Bow EJ, Kilpatrick MG, Clinch JJ (1999) Totally implantable venous access ports systems for patients receiving chemotherapy for solid tissue malignancies: A randomized controlled clinical trial examining the safety, efficacy, costs, and impact on quality of life. J Clin Oncol 17:1267
7. Biffi R, Pozzi S, Pace U et al (2001) Is there a real advantage in utilizing central venous ports in oncology surgery? An analysis of the cost-effectiveness ratio. Tumori 87:S74-S75
8. Biffi R, de Braud F, Orsi F et al (1998) Totally implantable central venous access ports for long-term chemotherapy. A prospective study analyzing complications and costs of 333 devices with a minimum follow-up of 180 days. Ann Oncol 9:767-773
9. Chenecky C (2001) Satisfaction versus dissatisfaction with venous access devices in outpatient oncology: a pilot study. Oncol Nurs Forum 28:1613–1616
10. Gallieni M, Pittiruti M, Biffi R (2008) Vascular access in oncology patients. CA Cancer J Clin 58:323-346
11. Kaste SC, Young CW (1996) Safe use of power injection with central and peripheral venous access devices for pediatric CT. Pediatr Radiol 26:499-501
12. Herts BR, O'Malley CM, Wirth SL et al (2001) Power injection of contrast using central venous catheters: feasibility, safety, and efficacy. AJR 176:447-453
13. Sanelli PC, Deshmuki M, Ougorets I et al (2004) Safety and feasibility of using a central venous catheter for rapid contrast injection rates. AJR 183:1829-1834
14. Amaral JG, Traubici J, BenDavid G et al (2006) Safety of power injector use in children as measured by incidence of extravasation. AJR 187:580-583
15. Rigsby CK, Gasber E, Seshadri R et al (2007) Safety and efficacy of pressure-limited power injection of iodinated contrast media through central lines in children. AJR 188:726-732

16. Ruess L, Bulas DL, Rivera O, Markle BM (1997) In-line pressure generated in small-bore central venous catheters during power injection of CT contrast. Radiology 203:625-629
17. Eisenhauer EA, Therasse P, Bogaerts J et al (2009) New response evaluation criteria in solid tumours: revised RECIST guideline (version 1.1). Eur J Cancer 45:228-247
18. Pittiruti M, Hamilton H, Biffi R et al (2009) ESPEN Guidelines on Parenteral Nutrition: Central Venous Catheters (access, care, diagnosis and therapy of complications). Clin Nutr 28:365–377

Removal of Totally Implantable Venous Access Device

35

Gennaro D. LaBella and Julius Tang

Abstract

Infection, thrombosis, catheter malposition, rupture and embolization associated less frequently with skin erosion make up the main reasons for TIVAD removal. This chapter describes the cause, treatment and prevention of these complications. The surgical technique for removing TIVADs is thoroughly described. Lastly, attention is placed upon air embolism, a potentially devastating complication associated with TIVAD removal.

Keywords

TIVAD removal • Infection • Thrombosis • Catheter malposition • Air embolism • Fowler position

35.1 Life of a Port

It has been estimated that a total of 150,000 totally implantable venous access devices (TIVADs) are implanted each year in the United States [1]. Some of these procedures are performed by surgeons in the operating room, and others are performed by interventional radiologists in angiosuites equipped with real-time imaging devices. The overwhelming majority of these ports were indicated for the management of patients diagnosed with malignant disease. Compared to central venous catheters, the advantages of venous access ports include decreased risk of infection, less labor required for topical dressing

G.D. LaBella (✉)
Hatton Research Center, Good Samaritan Hospital, Department of Medical Education, Cincinnati OH, USA
e-mail: labella84@hotmail.com

I. Di Carlo, R. Biffi (eds.), *Totally Implantable Venous Access Devices*,

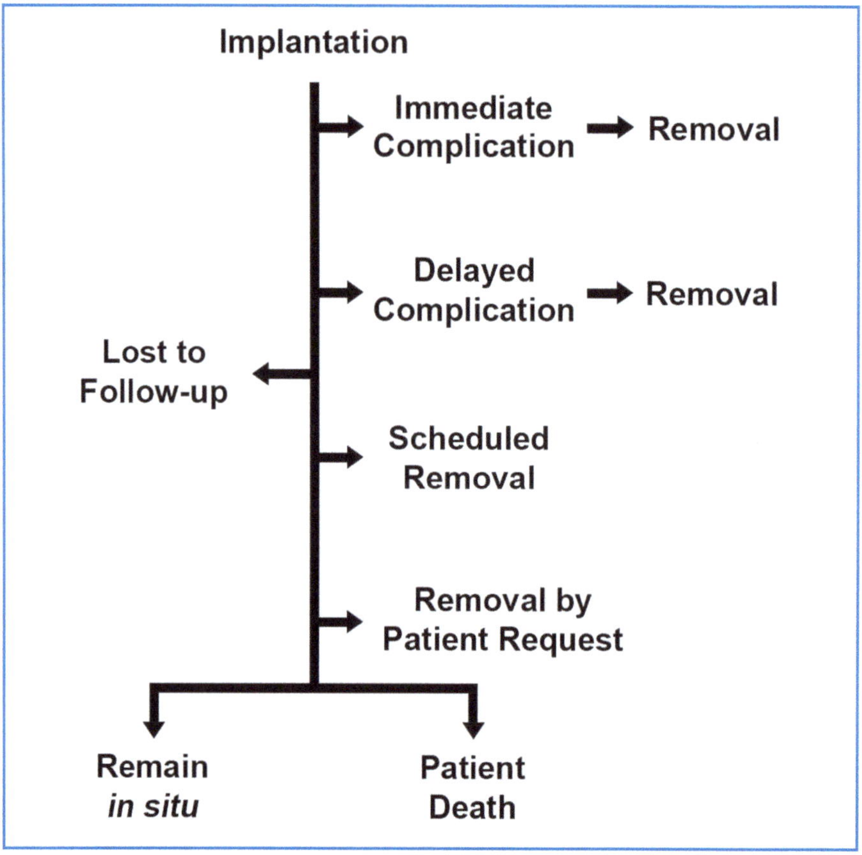

Fig. 35.1 Life of a port

changes, better patient comfort level, and better cosmetic result. Previous studies have also found that the overall cost for maintaining a venous access port was less than that for venous access catheters, therefore it is a more economic option for the healthcare system [2].

As shown in Figure 35.1, after implantation, a TIVAD will be expected to exhibit a variety of outcomes. It should be noted that the majority of TIVADs complete their functional roles without complications (87% in a series of 1500 ports with an average 284 days follow-up [3]). Among these complication-free TIVADs, some remain *in situ* either as a functional device or cause minor problems that are asymptomatic to the patient. Considering the fact that most TIVADs are implanted in patients diagnosed with cancer requiring chemotherapy, it is not surprising that many patients die with their TIVADs *in situ*. In a large series, the median patient survival after port placement was 387 days and the 3-year survival was 21% [4].

Like any implanted devices, TIVADs may cause problems that complicate the management plan. Some complications occur during the initial implantation procedure, such as disengagement between the catheter and port chamber [5], which may require immediate removal of the device. An attempt is often made to implant another device during the same procedure. Other complications occur in the delayed setting, which may be weeks or even months post-implantation. Many of these delayed complications can be managed without removal of the TIVAD, however occasionally explantation is the only reasonable option. The overall removal rate due to port complications is between 5.5% and 18% [5]. Most port-related complications occur after the first administration of chemotherapy [6].

Some care providers opt to schedule an elective TIVAD explantation procedure at the time of implantation [3]. This is done typically after the completion of the associated chemotherapy. It is also not uncommon to encounter a small subset of patients who request their TIVADs be removed, which is motivated by a drive to enjoy a psychological closure of their illnesses.

35.2 Reasons for Removal

35.2.1 Infection

Compared to the more old-school venous access catheter, TIVADs are associated with significantly less risk of infection. This advantage is also retained in the oncologic and AIDS patient populations [7, 8]. Compared to centrally placed ports, peripheral ports have an even lower infection risk [5]. However, throughout the literature, infection of the device has been cited to be the leading cause for device removal. In one series, the overall incidence of infection was estimated to be 4.8% [3]. Patients with solid tumors are less likely to be infected than those with hematologic diseases (6% vs. 8%) [3]. The severity of infection progresses in the following order: port pocket, catheter tunnel, catheter tip and port-related bacteremia.

Infection of the port pocket and the catheter tract most likely indicates direct inoculation or migration of organisms along the accessing needle [2]. Such infection is a rather uncommon event with incidence less than 1%. Administration of empiric antibiotic is appropriate; covering gram-positive cocci is important because the offending species are often found to be *Staphylococcus* species. Port removal is not warranted unless the infection progresses to systemic disease or is associated with thrombosis [5].

Unlike infections of the port and catheter, bacteremia is a much stronger indication for port removal. The incidence was around 2.4% [2]. Causative agents include *Staphlococcus aureus*, *Staphylococcus epidermis*, *Streptococcus lactaceae*, *Pseudomonas aeruginosa*, Klebsiella, *Escherichia coli*, and *Bacillus subtilis*. Bacteremia can be a much delayed problem. In one series, the median period between implantation and diagnosis of bacteremia was 165 days.

35.2.2 Thrombosis

Thrombosis of the catheterized vein is the second leading cause for TIVAD removal. The incidence has been estimated to be between 1.5% and 5.9% [2, 3, 9]. The cardinal complaint is ipsilateral arm swelling without neurologic deficit. The diagnostic work-up includes an initial screening by duplex ultrasonography followed by a confirmation test by contrast venography. Full anticoagulation is recommended and has been shown to fully treat the condition and prevent port removal [5]. It has been proposed that thrombosis of the catheterized vein is a progression of catheter obstruction. For thrombosis within the catheter, per catheter lytic therapy (urokinase) has been used with a 40% success rate. It has also been noted that a catheter tip above the level of T3 can be associated with major risk factor for thrombosis [10]. Thrombosis combined with ongoing infection are strong grounds for prompt port removal.

35.2.3 Catheter Malposition

The incidence of catheter malposition complication is estimated between 1.6% and 2.4% [3, 9]. There are two types of pathophysiology. One is heralded by the pinch-off sign on chest radiograph, which indicates the site of catheter leakage between the clavicle and first rib (Fig. 35.2). The other occurs in obese patients where the tip of the catheter migrates too peripherally due to tissue traction in the upright position. Placing the catheter tip deep in the right atrium is recommended in the obese patient population.

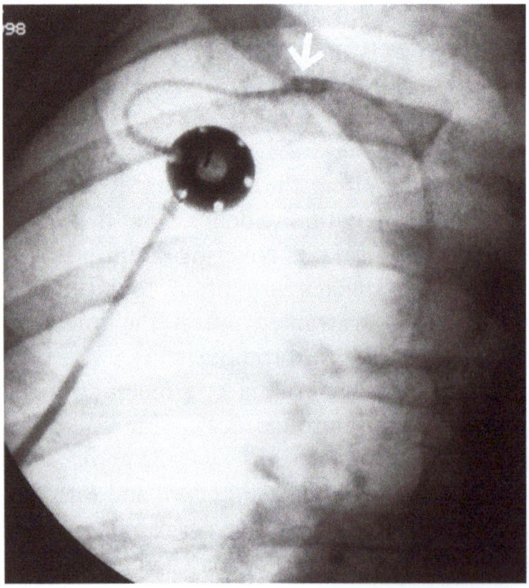

Fig. 35.2 Pinch-off sign (*arrow*) in a female patient (31 years). From [9], with permission

35.2.4 Other Problems

Catheter rupture and embolism caused by the fractured segments have been reported [2]. The incidence was 1.5% in a series of 328 patients. Clinical presentation included palpitations and chest discomfort, and the diagnosis was made by chest radiograph. Other cases were found incidentally on chest films ordered for cancer re-staging. All dislodged fragments were retrieved via venous transfemoral approach without additional morbidity. Device removal was not performed.

Skin erosion over the port is an uncommon event, reported as one occurrence in over 300 devices placed in one series [2]. A new implant is often needed at a different anatomic site. Ensuring a skin thickness of at least 1 cm over the port during implantation has been recommended to prevent this problem.

35.3 Surgical Technique

Due to the fact that many TIVADs are removed by surgeons who did not implant them, it is important to familiarize oneself with the type of device implanted, the anatomic location, and the vascular structures involved prior to the explantation procedure.

There are a great number of TIVADs available on the market. Nearly all of them include a silicone rubber catheter, a port chamber made from stainless steel, titanium or non-metal materials, and a silicone rubber septum for access. The differences between different device systems are limited to geometric shape and mechanical details.

In nearly all TIVADs implanted on the chest wall, the port chamber is embedded in the subclavicular fossa. However, there is no consensus regarding which side is preferred. Some prefer the non-dominant side (left side in most patients). Some prefer the right side due to a more linear course of the subclavian vein and SVC. Neither is there consensus regarding the priority of veins to be cannulated. One group of practitioners attempted the subclavian vein first and only used the jugular vein if the subclavian vessel could not be reached with the standard length needle. In another study, the external jugular veins were most commonly accessed. In very rare cases, the great saphenous vein was chosen after all upper body options were exhausted.

The vast majority of TIVAD implantation procedures are done by using local anesthesia without perioperative antibiotic prophylaxis. It can be easily argued that the explantation procedure can be accomplished by using the same standards. It is preferable to place the patient in the Trendelenburg position if it is tolerated. By doing so, one lowers the operative field below the heart, creating a greater intravascular-to-environment pressure gradient, which decreases the risk of air embolism. Incision is typically made through the old incision used for port placement. In very recently placed ports, the body typically

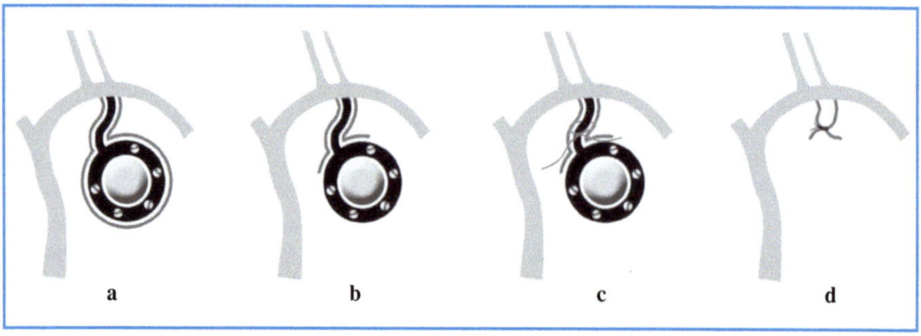

Fig. 35.3 Removal of a port

forms a fibrous sheath around the port chamber and the catheter (Fig. 35.3a). This sheath needs to be meticulously dissected without damage to the underlying hardware (Fig. 35.3b). It is particularly helpful to use a scalpel, instead of a pair of scissors, to dissect around the catheter-port-junction in order to avoid damage to the catheter. After this is accomplished, the visible part of the catheter is secured to prevent its dislodgement from the operative field. Attention is then turned to the possible presence of anchoring sutures around the port chamber. There has been much variability regarding whether and where to put these sutures that one must fully explore the entire circumference of the port to be sure. At this point, after ensuring the catheter is fully mobile in its tunnel, the surgeon may place a figure-of-eight stitch around the catheter exit site without tying it (Fig. 35.3c), then the catheter is pulled and this stitch is quickly tied down (Fig. 35.3d). Placing the figure-of-eight stitch prior to catheter withdrawal enhances the prompt closure of the catheter tract, therefore decreasing the risk of air embolism. The empty pocket is now inspected for hemostasis and the skin incision is closed in layers. It is not unreasonable to send the fibrous sheath for pathologic analysis [11].

35.4 Air Embolism

The phenomenon of air embolism deserves a separate and focused discussion because it is perhaps the most devastating complication associated with port removal. It is, however, an uncommon event. The exact incidence of air embolism occurring during TIVAD explantation has not been reported in the literature, yet it can occur in up to 10% of neurosurgical procedures with the patient in the supine position and up to 80% in the Fowler's (sitting) position.

Two conditions must coexist for air embolism to occur: (1) a direct communication between the intravascular compartment and a source of air; and (2) a pressure gradient favoring the transfer of air from the environment into the lumen of a blood vessel. Unfortunately, both conditions can be provided during removal of a port. The withdrawal of the catheter from its tract creates a passageway for

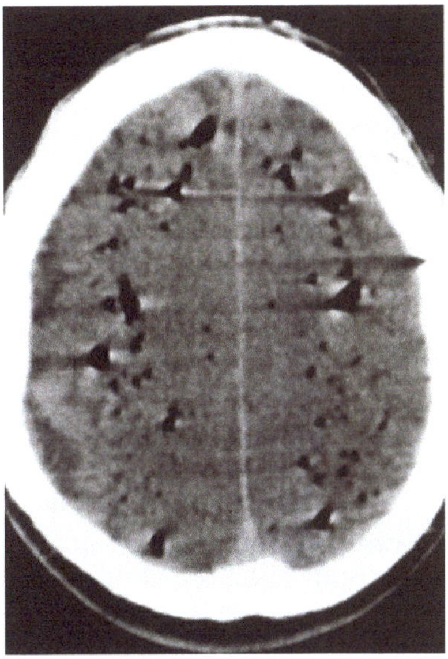

Fig. 35.4 Gas in both cerebral hemispheres with diffuse edema. From [15], with permission

air movement, and the position of the operative field above the heart (if patient not placed in Trendelenburg) creates the pressure gradient needed.

Because this discussion is limited to venous air embolism involving the superior vena cava and its feeding branches, the destination of the air emboli lies in the pulmonary vasculature. Patent foramen ovale, cardiac septal defect, and pulmonary arterial-venous malformation may provide opportunities for paradoxical embolism and involvement of the arterial vasculature. The lungs are known to be able to filter microbubbles of air from the venous circulation, however this filtration system can be overwhelmed. It is estimated that the fatal dose of air for humans is 300 mL to 500 mL of gas at rate of 100 mL/s. This can be introduced by a 14-gauge needle with a pressure gradient as low as 5 cm of H_2O [12].

Air embolism, especially in the operating room setting, largely remains as a clinical diagnosis and a diagnosis of exclusion. An almost universal presentation is dyspnea which may be accompanied by substernal chest pain. A sucking noise is occasionally audible to the operating surgeon. A fall in end-tidal CO_2 may be noticed by the anesthesia team. Chest radiograph is usually normal. A postoperative CT scan can detect only 10 to 25 percent of asymptomatic air emboli, however massive intraparenchymal gas of the brain can sometimes be quite impressive (Fig. 35.4) [13].

A number of maneuvers or prevention mechanisms can be used to decrease the likelihood of air embolism or its progression. They are listed below.

- Preoperative:
  - Treat hypovolemia;
  - Prophylactically place the patient in Trendelenburg position;

- Intraoperative:
  - When the diagnosis of air embolism is suspected, immediately place the patient in the Trendelenburg position, left lateral decubitus position (Durant's maneuver), or left lateral decubitus head down position. Since the pulmonary artery is towards the right side of the right ventricle, these maneuvers will increase the chance that the air bubble will be trapped within the right ventricle without distal migration;
  - If these maneuvers fail, chest compressions should be performed. The rationale is to force the air out of the pulmonary outflow tract and into smaller pulmonary vessels;
  - Attempt to aspirate the air if a central venous catheter is already in place. However, placing a new catheter for this purpose has been associated with limited benefit;
  - Start high-flow supplemental oxygen, which replaces the nitrogen in the air bubble to facilitate its absorption into the blood;
  - Discontinue nitrous oxide, because it has a tendency to diffuse from blood into the air bubble, enlarging its size.
- Postoperative:
  - Hyperbaric oxygen therapy, if available and started between 6 to 30 hours, may improve outcome [13, 14]. Early therapy is associated with greater benefit.

Despite advancements in treatment strategies developed in the late part of the last century, air embolism is still associated with 1-year mortality of 21%.

35.5 Conclusions

In the authors' experience, to avoid back-bleeding the simple removal of the port without stitching closed the tract of the catheter can lead to delayed bleeding and hematoma formation. Air embolism, although a rare complication, can also occur. Careful attention to hemostasis and closure of the sheath that forms around the capsule should eliminate this potential complication from TIVAD removal.

References

1. Sticca RP, Dewing BD, Harris, JD (2009). Outcomes of surgical and radiologic placed implantable central venous access ports. Am J Surg 198:829–833
2. Biffi R, de Braud F, Orsi F et al (1998) Totally implantable central venous access ports for long-term chemotherapy: a prospective study analyzing complications and costs of 333 devices with a minimum follow-up of 180 days. Ann Oncol 9:767–773
3. Kock HJ, Pietsch M, Krause U et al (1998) Implantable vascular access systems: experience in 1500 patients with totally implanted central venous port systems. World J Surg 22:12–16
4. Schwarz R, Groeger J, Coit D (1997) Subcutaneously implanted central venous access devices in cancer patients: a prospective analysis. Cancer 79:1635–1640

5. Vardy J, Engelhardt K, Cox K et al (2004) Long-term outcome of radiological-guided insertion of implanted central venous access port devices (CVAPD) for the delivery of chemotherapy in cancer patients. Br J Cancer 91:1045-1049
6. Ignatov A, Hoffman O, Smith B et al (2008) An 11-year retrospective study of totally implanted central venous access ports: Complications and patient satisfaction. Eur J Surg Oncol 35:241–246
7. Groeger JS, Lucas AB, Thaler HAT et al (1993) Infectious morbidity associated with longterm use of venous access devices in patients with cancer. Ann Intern Med 119:1168–1174
8. Muscedere G, Bennett JD, Lee TY et al (1998) Complications of radiologically placed central venous ports and Hickman catheters in patients with AIDS. Can Assoc Radiol J 49:84–89
9. Lorch H, Zwaan M, Kagel C, Weiss H (2001) Central venous access ports placed by interventional radiologists: experience with 125 consecutive patients. Cardiovasc Intervent Radiol 24:180–184
10. Puel V, Caudry M, Le Metayer P et al (1993) Superior vena cava thrombosis related to catheter malposition in cancer chemotherapy given through implanted ports. Cancer 72:2248–2252
11. de Gregorio MA, Miguelena JM, Fernandez JA et al (1996) Subcutaneous ports in the radiology suite: an effective and safe procedure for care in cancer patients. Eur Radiol 6:748–752
12. Ordway CB (1974) Air embolus via CVP catheter without positive pressure: presentation of case and review. Ann Surg 179:479
13. Armon C, Deschamps C, Adkinson C et al (1991) Hyperbaric treatment of cerebral air embolism sustained during an open-heart surgical procedure. Mayo Clin Proc 66:565
14. Groell R, Schaffler GJ, Rienmueller R, Kern R (1997) Vascular air embolism: location, frequency, and cause on electron-beam CT studies of the chest. Radiology 202:459
15. Valentino R, Hilbert G, Vargas F, Gruson D (2003) Computed tomographic scan of massive cerebral air embolism. Lancet 361:1848

Cost Issues

36

Robert P. Sticca, Bree D. Dewing and Joel D. Harris

Abstract

Costs associated with totally implantable venous access devices (TIVAD) are variable and depend on multiple factors. TIVAD costs can be categorized into four types, insertion, maintenance, removal and complications. Variation in TIVAD costs are due to regional and national variation in expenses, contractural agreements, healthcare system variation, cost bundling, and variable accounting methods. They can be difficult to reliably track and there is wide variation in the reported costs in the literature. Costs for complications of TIVAD insertion and use can be significant and add to the total cost of TIVAD. Despite the costs, the convenience and improved quality of life for patients who need long term venous access make TIVAD an important part of their treatment programs.

Keywords

Costs • Totally implantable access devices • Portacath • Central venous access • Complications

36.1 Introduction

The use of totally implantable venous access devices (TIVADs) has become routine in patients needing long-term venous access for a variety of indications, most commonly for oncologic treatment or blood product administration. While generally accepted as the standard of care for long-term venous

R.P. Sticca (✉)
University of North Dakota School of Medicine and Health Sciences,
North Dakota, USA
e-mail: robert.sticca@med.und.edu

access because of their reliability, convenience and ease of use, the actual costs of TIVAD can be difficult to evaluate. TIVAD costs can be divided into four principle categories including insertion, maintenance, removal and complications. Costs are defined as the actual expense of the goods or services that are used by the provider in TIVAD related expenditures. As in the case of most medical expenses, TIVAD costs are then passed on to the patients, through charges to the payor (either the patient or a third party payor). Charges are defined as the amount billed to the payor for services. The amount of reimbursement, or compensation for the charges, is highly variable and depends on the payor (private insurance, government insurance or patient) and the type of contractual agreement with the provider. In the USA the reimbursement for medical charges can range from 30–85% of the actual charges due to discounts and contractual agreements between the provider and the payor.

Table 36.1 gives the approximate costs and charges for insertion, maintenance and removal of TIVAD in the Midwestern USA in 2011 US dollars. These figures are listed for comparison. Because of the variability in costs and charges the figures shown in this table may not be transferable to other parts of the USA or other countries. Professional fees charged by the surgeon, interventional radiologist or anesthesiologist are reported in work relative value units (RVUs), which are the units used to quantify the value of the work product in the USA. RVUs are listed as a cost in this report as the surgeon or interventional radiologist fees are an expense paid to the providers for their services inserting and removing the TIVAD. The monetary value of each RVU may

Table 36.1 Current (2011) approximate costs and charges of TIVAD

Category	Costs (US $)	Charges (US $)
Insertion		
Patient charge	N/A	5,300
Single lumen port	175	Included in patient charge
Double lumen port	325	Included in patient charge
Operating room	800	Included in patient charge
Recovery	225	Included in patient charge
Anesthesia	Variable	855
Surgeon	6.04 RVU*	2,445
Interventional radiologist	6.04 RVU	2,445
Maintenance		
Patient charge	N/A	55
Supplies	5.50	Included in patient charge
Nursing	15	Included in patient charge
Removal		
Patient charge	N/A	105
Surgical supplies	25	Included in patient charge
Nursing	15	Included in patient charge
Surgeon	3.35 RVU	597

*Relative Value Unit.

vary by region or by individual institution within a region (currently in the US the value of each RVU ranges from $40-$60 for general surgery). As with hospital or clinic charges the reimbursement for the professional fees is often discounted or limited by third party payors. There are several inherent problems in collecting, analyzing and comparing costs of TIVAD, including the regional and international variation in costs and charges, the bundling of TIVAD costs with other treatment charges, variable accounting methods of costs and charges between institutions and healthcare systems, and the variation in allowed billable expenses in different locations and health systems. The types of costs associated with TIVAD placement and use and some of the difficulties in collecting and analyzing them will be discussed in this chapter.

36.2 Insertion Costs

Because of the multiple types of healthcare systems, payor arrangements and reimbursement methods, the actual costs and charges for TIVAD placement can vary significantly depending on the geographic location of insertion and use. The cost of insertion is determined by several factors including the type of port placed, the manufacturer of the TIVAD, the type of contract the TIVAD manufacturer has with the institution where the port is placed, the location of placement (operating room or interventional radiology suite), type of anesthesia used and technique of insertion. Several studies have demonstrated improved safety and efficacy with the use of fluoroscopy and ultrasound in the insertion of TIVAD, therefore these expenses are generally incorporated into the insertion costs of TIVAD [1-3].

While there are a wide variety of TIVAD types and manufacturers there is little objective evidence to indicate that any one type of port is superior to another [4, 5]. The variations in TIVADs include different materials for construction of the port or catheter, valved versus unvalved ports and manufacturers claims of superiority for a particular type of TIVAD. The type of port selected for use should be based on the best cost and service available to an institution. The one exception is the choice between single and double lumen ports. Double lumen ports traditionally carry higher complication and infection rates [6, 7] and cost almost twice as much as single lumen ports (Table 36.1), therefore they should only be used in selected circumstances when access to the central venous system for two different purposes is needed. Additional costs for TIVAD insertion include operating room or interventional radiology suite expenses, pharmacy charges (antibiotics), recovery room expenses and the professional fees for the surgeon, interventional radiologist and anesthesiologist (Table 36.1). In 2011 total costs and charges for TIVAD insertion in the USA are approximately $1500 and $8,500 respectively (Table 36.1). Reimbursement for TIVAD insertion is typically 30 to 43% of the charges or $2600 to $3650.

In addition to the variability in costs and charges caused by the differences

Table 36.2 Cost comparison of totally implantable access port (TIVAD) placement

Author	Institution	Cost	Charge (US$)
Biffi et al. (1998)	European Institute of Oncology	$1591 (USD)	Not reported
Bow et al. (1999)	University of Manitoba Study Control	$1988 (CAD) $2005	Not reported
Schuld et al. (2009)	Germany	Local $400.72 (EUR) General $484.86	Not reported
Sticca et al. (2009)	University of North Dakota	Not Reported	IR $5,301 Surg $4,553
Hancock et al. (2010)	University of Toronto	IR $20,762 (CAD) Surg $20,900 (what was included?)	Not reported

in health systems and payment methods, the cost of TIVAD insertion can also vary between professionals in different specialties who perform the insertion. In the medical literature there has been debate on which specialty can perform TIVAD insertion at lower cost with better outcomes, especially among surgeons and interventional radiologists. In the radiology literature there are several articles that have indicated radiologic placement of TIVADs can be done with improved outcomes and at a lower cost than surgical placement [8, 9]. A Canadian study published in 2010 by Hancock et al. found slightly lower costs with pediatric TIVADs inserted by interventional radiology versus operative insertion (Table 36.2) [10]. We studied the differences in billed charges and reimbursement of 368 TIVADs placed by surgery and interventional radiology in a Midwestern US community hospital. Of these, 276 were placed by interventional radiology with a mean charge and reimbursement of $5,301 (USD) and $1,660 (USD) respectively. This resulted in a 31% reimbursement for TIVADs placed radiologically compared to 43% for surgically placed TIVADs for which the average charge was $4,553 (USD) and reimbursement $1, 660 (USD) [11]. There was no statistical difference in the rate of complications from this study, with the surgically placed ports showing a trend towards fewer complications. Based on this study it was concluded that prior assertions of radiologically placed TIVADs being less expensive and resulting in fewer complications may no longer be valid.

Unfortunately, the limited literature on TIVAD insertion cost makes comparisons difficult due to lack of standardization of placement techniques, where the insertion occurs (interventional radiology suite versus operating room), access to and use of imaging guidance, type of anesthesia, involvement of anesthesia practitioners, experience of the physician performing the procedure and variation in professional charges. Available information from currently published sources on TIVAD is summarized in Table 36.2. These figures demonstrate the wide variability in reported costs for TIVAD insertion, making comparison and critical evaluation of these costs difficult.

36.3 Maintenance Costs

Costs for maintenance of TIVAD are related to the frequency of maintenance flushes and therapeutic use. The costs are similar for both functions of TIVAD and involve the cost of the preparation and access kit, the nursing time necessary to access the port and the heparinized solutions used to flush the port. Current guidelines recommend TIVAD flushing every 4 weeks when not in use [12-13]. Similar costs are also incurred after each therapeutic use, of which the frequency varies depending on the treatment regimen and type of use. Current costs in the US are $5 for the access kit, $15 for nursing time, and $0.50 for the heparin flush with a total cost of $20.50 (Table 36.1). The current charges for maintenance flushing are $55.

36.4 Removal Costs

TIVAD removal is commonly done as an outpatient procedure in an office setting. Some providers prefer to remove TIVAD in an operating room which significantly increases the costs. When done as an office procedure the costs are related to the surgical supplies used to remove the port and close the incision. There is a professional fee which is charged for port removal. In the US port removal costs and charges are approximately $225 and $600. These figures include the surgical supplies, nursing time and professional fees for TIVAD removal.

36.5 Complications Costs

In the current literature there are multiple detailed studies which elucidate the causes and prevention of complications related to TIVAD. A smaller body of literature is available which evaluates costs associated with port placement and removal. However, there remains a paucity of data regarding the costs associated with port complications. The few studies which made an effort to determine cost data for TIVAD related complications are often limited by confounding factors such as:

- additional procedures completed during the hospital stay;
- professional charges are often separated from institution charges;
- billed charges do not often represent actual costs or reimbursement;
- cost data is variable and studies reviewing costs more than 3-5 years prior significantly under represent current costs;
- costs cannot be generalized between health systems, both public and private as well as between countries with vastly different cost structures.

A 2004 study by Carlo et al. compared catheter tip occlusion and clotting of valved and nonvalved implantable ports [14]. During the first 180 days postimplantation, events of catheter tip occlusion or thrombosis requiring

Table 36.3 Costs associated with TIVAD complications [15]

Early complication	Treatment	n (%)	Cost ($US)/patient
Pneumothorax (<30%)	Observation	4 (1.2)	535
Pneumothorax (>30%)	Tube thoracostomy	6 (1.8)	1827
Early malfunction or obstruction	Revision of device	6 (1.8)	637
Late complication	**Treatment**	**n (%)**	**Cost ($US)/patient**
Catheter rupture or migration	Angiogram and retrieval	5 (1.5)	1182
Venous thrombosis	LMWH then warfain	5 (1.5)	1840
Pocket infection	Antibiotics	1 (0.3)	85
Skin erosion without infection	Reimplantation	1 (0.3)	474.50
Port-related bacteremia	Antibiotics alone	2 (0.6)	1145
Port-related bacteremia	Antibiotics and removal	6 (1.8)	2141

LMWH, low molecular weight heparin.

alteplase administration were identified in 39 of the 73 study patients. The cost of alteplase, nursing charges and infusion tubing totaled $480/event. Some of the events also required a chest radiograph to rule out anatomic complications such as catheter kinking which further increased costs.

A 1998 study conducted in Italy provided the most comprehensive look at total costs related to port complications [15]. Three hundred thirty-three ports were placed in 328 patients after diagnosis of a solid tumor. The patients were followed for a median of 237 catheter days. The number of early and late complications and associated costs are summarized in Table 36.3. Because these costs were reported over a decade ago, current costs for TIVAD complications are expected to be significantly higher. In 2010, Scaife et al. from the University of Utah reported that inpatient treatment including catheter removal in a single patient who developed a catheter related infection amounted to $49,000 [16].

Complications related to implantable catheters are relatively rare but they continue to occur despite refinements in technique, catheter care and management. They can add significant cost to the total cost of port placement and use. TIVAD complication costs can be difficult to analyze and compare due to many factors which impact the data. To date, few studies have evaluated the cost and impact of catheter related complications. Additional studies focusing on the cost of catheter related complications are necessary particularly when faced with the persistent rise in the cost of medical care and the possibility that caregivers and institutions are being threatened with declining reimbursement when treating catheter-related complications.

36.6 Conclusions

The costs associated with TIVAD placement and use are difficult to assess and compare due to multiple factors, but are considered reasonable and necessary for patients needing long-term venous access. The convenience and improved quality of life have made TIVAD an important part of the treatment program for many patients. Complications related to TIVADs can be costly and can significantly add to the total cost of TIVAD placement and use.

References

1. Hind D, Calvert N, McWilliams R et al (2003) Ultrasonic locating devices for central venous cannulation: meta-analysis. BMJ 327:361
2. Calvert N, Hind D, McWilliams R et al (2004) Ultrasound for central venous cannulation: economic evaluation of cost-effectiveness. Anaesthesia 59:1116–1120
3. Bold RJ, Winchester DJ, Madary AR et al (1998) Prospective, randomized trial of Doppler-assisted subclavian vein catheterization. Arch Surg 133:1089–1093
4. Biffi R, De Braud F, Orsi F et al (2001) A randomized, prospective trial of central venous ports connected to standard open-ended or Groshong catheters in adult oncology patients. Cancer 92:1204–1212
5. Pratt RJ, Pellowe CM, Wilson JA et al (2007) epic2: National evidence-based guidelines for preventing healthcare-associated infections in NHS hospitals in England. J Hosp Infect 65[suppl]:S1–S64
6. Dezfulian C, Lavelle J, Nallamothu BK et al (2003) Rates of infection for single-lumen versus multilumen central venous catheters: a meta-analysis. Crit Care Med 31:2385–2390
7. Farkas JC, Liu N, Bleriot JP et al (1992) Single versus triple-lumen central catheter-related sepsis: a prospective randomized study in a critically ill population. Am J Med 93:277–282
8. Funaki B, Szymski GX, Hackworth CA et al (1997) Radiologic placement of subcutaneous infusion chest ports for long term central venous access. Am J Radiol 169:1431-1434
9. McBride KD, Fisher R, Warnock N et al (1997) A comparitive analysis of radiologic and surgical placement of central venous catheters. Cardiovasc Interv Radiol 20:17-22
10. Hancock HR, Connolly BL, McMahon M et al (2010) Cost-effectiveness analysis of implantable venous access device insertion using interventional radiologic versus conventional operating room methods in pediatric patients with cancer. J Vasc Interv Radiol 5:677-684
11. Sticca RP, Dewing BD, Harris JD (2009) Outcomes of surgical and radiologic placed implantable central venous access ports. Am J Surg 198:829-833
12. Bishop L, Dougherty L, Bodenham A et al (2007) Guidelines on the insertion and management of central venous access devices in adults. Int J Lab Hematol 29:261–278
13. Infusion Nurses Society (2006) Infusion nursing standards of practice. J Infus Nurs 29[suppl]:S1–S92
14. Carlo JT, Lamont JP, McCarty TM et al (2004) A prospective randomized trial demonstrating valved implantable ports have fewer complications and lower overall cost than nonvalved implantable ports. Am J Surg 188:722-727
15. Biffi R, de Braud F, Orsi F et al (1998) Totally implantable central venous access ports for long term chemotherapy. Ann Oncol 9:767-773
16. Scaife CL, Gross ME, Mone MC et al (2010) Antibiotic prophylaxis in the placement of totally implanted central venous access ports. Am J Surgery 200:719-723

Quality of Life and Patients Satisfaction

37

José Luis Fougo

Abstract

Although not scientifically proven yet, there are patient-driven data that suggest that TIVADs have brought gains to the quality of life of oncologic patients.

Keywords

Quality of life • Morbidity • Outpatient

37.1 Introduction

The clinical application of totally implanted venous access devices (TIVADs) started in 1982 [1].

At the time, surgeons used to implant TIVADs in the main operating room, under general anesthesia, in an inpatient regimen, and with the aid of perioperative radiography (C-arm); patients had to meet all the requirements of the pre-anesthetic protocol (blood tests, electrocardiogram, 6 hours of fasting).

Requests for placement of TIVADs were scarce. However, healthcare professionals were aware that the need for frequent venipuncture in cancer patients, as well as the irritating effect of cytostatic agents, lead to strong inconvenience and to venous thrombosis and sclerosis. Therefore, the need for a permanent access to a central vein plays a leading role in current oncology.

J.L. Fougo (✉)
Breast Centre and Department of General Surgery,
Hospital de São João,
Porto, Portugal
e-mail: joseluisfougo@gmail.com

I. Di Carlo, R. Biffi (eds.), *Totally Implantable Venous Access Devices*,

Over time more aggressive treatment regimens were emerging; in addition, the development of home care chemotherapy treatments, with elastomeric infusion pumps, has driven demand for the placement of such devices.

TIVADs have several advantages over peripheral venipuncture and other types of central vein devices, such as short-term central venous catheters or long-term Hickman or Broviac catheters. These include easy access to blood samples, low rates of catheter-related infections, easy puncture and perfusion, full protection of the device through the skin, reduced cosmetic impact, diminished impact on the daily life activities (such as bathing), easy placement and removal, allowance of home treatments and feeling of security [2-4].

Hickman/Broviac lines are long-term intravenous catheters that are partially tunneled under the skin, from the entry site to the vein puncture site; moreover, they are manufactured with a cuff near the entry site, which secures the catheter to the skin and protects the patient from bacterial migration. They are mainly used for chemotherapy treatment purposes, but they may be used for dialysis or aphaeresis. Their major handicap is the fact that a part of the catheter is external and requires patient care and frequent dressings.

Nevertheless, TIVADs have some drawbacks. They are not free from complications, which may be over 40%. Although considered a simple procedure, TIVAD placement (as well as utilization and maintenance) requires care and precision. Each step of the procedure may induce distinct types of complications. A defective procedure may have direct impact on the quality of life of the patient (possible hospital admission to treat a pneumothorax, possible chronic pain owing to brachial plexus injury, possible device replacement, eventual requirement of coumadin anti-coagulants, etc.) or indirect, as the chemotherapy treatment may be delayed due to TIVAD problems. In order to avoid these troubles, TIVAD placement and handling should be organized by experienced teams of surgical oncologists and cancer nurses.

Some of the disadvantages may be detailed as follows: pain in the act of puncturing, unsightly scars, the need for regular (monthly) heparin flushing, the need for a final surgical intervention for the removal of the device, beyond its intrinsic morbidity.

Adequate use of the device is crucial for the cancer patient. Port puncture should be done under strict sterile conditions [5]. After each use, the port and the catheter should be flushed to clean any kind of precipitate sediments and to prevent clot formation, both of which will impair the future proper use of the TIVAD.

37.2 Use of TIVADs Nowadays

Today, TIVADs may be inserted in an outpatient setting, under local anesthesia and without perioperative radiological control. The growing calls for the insertion of TIVADs, the local logistics, and the feeling that we should simplify the patient's life have forced these changes in surgical practice. These

Table 37.1 Patient questionnaire to assess changes in TIVAD implantation

Table Query	Yes (%)	No (%)
Were you well informed about the surgical procedure?	85	15
Did you feel supported during the operation?	89.5	10.5
Was the procedure painful?	21.2	78.8
Did the procedure take too long?	11.2	88.8
Were you provided with adequate information about the catheter?	88.1	11.9
Would you repeat the procedure under local anesthesia?	83.6	16.4
Would you repeat the procedure as an outpatient?	85.1	14.9
Would you counsel a friend or relative to undergo such a procedure under the same conditions?	91	9
Were your preoperative fears and expectations realized?	29.9	70.1
Did the TIVAD affect your daily living?	6.1	93.9
Did the TIVAD facilitate the treatment?	98.5	1.5

changes were analyzed in a prospective and observational cohort [6]. To assess the impact of these changes, from the standpoint of the patients, we conducted an anonymous survey in a consecutive series of 100 patients. We obtained complete answers from 67 patients, and the results (Table 36.1) validated the changes [7].

This outpatient surgery setting minimally interferes in the patient's daily life. The implantation through the internal jugular vein achieved acceptable morbidity rates, well within the range of actual published morbidity rates [8, 9].

Although it stands to reason that TIVADs improve quality of life and the satisfaction of oncologic patients during the treatment process, we could find no clear published data to support this. Bow et al. [2] developed a randomized study to compare the outcomes (safety, efficacy, costs and quality of life) of two distinct vein accesses: peripheral vein vs Port-a-Cath. They verified that ports (TIVAD) are safe and effective, but lack a positive impact on quality of life, despite the reduced anxiety, pain and discomfort associated with the port access. The drawback of this study may be related to its design, since TIVAD carriers kept receiving peripheral venous punctures and finger-pricks for blood tests. Costs for the TIVAD placement and use were considered to be four times higher than for peripheral access.

The choice of the central vein, as well as the choice of the technique to implant the device, may generate different rates of morbidity [9] and hence may impact positively or negatively on quality of life. To address this issue, Biffi et al. [10] carried out a randomized study to assess the impact on quality of life of three different TIVAD placement approaches: percutaneous landmark to the internal jugular vein, ultrasound-guided to the subclavian vein and surgical cutdown to the cephalic vein. In terms of quality of life, none of the techniques demonstrated advantages over the others.

Another patient query-based study was published by Kreis et al. [4]. Patients answered a 26 question survey on port-related aspects of everyday life. The authors received positive feedback from patients, supporting TIVAD placement and use among cancer patients. They highlighted the need for a prompt removal of the device after the end of the chemotherapy.

The common techniques for TIVAD placement are safe and effective and can be done in a simple way, minimally interfering with patient routines. The TIVAD also provides a way for safe drug perfusion, in the hospital or at home. In spite of its intrinsic morbidity, higher costs and the absence of clear published evidence of improved quality of life, there are patient-driven data, together with the daily experience of healthcare professionals (placement and use of TIVADs) that indicate improvements in the quality of life and satisfaction of cancer patients. The time may have come for a definitive study to confirm these issues.

References

1. Niederhuber JE, Ensminger W, Gyves JW et al (1982) Totally implanted venous and arterial access system to replace external catheters in cancer treatment. Surgery 92:706-712
2. Bow EJ, Kilpatrick MG, Clinch JJ (1999) Totally implantable venous access ports systems for patients receiving chemotherapy for solid tissue malignancies: a randomized controlled clinical trial examining the safety, efficacy, costs and impact on quality of life. J Clin Oncol 17:1267-1273
3. Teichgraber UK, Kausche S, Nagel SN, Gebauer B (2011) Outcome analysis in 3160 implantations of radiologically guided placements of totally implantable central venous port systems. Eur Radiol 2011 DOI: [Epub ahead of print] doi:10.1007/s00330-010-2045-7
4. Kreis H, Loheberg CR, Lux MP et al (2007) Patient's attitudes to totally implantable venous access port systems for gynecological or breast malignancies. Eur J Surg Oncol 33:39-43
5. Vescia S, Baumgartner AK, Jacobs VR et al (2008) Management of venous port systems in oncology: a review of current evidence. Ann Oncol 19:9-15
6. Araújo C, Silva JP, Antunes P et al (2008) A comparative study between two central veins for the introduction of totally implantable venous access devices in 1201 cancer patients. Eur J Surg Oncol 34:222-226
7. Fougo JL (2008) Cateteres venosos centrais de longa duração: considerações práticas sobre a sua colocação, utilização e remoção. Lidel-edições técnicas, Lda, Portugal
8. Di Carlo I, Pulvirenti E, Mannino M, Toro A (2010) Increased use of percutaneous technique for totally implantable venous access devices. Is it real progress? A 27-year comprehensive review on early complications. Ann Surg Oncol 17:1649-1656
9. Teichgraber UK, Pfitzman R, Hofmann HA (2011) Central venous port systems as an integral part of chemotherapy. Dtsch Arztbl Int 108:147-154
10. Biffi R, Orsi F, Pozzi S et al (2010) No impact of central venous insertion site on oncology patients' quality of life and psychological distress. A randomized three-arm trial. Support Care Cancer 2010 DOI: [Epub ahead of print] doi:10.1007/s00520-010-0984-9

Legal Aspects

38

Rita Celli

Abstract

The Author first examines the essential juridical aspects of the doctor/patient relationship and the foundations of medical professional liability. She thus comes to the observation that specialists are not exempt from a certain professional risk, especially in relation to the delicacy of the main evaluation contests, she also underlines the difficulty of translating a biological fact into specific elements of juridical significance.

The professional liability of the clinician is thus examined on the basis of paradigmatic cases taken from personal experience and of indications supplied on legal doctrine and jurisprudence.

In conclusion, specific attention is drawn to the indications provided by the current codes of medical ethics on the tasks and functions of clinical profession.

Keywords

Totally implantable vascular access device • Medical liability • Complications • Diagnostic error • Informed consent • Healthcare • Medical profession • Malpractice • Medicolegal opinion • Professional obligation

38.1 General Principles

Individual and systemic errors inevitably occur in the delivery of health care, and they can be more frequent if daily surgical practice is characterized by a

R. Celli (✉)
Medico Legal Institute. University of Turin,
Turin, Italy
e-mail: ritacelli@alice.it

I. Di Carlo, R. Biffi (eds.), *Totally Implantable Venous Access Devices*,

high complexity of the operative procedures, while time pressure on the staff continues to increase [1]. The clinician - patient relationship has historically undergone many transformations, and recently a sort of imbalance has occurred, leading to a critical attitude towards medical practice, which on occasion has manifested in open conflict.

Because medical ethics has partly evolved as a critical reaction to the old paternalism, the clinician - patient relationship is no longer characterized by the old line *doctor knows best*, but rather by other catchphrases such as *partnership in care*. It is now widely accepted that clinicians should involve patient in the clinical decision making, rather than dictate what is in the best interests of patients.

Liability, informed consent, malpractice and medicolegal opinion are terms and concepts which are increasingly cropping up in the clinicians daily working life. They characterize weighty subjects of debate which are taking place either in scientific meetings or confidential *offstage* talks among colleagues. Therefore, clinicians need to be well informed about the regulations related to their profession, even when the proposed procedure is the implantation of a long-term central venous device.

38.2 Informed Consent

Informed consent may be defined as "the legal term describing a patient's voluntary agreement to a doctor performing an operation, arranging drug treatment, or carrying out diagnostic tests" [2] . It may also be defined from the medical ethicist's point of view as a "voluntary, uncoerced decision made by a sufficiently competent, autonomous person on the basis of adequate information and deliberation to accept rather than to reject some proposed course of action that will affect him or her" [3]. The successful relationship between clinicians and patients undeniably depends on trust [4]. To establish trust, patient autonomy must be respected, including his/her right to decide whether or not to undergo any medical treatment, and information must be given to enable patients to make their own decisions.

Once accepted that surgeons must obtain consent from patients before carrying out any procedure, no matter how minor is, the main elements of a proper informed consent in surgery include:

1. Explanation of the procedures to be followed and the purposes of each.
2. Description of any attendant discomfort and risk that can be expected.
3. Description of any benefit that can be expected.
4. Disclosure of any appropriate alternative procedures.
5. Instruction that the person is free to withdraw his consent or to discontinue treatment or participation in the project or activity at any time, without prejudice to the subject.

A large number of editorials appear to underline and embrace the so-called *moral consensus*. In many countries the law endorses the moral importance of respect for patient autonomy within the field of medicine. A patient has a right to determine his own medical treatment and that right is superior to the surgeon's duty to provide necessary care. No surgical 'ethics' can deviate from this position. The constitutionally protected right of the individual patient should be paramount at all times, and a citizen's right cannot be abridged with the intention of protecting him. Patient's choices must not be coerced by other third parties (e.g. relatives). Country-specific medical councils have the power to de-register any clinician found to be in breach of these principles. To avoid a claim of physical abuse, the consent to treatment must be based on information *in broad terms* about the nature of and reason for proposed treatment choices.

Leaving aside breaches of professional obligation so obvious that they speak for themselves , what has just been stated above has been determined by law and medicolegal tests. For example, in the UK the Bolam test is well known [5, 6], whereby expert witnesses are asked to confirm the appropriateness of a particular aspect of medical care. However, in many other countries the same activity is regarded as appropriate if the experts (usually medicolegal but not only) convince the court that a relevant reasonable body of professional opinion would approve the course of action that was actually taken. Therefore, consent assessed as appropriate by the law in many industrialized countries is usually judged by a *professional standard*.

Legally effective consent should be considered as consent expressed freely and spontaneously on the basis of full, fair and truthful information regarding the motivations that indicate a particular therapy, as well as the cognitive purposes it is intended to pursue through the therapy and any related risks.

At the same time, patients must be able to provide consent: to be able to understand, remember, deliberate about, and believe clinical information given to them about their specific treatment options.

Some clinicians have found it difficult to embrace this professional and legal consensus. Authors often argue that some patients want little or no information about therapeutic risks and that the standard of the disclosure should not be applied to them. They believe that patients should be asked about how much information they want and given it accordingly. They dispute that in such circumstances, competent patients may feel unable to understand the information they require to give proper consent. Of course, if patients are incompetent, then the issue of consent does not arise. Competent patients are sometimes unable to understand clinical information, especially information about risks. Equally, some patients explicitly state that they want their clinician to make the final decision about their care and that is fair. The fact that patients may say that they want their clinicians to make final decisions about their care does not mean that they do not want to be involved in it. In fact, such patients may be simply be stating the obvious - that clinicians must still make the final decision to proceed with treatment after informed consent has been given [7].

In discharging the responsibilities to determine the best interests of incompetent adults, it is appropriate for clinicians to consult acceptably nominated representatives. To be effective, such consultation demands a level of disclosure of information, analogous to that pertaining to informed consent.

A model of informed consent could be reasonably the following:

I, the undersigned......... declare my acceptance of the treatment proposed. I also declare that I have been exhaustively informed of the motivations underlying the decision to undertake said treatment, the purposes of the treatment pursuable through said treatment and, finally, the nature of the risks that can occur both during the implant or as a consequence of the positioning of the device itself.

More detailed model of informed consent for central venous catheterization and TIVAD implantation can be obtained at GAVeCeLT website (www.gavecelt.org), the Italian Study Group for Long Term Central Venous Access [8]. The information associated with a surgical procedure can be exchanged verbally, in writing, by video, or by computer technology. In this respect, large differences exist between countries. The US and Italy demands a patient signature, whereas a note in the patient chart is sufficient in the UK. In the Netherlands, doctors are not strictly required to obtain written consent.

38.3 Medical Liability

The issue of professional liability has certainly been characterized lately more by *passion than reason*, but it must always be distinguished from imputability, which suggests a correlation between a subject and the negative outcome of the subject's action.

A large number of cases of litigation involving medical actions claim a positive conclusion, i.e. recovery. Put simply, we could say that liability arises from professional action in a context where the patient's growing awareness that he has the right to know and make independent decisions about his state of health meets autonomous medical discipline (i.e. cognitive and evaluation skills), professional ability (i.e. professional applicational skills), and behavioural principles (i.e. personal skills).

Medicine has been defined as an applicational science because it is characterised by the epistemological canons of science, given its ability to measure scientific phenomena. It applies its own canons to variable subjects with probabilistic results. We cannot ignore that medical intervention must always be based on the theories ruling at the moment in which we operate, and on the scientific theories which at that moment in time are held to be true. Federspil and Vettor [9] were well advised to stigmatise the current situation when they stated:

- medicine is uncertain knowledge in a state of constant flux, like all scien-

tific knowledge;
- in formulating a diagnosis the physician can only rely on probabilistic considerations. Therefore no diagnosis is ever absolutely certain, but is characterised by a certain probability.

Clinical medicine is therefore characterised by probability and it is thus that the physician becomes more exposed than other professionals to the possibility of being wrong. We are therefore dealing with a mistake characterized by a failure in quality as a result of the physician having acted with *negligence* (identifiable with carelessness, lack of solicitude, namely with passive behavior that translates into the omission of certain precautions), *imprudence* (insufficiently reflecting on what can be done, acting rashly without respecting others' interests) or *incompetence* (lack of aptitude in the exercise of a professionally qualified activity; this is identified with inadequate training, ineptitude, unfitness for the profession, absence of the basic knowledge indispensable for the exercise of the medical profession; this is closely related to the evolution of science and experience) or failure in a specific quantity or degree of error.

When defining and evaluating error, an indispensable feature is precise structural analysis capable of defining the fine borderline between error proper (i.e. purely technical error) and professional error (i.e. error that has legal relevance) [10-15]. Malpractice means identifying the technical action that has gone wrong, whether it is the cause of an error of omission or of commission, due either to a lack of knowledge or culture, or to the ill-considered or irresponsible or inadequate application of diagnostic methods, or techniques, or approaches fitting for effective medical culture.

Malpractice may be due to diagnostic error, when, notwithstanding the evidence of a disease, the physician errs out of negligence, imprudence or incompetence in interpreting the clinical case, failing to accurately classify its probable outcome as laid down by the science of the time.

The error may be due to a shortcoming in skill (obligation to operate competently); the specialist is expected to use cultural and technical means on a par with the level of teaching imparted at specialization schools, for the attainment of specialist qualifications and the obligation always to keep up to date. Within the realm of prudence (obligation to foresee situations of danger or damage connected with the operation) the utmost must be demanded from the application. The same goes for diligence as an obligation to assist the patient with due treatment and attention. The failure to apply these concepts leads to an attitude that is in clear contrast with the minimum of training and experience required of anyone qualified to exercise the medical profession. Lastly, another field for error is the physician's choice of treatment. Very often this is attributable to diagnostic error, on occasion to an operational error.

The profound difference between error and culpability has been correctly underlined. This says that a certain degree of error cannot be eliminated from any human endeavour, even more so from highly technological activities in which error becomes negligence when medical performance is unacceptably below the standard that should be demanded of a specialist in the subject.

Activities related to vascular access devices and infusion therapy have to take into account the new distinction between *error* in the solution of any scientific problem and *mistake* in attaining a result. In a medical situation the latter becomes a mistaken classification of the patient in the context of consolidated knowledge, namely an incorrect prediction of the possible evolution of the disease and, finally, the mistaken attempt to control and correct the course of the disease and its complications.

38.4 Implantation of TIVADs

The activity of the physician carrying out the implant of a TIVAD is subject to the respect for numerous procedures in matters of implantation that possess essential value. The implantation of a vascular access for infusion therapy is related with calculated risks, that make them acceptable in the field of the clinical activities. The accurate preoperative evaluation of patients, as well as the adherence to internationally-recognized clinical guide-lines are able to minimize procedural and late complications [16]. A paramount importance has also the good knowledge of the specific characteristics of the device to be used.

Lastly, it should be born in mind that concern over possible medico-legal implications or misunderstanding of the problem can produce an *escape reaction*, which can lead the clinician to refuse the implantation of the device.

References

1. Kohn KT, Corrigan JM, Donaldson MS (1999) To err is human: building a safer health system. Washington, DC, National Academy Press
2. Peters M (2008) The British Medical Association illustrated medical dictionary, 2 edn. Dorling Kindersley, London, p 142
3. Gillon R (1985) Philosophical medical ethics. Wiley and Sons, Chichester, p 113
4. Doyal L (2002) Good clinical practice and informed consent are inseparable. Heart 87:103?106
5. Shanmugam K (2002) Testing the Bolam Test: consequences of recent developments. Singapore Med J 43:7?11
6. Bolam v Friern (1957) Hospital Management Committee. I WRL 582
7. Leclercq WK, Keulers BJ, Scheltinga MR et al (2010) A review of surgical informed consent: past, present, and future. A quest to help patients make better decisions. World J Surg 34:1406-1415
8. Consenso informato ed accessi venosi centrali - documento GAVeCeLT. Released: Fri, 02-Dec-2005. Available at www.gavecelt.org
9. Faden RR, Beauchamp TL (1986) A history and theory of informed consent. Oxford University Press, USA
10. Barnett v Chelsea & Kensington Hospital (1968) I All ER 1068
11. Whitehouse v Jordan (1981) I All ER 267
12. Sidaway v Bethlem Royal Hospital Governors (1985) AC 871
13. Maynard v West Midlands Health Authorithy (1985) I All ER 635
14. Bolitho v City and Hackney Health Authority (1997) 4 All ER 771

15. Palmer v Tees Health Authority (1998) All ER 180 and (1999) Lloyd's Medical Reports 151 (CA)
16. Pittiruti M, Hamilton H, Biffi R et al (2009) ESPEN Guidelines on Parenteral Nutrition: central venous catheters (access, care, diagnosis and therapy of complications). Clin Nutr 28:365-377

Future Investigation

39

Roberto Biffi and Isidoro Di Carlo

Abstract

Development of new teaching tools in the field of central venous access, especially with the use of computerized programs and simulators, will be able in the near future to improve the skill and practical training of young doctors. Three-dimensional multiplanar and volume-rendered views are now allowing the simultaneous view of the neck anatomy in 3 orthogonal planes, with the potential to confer a safety benefit to the patients. A number of measures have been implemented to reduce the risk of infections, including maximal barrier precautions during catheter insertion, catheter site maintenance, and hub handling. New technologies and materials will be available in the near future, and will need appropriate trials. Implementation of educational interventions has proven to significantly decrease infection rates, and this will help support a culture of zero tolerance for infection. Thrombosis still remains a major problem. Areas that warrant further research include the benefit of prophylaxis in the ambulatory setting, the risk/benefit ratio of prophylaxis for hospitalized patients with cancer, an understanding of incidental venous thromboembolism, and the impact of anticoagulation on survival. Future prevention studies should aim to achieve a better understanding of the risk factors for thrombosis, thus contributing to a better definition of the patient population at risk; certain patient groups, including those with a hematologic malignancy undergoing intensive chemotherapy, as well as those with hereditary thrombophilia or with a history of unprovoked thrombosis, may have an elevated risk of developing this complication, making them reasonable candidates for prophylaxis.

R. Biffi (✉)
Division of Abdomino Pelvic Surgery, European Institute of Oncology,
Milan, Italy
e-mail: roberto.biffi@ieo.it

I. Di Carlo, R. Biffi (eds.), *Totally Implantable Venous Access Devices*,

Keywords
Three-dimensional view • Catheter-related blood stream infection (CR-BSI) • Targeting zero • Thrombosis • Thrombophilia

39.1 Implantation Techniques

The advantages of ultrasound (US)-guidance for placement of central venous catheters (CVCs) have been demonstrated in many randomized trials and confirmed by all the meta-analyses on this subject. There is now strong evidence to indicate that US-guided insertion of central catheters is more effective and safer than blind techniques in both adults and children. An additional improvement could derive from the use of realtime 3-dimensional US for insertion of a central venous catheter. An HD11 XE™ US system with a V8-4 transducer (Philips Medical Systems, Bothell, WA) was recently used in a surgical patient [1] and this experience was published by UK authors. Three-dimensional multiplanar and volume-rendered views allowed simultaneous view of the neck anatomy in 3 orthogonal planes. Needle entry into the vein and subsequent catheter placement could also be visualized. The authors were able to rotate the views in realtime, thereby enabling visualization of the catheter within the lumen of the vein. The ability to see simultaneous realtime short- and long-axis views along with volume perspective without altering transducer position is a significant development, with the potential to confer a safety benefit to the patient. Possible limitations can derive from processing power and transducer size, which are expected to be overcome with advancing technology.

Another important issue will be the development of new teaching tools in this field, with the use of computerized programs and simulators able to improve the skill and practical training of young doctors.

Until these developments have spread, the surgical approach and the percutaneous US-guided insertion remain the safest methods of avoiding immediate complications. Due to the anatomy with the surgical approach these complications can be avoided even by inexperienced operators, whereas US-guided insertion needs expert hands.

39.2 Complications

Important complications like thrombosis and infections are still associated with permanent CVCs, especially in oncology, which may lead to device loss, significant morbidity, increased duration of hospitalization and additional medical costs. Nowadays most infections can be prevented. A number of measures have been implemented to reduce the risk of infections, including maximal barrier precautions during catheter insertion, catheter site maintenance, and hub handling. New technologies and materials will be available in the near future, needing appropriate trials. Development of a new bifunctional coating concept that can be applied to make CVC surfaces antimicrobial and antithrombogenic at the same time was recently proposed [2]. The novel coating consists of a moderately hydrophilic synthetic copolymer of N-vinylpyrrollidinone (NVP) and n-butyl methacrylate (BMA), containing embedded silver nanoparticles (AgNPs) and sodium heparin. AgNPs were shown to strongly inhibit adhesion of *S. aureus* (reference strain and clinical isolates), and heparin not only rendered surfaces practically non-thrombogenic, it also contributed synergistically to biocidal activity.

Central line-associated bacteremia is a key issue for future perspectives, due to morbidity/mortality related rates and increased costs. It has been estimated that infections are associated with increased length of stay in intensive care units of up to 6 days, increased hospital length of stay of approximately 21 days, attributable mortality of approximately 35%, and incremental costs of approximately $56,000 per infection. The Center for Medicare and Medicaid Services recently declared that central venous catheter-associated bloodstream infections are preventable and no longer reimbursable. The new penalty paradigm creates substantial economic incentives for hospitals to eliminate infections. Future actions will explore preventions as well as treatment. Implementation of educational interventions has been proven to significantly decrease infection rates, and this will help support a culture of *zero tolerance* for infection. The first step will be to increase theoretical knowledge and improve practices regarding catheter care with educational programs directed at doctors and nurses. A recent survey by means of a questionnaire in a teaching hospital showed that only 13.6% of the doctors answered all questions correctly [3]. Moreover, a survey was carried out to determine the prevalence and appropriateness of antimicrobial therapy in the Netherlands [4]; in 16% of the patients antibiotic treatment was considered inappropriate.

Immunocompromised patients suffering from cancer, transplantation, and dialysis patients with a long-term vascular access may mostly benefit from antibiotic-releasing catheters. So far, many of these devices have demonstrated the ability to limit their antimicrobial activity to 10-14 days after implant, with substantial inability to prevent fungal colonization / infections. A study with 223 adult surgical patients randomized to receive either a rifampicin-miconazole-impregnated CVC (n=118) or a standard CVC (n=105) showed that antimicrobial CVCs are able to reduce catheter colonization (CC) and catheter-related local infection (CRI) significantly, even at long-term catheterization [5]. Subgroup analyses showed a pronounced reduction of CC and CRI in male, overweight and oncology patients. Important covariates were skin colonization for CC and oncologic disease for CRI. Odds ratio (OR) for reducing CC was 0.076 (95% CI: 0.016–0.360) and CRI was reduced from 26% to 2.3% (p=0.001) in the cancer subgroup. *Ex vivo* long-term antimicrobial activity of modified catheters exceeded 4 weeks.

Thrombosis still remains a major problem. When device-related deep vein thrombosis occurs, it seriously complicates the clinical management of the patient because of the need for anticoagulant treatment and sometimes the need to achieve another central line. It may be particularly troublesome in a patient who already has compromised venous access because of multiple courses of chemotherapy. There is broad consensus regarding the importance of thromboprophylaxis in hospitalized patients with cancer, including prolonged prophylaxis in high-risk surgical patients. Prophylaxis is not currently recommended for ambulatory patients with cancer (with exceptions) or for central venous catheters. Areas that warrant further research include the benefit of prophylaxis in the ambulatory setting, the risk/benefit ratio of prophylaxis for hospitalized patients with cancer, an understanding of incidental venous thromboembolism, and the impact of anticoagulation on survival. Future prevention studies should aim to achieve a better understanding of the risk factors for thrombosis, thus contributing to a better definition of the patient population at risk; certain patient groups, including those with a hematologic malignancy undergoing intensive chemotherapy, as well as those with hereditary thrombophilia or with a history of unprovoked thrombosis, may have an elevated risk of developing this complication, making them reasonable candidates for prophylaxis. Currently available prophylactic agents are not optimal for the prevention of thrombosis, especially in the cancer patient. Future studies should be adequately powered and evaluate the effects of newer factor Xa inhibitors or direct thrombin inhibitors.

39.3 Quality of Life

More studies are needed to investigate the issue of patient satisfaction and quality of life and their relationships with the device adopted for long-term use, a topic rarely studied so far. There is only limited information available on patient satisfaction with different types and sites of central venous long-term accesses, while the perceived advantages/disadvantages of the type and site from the patient's perspective has rarely been investigated in a randomized trial; very few studies have focused on the impact of central venous insertion site on quality of life. Whereas patients and their families still currently play a minor role in the selection of a vascular access device at the onset of treatment, patient satisfaction should be a major issue in the clinical setting of cancer palliation.

39.4 Open Issues and Future Development

There are still numerous controversial aspects to the problem of power injection, and they mainly concern the cost-effectiveness ratio. In particular, there are no studies of adequate statistical power and good scientific quality (Randomized Clinical Trials - RCTs) comparing a *power on principle* strategy (i.e. always and in any case inserting a *power injectable* port and using it for all radiologic exams) vs. a *peripheral venous access device on principle* strategy (the use, always and in any case, of a peripheral venous access device for the execution of CT exams, both in patients without implanted port and in patients with non-*power injectable* ports). The endpoints of this type of study should be patient satisfaction, including issues concerning comfort and quality of life (anxiety, pain, etc.), as well as the direct costs of the two different strategies (in the case of the *power injectable* port with *power injectable* non-coring needles, could a higher *raw* cost be offset by possible savings on patient management?).

A second aspect that should be studied is the impact of using a power injectable port on the quality of the images. This might be of significance, for example, in oncologic patients with hepatic lesions. In such cases, it is essential to have an optimal standardized sequence of the different CT phases (the so-called *3-phase*). The dual blood supply of the organ and the need to complete the scan before the balance between the intra- and extravascular compartments occurs make the liver unique. The use of a *power injectable* technology, especially for RECIST assessments, could be more cost-effective than peripheral access.

References

1. Dowling M, Jlala HA, Hardman JG, Bedforth NM (2011) Real-time three-dimensional ultrasound-guided central venous catheter placement. Anesth Analg 112:378-381
2. Stevens KN, Croes S, Boersma RS et al (2011) Hydrophilic surface coatings with embedded biocidal silver nanoparticles and sodium heparin for central venous catheters. Biomaterials 32:1264-1269
3. Koutzavekiaris I, Vouloumanou EK, Gourni M et al (2011) Knowledge and practices regarding prevention of infections associated with central venous catheters: A survey of intensive care unit medical and nursing staff. Am J Infect Control [Epub ahead of print] doi: 10.1016/j.ajic.2010.11.003
4. Willemsen I, van der Kooij T, van Benthem B et al (2010) Appropriateness of antimicrobial therapy: a multicentre prevalence survey in the Netherlands, 2008-2009. Euro Surveill 15. pii:19715
5. Schierholz JM, Nagelschmidt K, Nagelschmidt M et al (2010) Antimicrobial central venous catheters in oncology: efficacy of a rifampicin-miconazole-releasing catheter. Anticancer Res 30:1353-1358

Subject Index

MIX
Papier aus verantwortungsvollen Quellen
Paper from responsible sources
FSC® C105338

If you have any concerns about our products,
you can contact us on
ProductSafety@springernature.com

In case Publisher is established outside the EU,
the EU authorized representative is:
Springer Nature Customer Service Center GmbH
Europaplatz 3, 69115 Heidelberg, Germany

Printed by Libri Plureos GmbH
in Hamburg, Germany